CRITICAL MASS

Bicycling's Defiant Celebration

Edited by Chris Carlsson

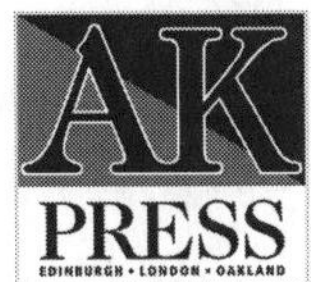

This book is dedicated to all the people who "got it"
and made Critical Mass their own.
Critical Mass is an exhilarating opportunity
to make something rare and new (again) every month.

Some photos and short pieces in this book are unattributed. My apologies to any writers or photographers who were inadvertantly left out. Many things have arrived at my office over the past ten years and some of them made it into this book, even if I wasn't sure who sent it or wrote it or took the picture. —Chris Carlsson, editor

ACKNOWLEDGEMENTS: Far too many people deserve mention for the phenomenon of Critical Mass to be able to list them all here. Nevertheless, the San Francisco experience would not be what it is without the crucial involvement of Jim Swanson, Markus Cook, Kash, Joel Pomerantz, Steven Bodzin, James Kern, Dierdre Crowley, Travis Moraché, Ted White, Stuart Coulthard, Kathy Roberts, Donald Francis, Dave Snyder, Emily McFarland, and many others (apologies to anyone who isn't named and should have been)... of course there are dozens of people in cities across the world who have made Critical Mass a part of their cities' lives, and they deserve recognition and appreciation too. Beth Verdekal was a huge help organizing ten years of sprawling files that have accumulated here since the early days of Critical Mass, in addition to her buoyant involvement over the years. Glenn Bachmann, Ben Seibel, James Sederberg, and Hugh D'Andrade all helped with proofreading, indexing, and general oversight. All the contributing writers worked hard and cooperatively to reach the final versions you will read here. Thanks for their patience, commitment and openness. Thanks to Jym Dyer, Michael Bluejay, Damon Rao, and Kevin Cole for compiling their awesome websites listing Critical Masses all around the world. This book would be a very different volume without the contacts their work made possible.

Front Cover by Mona Caron
Back Cover photo by Chris Carlsson (San Francisco Critical Mass, July 2001, looking north on Battery Street towards Clay Street)

Typesetting and Book Design by Chris Carlsson, Typesetting Etc., San Francisco

ISBN 1-902593-59-6
A catalogue for this title is available from the Library of Congress
1. Bicycling—transportation politics. 2. Bicycling—urban studies. 3. Anarchy—political movements.
I. Carlsson, Chris 1957- II. Title

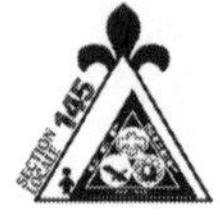

AK Press, PO Box 12766, Edinburgh, Scotland EH89YE www.akuk.com
AK Press, 674A 23rd Street, Oakland, CA 94612 www.akpress.org
Printed in Canada

Table of Contents

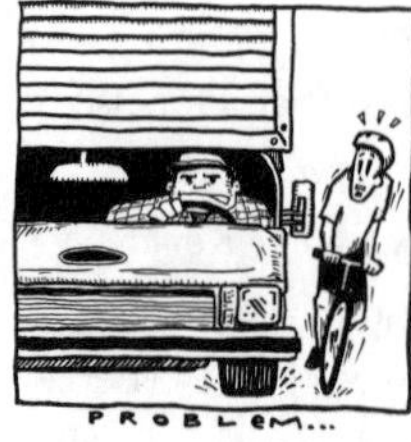

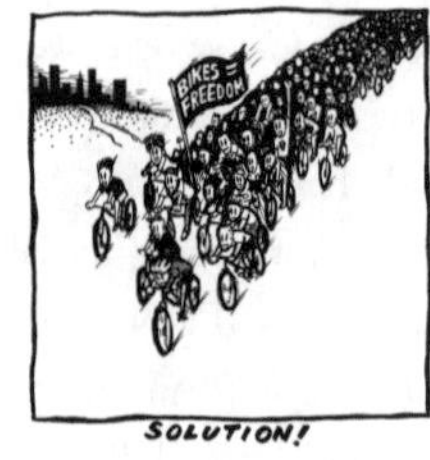

HUGH D'ANDRADE

INTRODUCTION

Critical Mass—the name inspires passion and loathing. Originally a term applied to nuclear fission, it has become a rallying cry for bicyclists, rejecting the priorities and values imposed on us by oil barons and their government servants. But Critical Mass bicycle rides are no protest movement as we commonly imagine. Instead, riders have gathered to *celebrate* their choice to bicycle, and in so doing have opened up a new kind of social and political space,

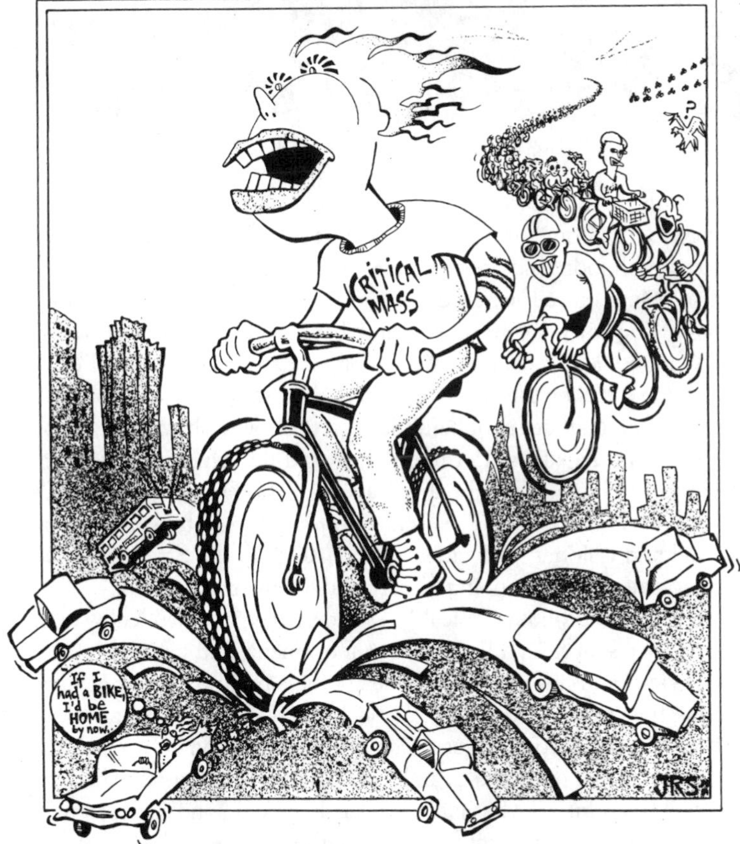

JAMES R SWANSON

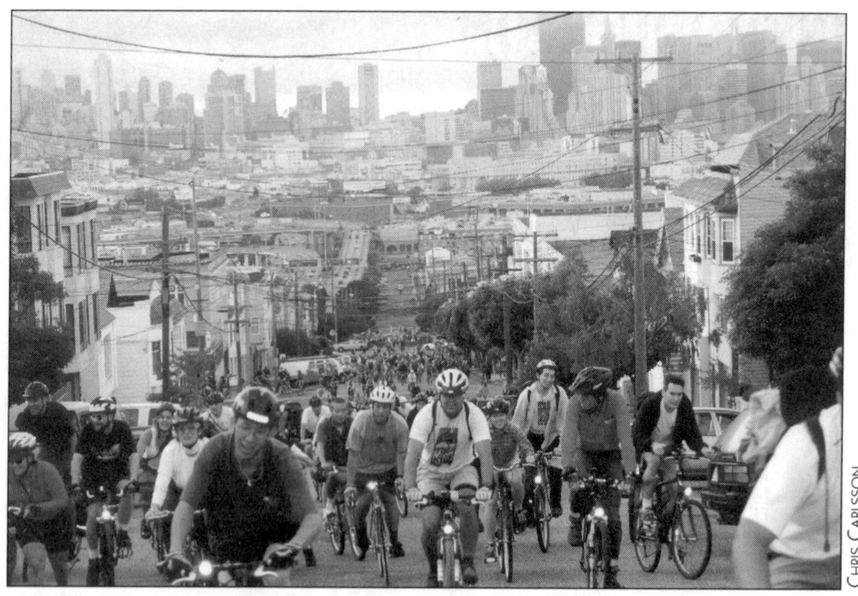

Critical Mass chugs up San Francisco's Potrero Hill, August 1998

unprecedented in this era of atomization and commodification. Bicyclists are reclaiming city life from San Francisco to St. Louis, Melbourne to Milan, Berlin to Bombay, and hundreds more cities across the planet.

Critical Mass started in the dark days of 1992 not long after Bush #1 had manipulated Iraq into becoming the new boogeyman, massacred thousands in the Gulf War and declared a New World Order. Critical Mass had already spread to over a dozen cities by the time the Zapatistas rose on New Year's Day in 1994 (against the "free market" neoliberal deal NAFTA was shoving down Mexico's throat). Since the Zapatista uprising, the myriad movements contesting corporate globalization have grown in the shadow of the famous "irrational exuberance" of the 1990s. Alternative seeds have sprouted into thickening branches of oppositional and visionary movements, from Reclaim the Streets to community gardening to the summit-hopping Turtles and Teamsters.

In the pages that follow, Critical Mass is described and defined by many voices. Critical Mass is far from a homogenous movement, and its participants have a diversity of views and missions. Inevitable conflicts that necessarily arise in public get an airing here too. The beauty of Critical Mass—one of them, anyway—is the chance it provides for people to face each other in the simmering cauldron of real life, in public, without pre-set roles and fixed boundaries. Naturally this leads some people to feel that Critical Mass fails to meet their goals, and such sentiments can be found among the writings that follow. Nevertheless, where else in our society has there been such a remarkable opportunity to test one's own theories and ideas in public, in a chaotic and unpredictable real life context? I will leave it to our many contributors to flesh out the details of the Critical Mass experience, its pros and cons, its beauty and its occasional ugliness. As several writers take pains to point out, no one can claim to have the "truth" when it comes to Critical Mass. Each person is equally capable of offering a perspective, a definition, a manifesto, a purpose. And it's in that openness that Critical Mass continues to thrive, ten years after its birth in San Francisco on a warm September evening in 1992.

This book came together rather abruptly during the early spring of 2002. After sending out a solicitation around the world, I was happily deluged with wonderful material. I spent the bulk of April and half of May intensely editing and working with contributors, then designing and producing the book. Thanks to AK Press for taking on the publisher's role, and promising to get the book out in time for our Tenth Anniversary celebration on September 27, 2002.

At the outset I wanted this book to be a global history of the amorphous phenomenon we call "Critical Mass." Dozens of contributors define this mysterious social movement in a charming cacophony of voices and perspectives. But this is less a history book than a solid resource for future historians. Nearly all the contributors are themselves participants, each writing from his or her own experience within Critical Mass in cities across the planet. In some ways we emulate the old saga of the blind men and the elephant, each of us describing the part of the experience we know best, which is in turn shaped by our preconceptions, hopes and fears.

Iain Boal's "The World of the Bicycle," and Hank Chapot's "Great Bicycle Protest of 1896" show how fuzzy the notion of a beginning is, when it comes to mass bicycle rides with a political-social purpose. Unfortunately, participants and outsiders have often fallen for the myth that Critical Mass was started by one person.

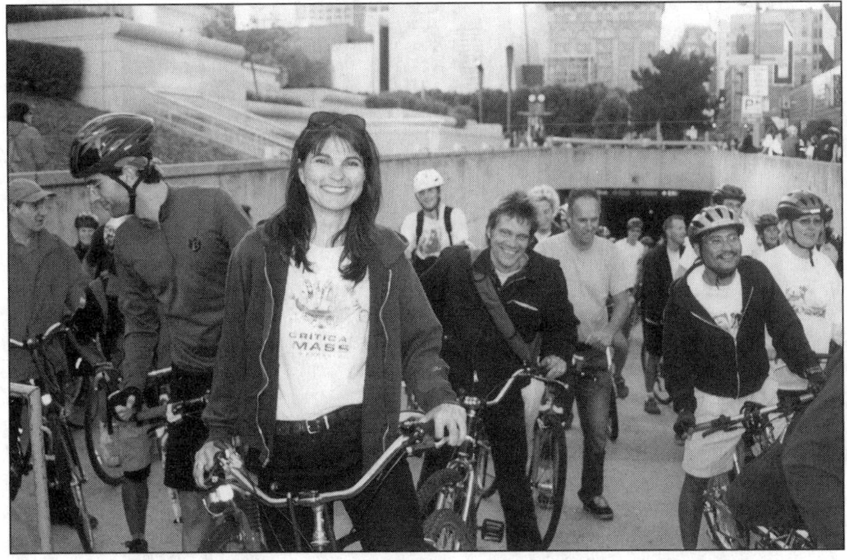

CHRIS CARLSSON

Critical Mass emerging from a sudden rush through the underground Moscone Convention Center , August 2000.

Due to our cultural predisposition to attribute all events to the exemplary efforts of one or more heroic individuals (usually "great men"), the mythical history of Critical Mass has become something like "it all started with Chris Carlsson going to the SF Bike Coalition in August 1992." While I did go to that meeting and make a suggestion for a spontaneous, monthly gathering of bicyclists, this idea was by no means mine alone. It is patently absurd to attribute any social movement to the good idea of a single individual. In fact, many of us had been discussing this idea for the better part of six months prior to its presentation to a (less-than-enthusiastic) SF Bike Coalition meeting. The concept evolved over this time, with multiple input and influence from many people, and plenty of others who never took part directly in the conversations.

Social movements don't erupt from individuals, and individuals don't have ideas that are solely theirs. We are all shaped and influenced by our social conditions; our sense of what's possible and what we do about it is shaped IN ACTION WITH EACH OTHER. No better example exists of this larger dynamic than Critical Mass itself.

—*Chris Carlsson*

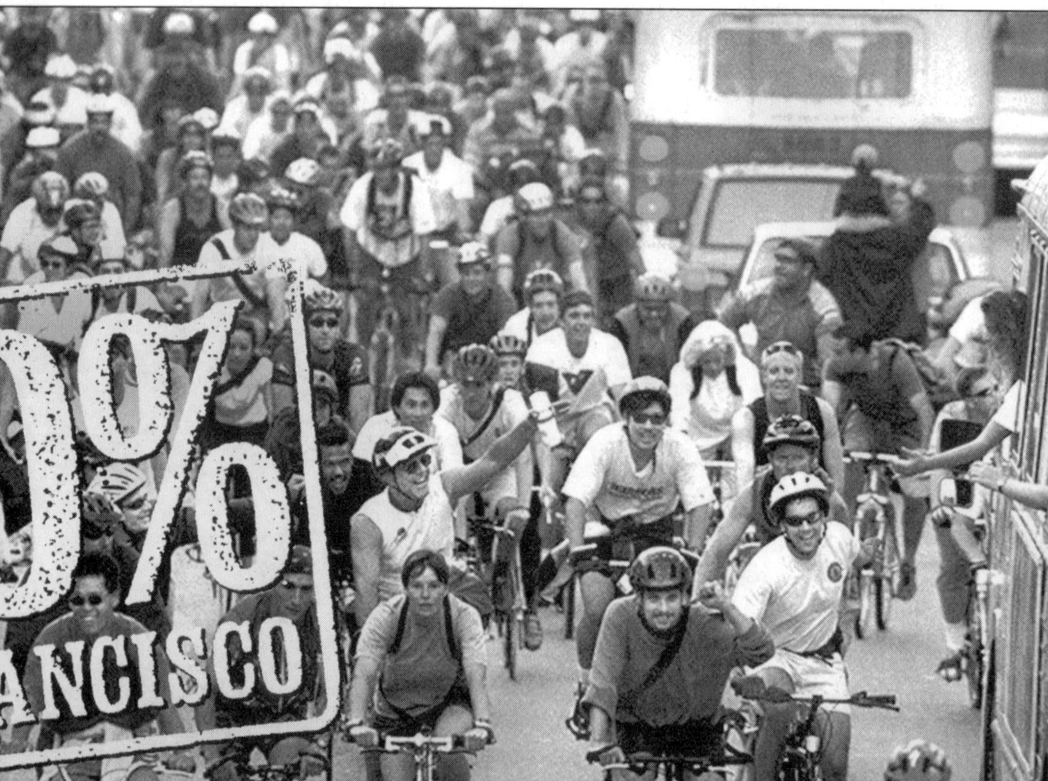

LIZ HAFALIA

San Francisco Critical Mass August 1996: The *SF Chronicle* used this image to advertise *itself* as authentically San Francisco!

SWEET SOUNDS, SWEETER SMELLS

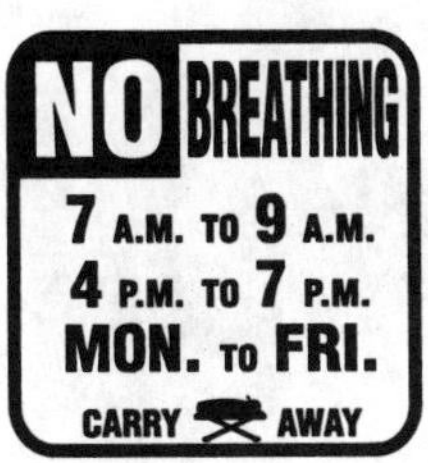

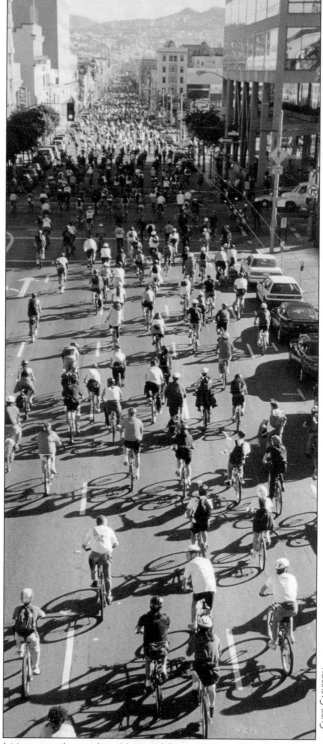

CHRIS CARLSSON

Critical Mass westbound on Howard Street in San Francisco, June 1996

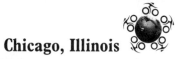

Chicago, Illinois

THE POWER IS HERE

BY TRAVIS HUGH CULLEY

Excerpt from *The Immortal Class: Bike Messengers and the Cult of Human Power* (Villard Books, New York: 2001)

Pulling into Daley Plaza I came upon a motley crowd. Bike messengers who looked like tired camels sat on their bikes, laughing and talking with riders dressed in suits who wore small Velcro straps around their ankles. Some guys with long beards and knitted hats wore signs that read slogans like "ONE LESS CAR" and "FUELED BY POTATOES." These greenies rode in harmony with young executives, schoolteachers, business owners, lawyers, stockbrokers. Many ages were represented. Children sat comfortably in plastic pannier seats, their round helmets tipping to one side.

There were a few older people there as well. There was Bill, on his 1960s steel clunker, who had kept to his 1960s sense of social responsibility rolling smooth. There was a woman my grandmother's age, still working as a teacher in Hyde Park. In her late 70s, she had ridden eight miles just to get to the Loop, and had at least fifteen more miles to go before she'd make it home again. Then there was Jim Redd. A man in his fifties, whose white hair and leathered hands could not conceal his youthfulness. He was strong and tall and he glowed with joviality. He stood on the stone pediment that footed Chicago's famous Picasso sculpture throwing rolls of blue crepe paper into a crowd of hundreds. People in the crowd scooped up the flying tape and began to tie it around their bars or lace it into the spokes of their bicycles.

I set my bike down, wondering for a moment if I should lock it up. Around me, sitting on their sides or in piles, were hundreds of bikes, twenty-dollar beaters, two-thousand-dollar road bikes, four-thousand-dollar Y-frame mountain bikes left upturned on their seat and handlebars. None of them were locked. In a rare act of conformity I dropped my old machine on the granite courtyard and stepped up to the white haired guy and asked if he was the guy in charge.

"No one is in charge! Are you kidding! That would spoil all the fun," Redd laughed, turning away to toss more decoration.

A clean-cut man with a red cheeks and bright blue eyes handed me route maps that would steer the demonstration through the city and

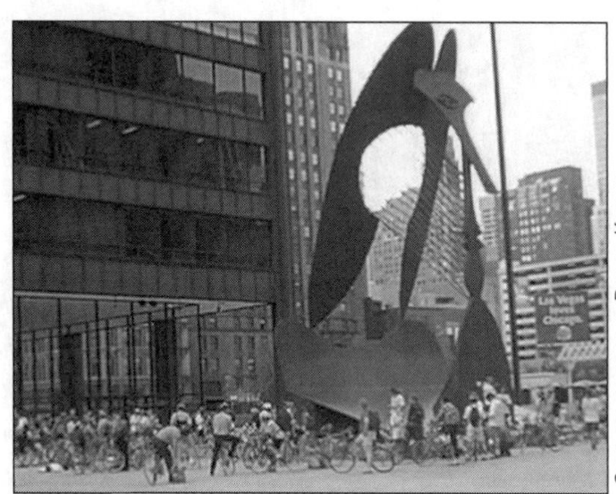

CHICAGO PHOTOS BY DANIEL KOPALD

Massing at Daley Plaza, Chicago, May 1998

lead us to the intersection of Clark and Belmont—an intersection on Chicago's hip north side. His only words to me were: "This'll wake 'em up." I found out his name was Michael Burton; he'd once been a bike messenger but now he was working for the Statewide Housing Action Coalition.

I saw a man with long silky brown hair and a thick beard. He had a boyish, saintly face and a helmet painted like a walnut. "Jimbo" he said outright, shaking my hand. I gave him my name and in exchange I got a little orange flyer, advertising the next *Critical Mass* ride.

"Critical Mass?" I asked. "Is that what they call this?"

"Uh, yep." He said simply as he walked away.

In the next instance I received a flier for the A-zone, an anarchist/activists network. Then I received an invitation to a party that was being thrown by DJ Esperanto. I received a flier advocating a big presence at the Police Brutality Demonstration in October. Then I received one about Rolando Cruz, Mumia, an underground film project. The offerings went on and on, until my hands were filled with colored paper. I balled it all up, looked at a young woman with shining curly hair who was straddling a mountain bike. "What the hell is this about?" I asked her, shoving all the fliers in my bag, overwhelmed.

She looked back with a big smile, held up a pack of fliers cut vertically that were tied together with a zip cord: "Did you get one of these?"

"What can it possibly be that I don't already have!"

She laughed, scooted her bike closer and handed me the whole pack of fliers. "These are for the people we'll see. It just tells them what the ride is about."

"Now that is what I need. I have no idea what this is about."

The young woman, whose name was Katherine, said, pondering a little, "I think it is about bikers who are tired of getting run over."

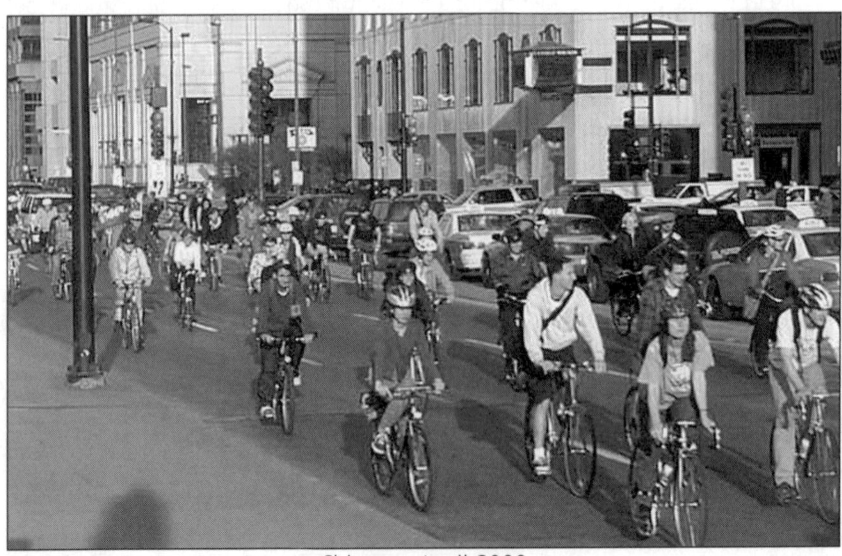

Chicago, April 2000

"I can relate," I replied.

Cheers from the crowd greeted one special guest. He rode a big Schwinn cruiser from the fifties with an old leather springy seat, wide handlebars, and fat tires. Mounted on his bars was an old brass horn with a big black rubber bulb. He wheeled around the massive sculpture, squeezing the fat bulb, making the horn sing over the crowd. Katherine called him BigHorn and said she thought his name was Eric.

"Okay. BigHorn it is."

Other instruments came to life accompanying the tooting trumpet that circled the crowd. There were tambourines, bike bells and ear piercing air horns. One guy had a collage of cowbells attached to his bars and yet another had drum cymbals delicately straddling his front tire. He held a drumstick and he could reach down and crash the symbols as he rode. One biker played a mounted conga with his right hand while he steered with the other. For a moment I couldn't stop laughing. I was entranced by the inventiveness of these demonstrators and their demeanor. They were serious but they were not angry. They were just having a good time, as if the work of grassroots activism had gotten somehow confused with celebration. I told Katherine how impressed I was, but she interrupted to say emphatically that this was not just a *local* thing. Apparently it happened all over the world, though it had only recently caught on in Chicago.

"All over the world?"

"Yes, simultaneously, the last Friday of the month, all over the world." She clarified that dates changed a little bit here and there but basically it was the same. She listed cities like Sydney, Berlin, Zurich, Paris, London, Tokyo, Kyoto, Austin, Phoenix, Seattle, New York, D.C., Portland, and Atlanta. The movement started in San Francisco where she said they have gotten over 10,000 people in their rides, completely dominating the city traffic. "It is local but it is a different kind of local. It is everywhere, *locally*."

I introduced myself to a couple of guys that appeared to be near the core of the activist group. I was surprised to find that they were not throwback radicals simply trying to eradicate the automobile from the world. This core group, as radical as some of their ideas seemed, were talking, arguing and then agreeing upon safe and conservative ideas for the mass.

Amid this group was a conservative looking guy named Gareth. He wore a tie, spoke with clarity, and advocated his ideas with an acute appeal to reason. "If you ask me, I would say lets get the mass on the highway and head out toward the airport. That's where our audience spends most of their time in transit," he reasoned. "For a stretch of a mile or two, what could they do? Come after us? I don't think so. They would just see us zipping past and they would get a flier jammed in their wipers, big deal."

Gregg Gunther, a tall and serious looking cyclist who wore a bright pink jersey covered with yellow happy faces, tempered Gareth's idea. "First things first," he said. "We need to take back the streets we have a right to; Logan, Clybourne, Clark—*city streets*. The people who are using these local streets might not be the suburban conservatives that we love to hate but these people can bike to work. They just don't know that they can."

"I don't see what's so *conservative* about suburbanites," Gareth interjected.

"That's where there are whole closed off neighborhoods of white republicans with 2.5 kids and all that."

"Suburban may be traditional but traditional is not conservative. The conservatives are right here *conserving*. That's why I say we need to have some suburban influence. But you make a good point: if city people can bike or access a train, you're right, we should encourage them to do that."

"Not that the highway is a bad idea," a guy named James, asserted.

"But it's too involved," Gareth agreed.

"Right. You're not asking them to bike, you're asking them to sell the car and move and change their whole lives—and that's a tough pull."

A horn sounded through the square like a trumpet. BigHorn was circling the sculpture, blowing on a little plastic bugle. In minutes, there were hundreds of cyclists following him, giving catcalls and weaving in and out of each other. For a moment I stood up on the sculpture's step-like platform. The sea of riders moving in circles was momentarily overwhelming, like seeing the swell of waves rise above the bow of a ship. From the ledge of the Picasso, I mounted my bike, pulling into the current of moving bicycles, becoming swarmed by the sound of their bike bells and air-horns. The ride had begun.

Cycling in a group of three hundred people is an incredible feeling, but the first time, it was a little weird. I was used to biking hunched down in an act of perpetual defense. But now there were all these people to talk to. It turned out that BigHorn and I had put in hours at some of the same stores to fund our creative endeavors.

"You got to make a living." He laughed, recognizing a curious social paradox. "If you can't make a living, how can you get any work done?" We compared notes about the ways that we had to work to support our careers. "And everything you earn goes right back to the world in materials, in time, in labor. You work to give it all away again."

"You have to sacrifice everything to contribute anything at all," I agreed.

"Totally! You've got to have a suicide reflex, a will to sacrifice all of your harvest, all of the time. If you don't, you won't ever have a chance to succeed. If you are not out there spending everything, how can you possibly earn anything?"

"I think I am going to throw myself in the fire and get it over with," I said lightly.

His laugh ripped through me, a laugh that was neither an agreement nor a disagreement. He had a fuzzy goatee and boyish face, and he smiled as his knees rose and fell smoothly with the traffic. He stretched his fingers out across the plastic handgrips of his old cruiser and extended his right palm to me. Our fingers met gently in a slow-motion high five that rolled smoothly from palm to palm. "Rock on," BigHorn said slyly.

A black kid in short hair and blonde beard rode up and piped in, "It's like

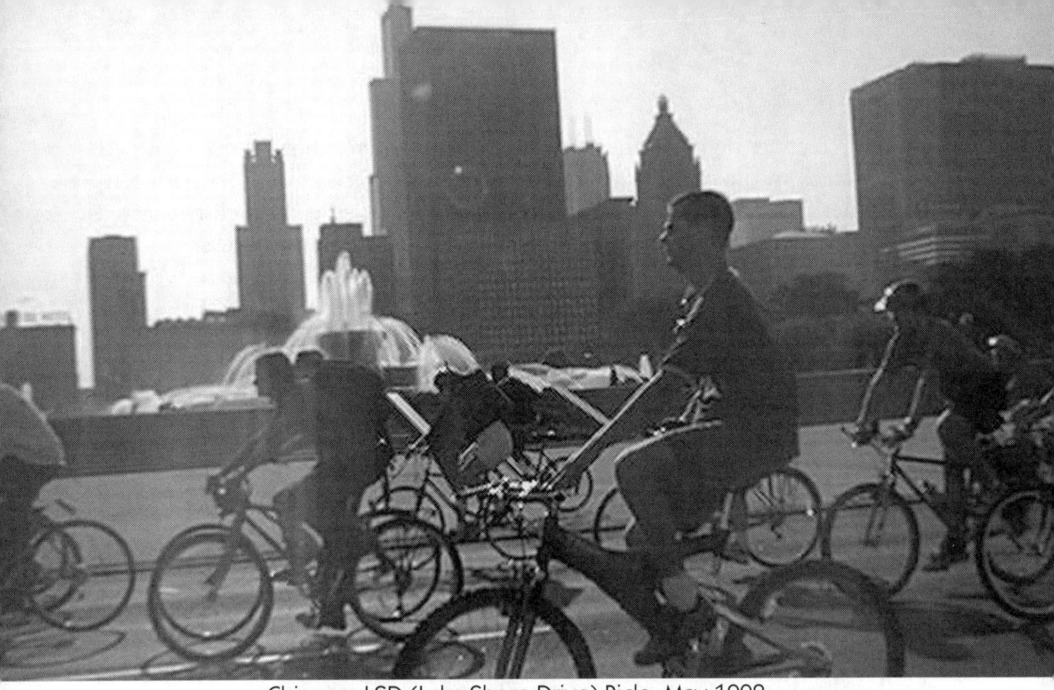

Chicago, LSD (Lake Shore Drive) Ride, May 1998

we're being told you can be anything in this country *but* creative, anything *but* different, anything *but* genuine. We are not forced into slavery. We're forced into minimum wage and we live in ghettos, left to fight over little pieces that are left for us like rats in a can. That's why the middle class drives cars and lives in the 'burbs. It's protection from the dirty and the poor and the people that are different. They put sanctions on the city, Man!"

Soon there were at least ten people supporting his speech by listening closely. "Do you know how many people are struggling just to make their own work come alive? Their life's work? Fuck music, fuck art. I'm talking about raising a child!" He started riding with both fists in the air. "I'm going to take this country, Man! I'm going to take it back!" Then he hurried off toward an oncoming taxicab and slipped one of those vertical fliers through its half-open back window. "The power is here, *brotha*," he told a passenger as the Mass carried on.

The women on the ride seemed especially excited. They smiled brightly and sat upright. Adrianna, a former courier, who had horns coming out of her silver helmet, exulted that it was great to ride in this kind of group. She complained that she was so used to being honked at, touched and told to get off the road that it made her sometimes hate riding. She told me about an incident that took place only a week back. A woman came up behind her in a car, hit her back tire and knocked her off the road. If Adrianna hadn't shouted at the driver she would not have even stopped! When she did stop, Adrianna found that she could have a rational conversation with her.

The motorist's testimony was that she just didn't know what else to do. "You were on the road. How *should* I get past you? " Adrianna quoted the driver. "What am I supposed to do?"

"Finally!" Adrianna said about the demonstration, someone was speaking out to protect *her* rights on the road, and to teach drivers how to *share space*. "I am not stuck in the sixties but I am not necessarily stuck in the twentieth century either. Roads were not made for automobiles!" A group of cyclists cheered her protest and she shook her head trying to hide her blushing cheeks.

At this point, the mass was only moving about seven miles an hour. We were trying to stay together because in demonstrations like these, strange things were known to happen. If the density of the group ever got too drawn out or diminished, I was warned, motorists would be tempted to push holes through the crowd. In other cities cars had charged through the mass at the expense of the two or three bikers who were in their way. At one point in a Philadelphia mass, a courier was run over and dragged about a hundred feet along the South Street Bridge. When his bike disconnected from beneath the car, the motorist just drove away.

Shocked by stories like this, I began to ride up a few blocks ahead of the mass, wondering how it is we let such hatred grow into our own cities. Roaming through my mind to find a suitable explanation, I noticed that I had traveled nearly seven blocks ahead of the mass. A little shocked by having so mindlessly ridden ahead, I decided to stop and let the group catch up with me. It was then that I realized I was standing in the middle of an intersection.

Lines and signs marked the street lanes explicitly for automobiles. The pedestrians were sanctioned to cross, inside carefully drawn white lines. I was somewhere in between, unsure of which directions to follow.

Traffic going north and south was thick and aggressive. Cars were speeding around me at thirty or more miles an hour. Contact with anyone of them could have been fatal. A truck, flashing a left blinker, stopped and sat on his horn. He looked at me through a dirty windshield and tried to yell something. I knew that 300 cyclists were a few blocks back and gaining. I thought, *What if I don't respond? What would that make me? Some kind of engineering obstruction? A malfunction? Would the driver get out and hunt me down or seek to punish me for assaulting his schedule? For tying up the tracks? Would he take or destroy my property? Would he kill me?*

I am a human being. I am not some machinist's error. Let him do what he's got to do.

With that, I dumped my bike, lay down in the street with my arms spread wide, and looked up at the miracle of life as seen in the reflection of a blue sky. At a café on the corner I saw two women hiding behind the thick plate glass stand up excited and curious. They had no idea what was going to happen here, and neither did I.

The trucker was cursing at me through his closed window, revving his engine. Other cars approached, one going south and one going north. They both came to a stop, clogging all the traffic behind them. I could hear the truck's wheels turn toward me. Then I began to hear the approaching cries and cheers from the bike parade as they approached the unsuspecting audience. As I looked up at the small clouds rolling past, the first few bikers' shadows started passing through them shouting "Yeah, dude!," "Go for it, Man!" etc. I pressed my ankles together so as to be narrow as possible, lifted my hands up in the air and shouted back in full voice—no words, just sheer celebration.

One after another, flying overhead, passing through the blue sky, bikers leaned down and started slapping hands with me. Some of the skin was soft, some of it hard. Some of the hands were white, and some of them black. Some were the hands of men, some were of women—but none of that mattered. Everyone touched my palms and fingers, shouting and celebrating to reclaim the street, to make it human again.

I lay there beneath the mass utterly amazed, watching the shadows pass overhead. I could hear the freewheels spin and the whirl of rubber traction hissing in the air as they passed. I shut my eyes while the last hundred bikers flew past and touched my upraised hands. When the storm passed, I found myself at the back of the pack. My palms tingled. My fingertips were sore. Digital Dan Kopald hung back to make sure I got up okay and that I was in order. He proved to me that these were not just weirdo's letting weirdo people do weirdo things. These people cared.

I leaped to my feet, my eyes open with excitement. He laughed at my stunt and uprighted my bike for me. I climbed back onto my pedals and sprinted into the crowd again.

At the next intersection I did a headstand, and as the bikers passed again I shook my legs around crazily. This time someone else was at the back of the crowd to stay with me. I thanked them, mounted up, and sprinted off ahead of the group again. At Wellington Avenue, I grabbed the seat of my bike and held the entire thing in the air with one hand. The front wheel leaned to one side in a soft repose. The handle bars twisted high above my head like the arrogant posture of a Civil War monument. Beyond the spokes and thin pipes of my simple instrument I could see that perfect blue sky. Lines of white clouds were drawn softly overhead as if they were carried by cherubs and hundreds of cyclists passed this time in a blur of color beneath the bicycle, as if it was a flag in a battle front.

At Belmont, where the rolling demonstration came to an end, I was walking in circles with my bike still held in the air. Around me in every direction, crowds of other bikers held their rides in the air triumphantly. The demonstrators were circling and shouting, using the street as a stage. None of the traffic disturbed us. Cars, pedestrians, and cyclists stood in amazement as far as the eye could see.

This was the theater I had come to Chicago for. *This* was the point where theater could change the way people think and live. This was a mission achieved, a performance well worth its acclaim—and, I was only one small part of its whole.

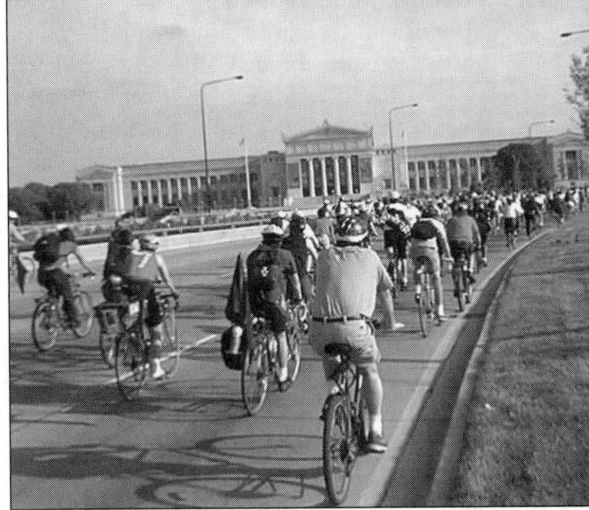

Chicago CM at the Field Museum, May 1998

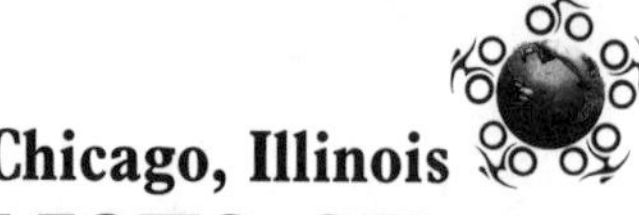

Chicago, Illinois

RUGGED INDIVIDUALISTS OF THE ROAD UNITE!

BY MICHAEL BURTON

The bicycle commuter in Chicago is like a cattleman riding the lonely range. While the City of Broad Shoulders would appear on the surface to have little in common with the land of big sky, urban cycling connected me to the rugged individualist roots of my frontiersman ancestry.

But urban cycling had failed to connect me with another quintessential experience of my American forefathers— that of community. Alexis de Tocqueville captured this early American spirit of community engagement in his landmark 1835 work *Democracy in America*: "Americans of all ages, all stations of life . . .are forever forming associations . . .In democratic countries knowledge of how to combine is the mother of all other forms of knowledge; on its progress depends that of all the others."

My daily commute was a solitary affair within the city's congested confines. During my first five years, pedaling was seldom interrupted by social interaction, save the occasional honk of an irate motorist, leaving my mind free to reflect and contemplate. But without a broad connection to a progressive community, my affinity for urban cycling seemed little different in the larger social context than the indulgent consumption of the isolated SUV driver.

Granted, I wasn't polluting, conspicuously wasting scarce petroleum resources, or storing undo amounts of cellulite in my buttocks as SUV owners tend to do, but I wasn't overtly contributing to society's progress, either. Merely not contributing to the problem was not enough. I longed to connect with the American democratic spirit described by de Tocqueville that advanced the common well being through collective social action.

As the bicycle became a central part of my life, there was no apparent avenue for connecting with others who shared my political, practical and romantic devotion to urban cycling. Existing Chicago cycling institutions had little to offer the street level urban cyclist. The city's bicycle federation emphasized a bureaucratic approach, valuing political bedfellows over grassroots empowerment. The city's cycling club was largely an association of weekend recreational enthusiasts. Messenger groups were spirited but narrow in their focus.

A three-month stint as a bike messenger, a job that valued stoic machismo interspersed with feats of physical frenzy, further reinforced parallels of the isolated cowboy to the urban cyclist. I took it for granted that urban cycling for me would remain a solitary sanctuary.

This notion abruptly changed in the summer of 1997 when I read a *Chicago Tribune* article off the AP wire about a San Francisco Critical Mass ride. It described how 5,000 cyclists rode together and asserted a positive urban vision of cycle-dominated streets. The article spurred me to dream about a utopian city free of the con-

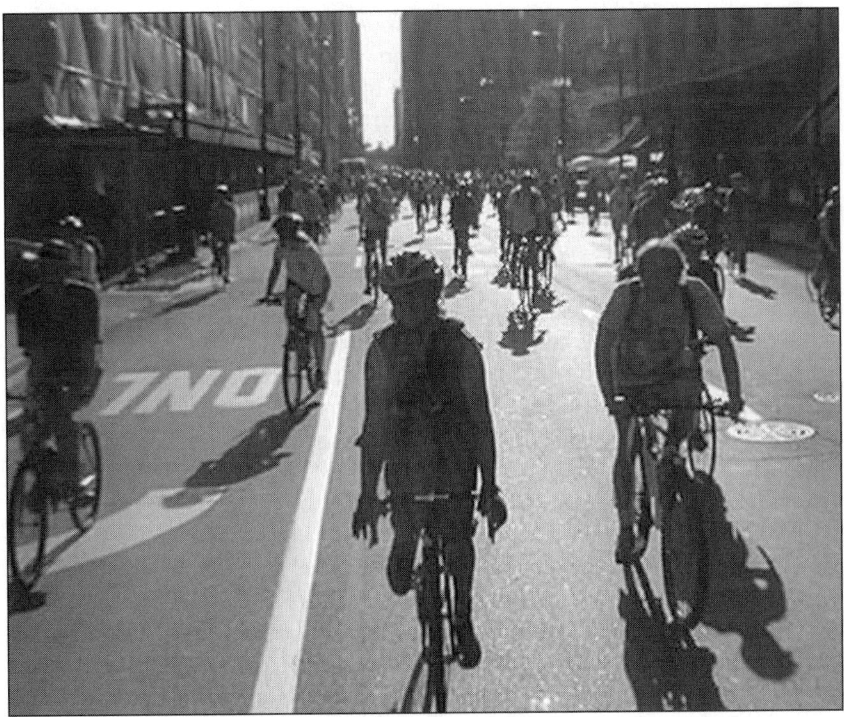

Chicago, May 1998

stant noise, pollution and dangers poised by over reliance on the private automobile.

I schemed with John Greenfield of the Windy City Messenger Association about starting a Chicago Critical Mass. We both agreed that the time was right and that Chicago desperately needed something to bring urban cyclists together. We choose a date and began spreading the word. A few days later, at a Chicago Messenger Band night at Phyllis' tavern, I met Jim Redd—a 56 year old software designer and bike commuter, who was passing out fliers promoting another date for a Chicago mass ride. He was driven by a concern for his son's safety, who worked as a bike messenger, and by a passion for social justice. We quickly joined forces, began aggressively promoting the ride and called together a meeting to coordinate our efforts.

The planning meeting for the ride brought together a disparate group into a funky Wicker Park cafe. Jimbo Daniels and Jim Redd's son, Adrian, a svelte 20 year old, were messengers. Three or four women from the local anarchist collective, the A-Zone, who had "organized" a few Chicago CM rides over the years that had been plagued by police harassment and arrests, offered their experience. And three bike commuters—Jim, me, and my friend Josh, a brewer at the local microbrewery—rounded out the stumbling group of would-be visionaries.

Jim started the meeting by passing out a draft flier for distribution to riders. The flier had "The Rules" written at the top and listed a few common sense guidelines like "don't get aggressive with the cops," and "smile a lot." The flier prompted a lecture from the A-Zone women on individual autonomy, and Jim, a little cowed but still enthusiastic, agreed to tone it down.

We plotted out a route and speculated that it would take well over a hundred cyclists in order for the ride to be too big for the police to shut down. Could we draw that many people for such a seemingly intangible issue as cyclists' rights, when it could quite possibly lead to some head bashing and arrests courtesy of Chicago's finest?

Though Chicago has a proud history of progressive social action, it also has a past checkered with overzealous police response to these movements. The spectre of the wrongful executions of the Haymarket Martyrs, union leaders who fought for the 8-hour workday in the 1880s, still weighs heavily on Chicago activism. The term "police riot" was coined in Chicago during the 1968 Democratic Convention as the First Mayor Daley quipped, "The policeman isn't there to create disorder, the policeman is there to preserve disorder," giving the cops *carte blanche* for indiscriminate head bashing of demonstrators.

Perhaps fear of overzealous police activity had kept previous Chicago Critical Mass rides from garnering more than a few dozen riders or sustaining itself beyond a consecutive month or two. Or maybe it was Chicago's shot-and-a-beer, pragmatic nature that had doomed the previous incarnations of Critical Mass from taking root. We worried that the naysayers who scoffed at our fliers, reminding us that we weren't living in San Francisco, would be right and our efforts were destined to fail.

While we were concerned about the police reaction to the Mass, our motivations for staging the ride went beyond merely provoking the police. While it

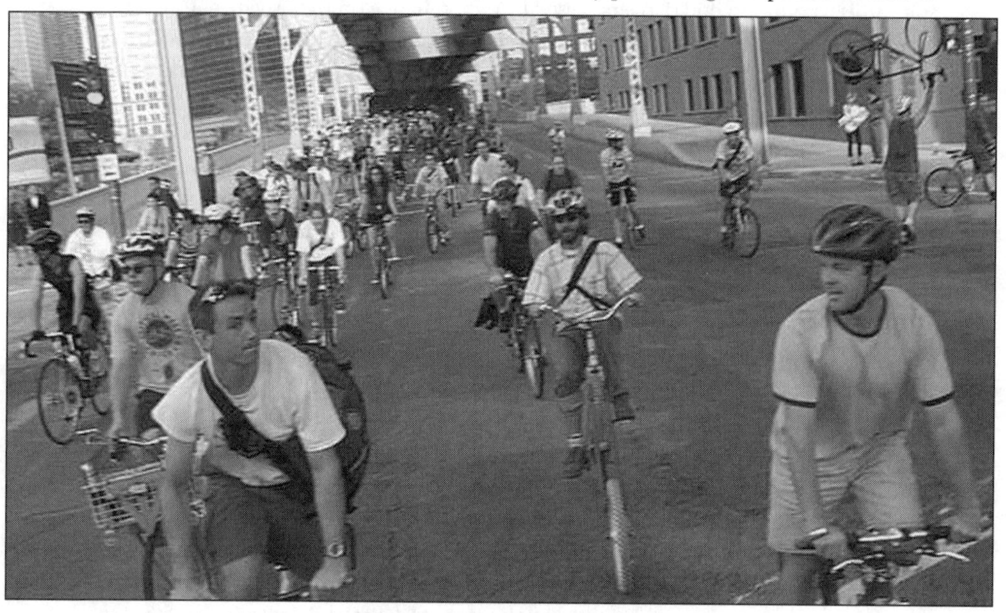

Chicago, under the El, August 2000

is not possible to speak for the motivations and intentions of a large, diverse group without an agreed upon mission such as a Critical Mass, to me the ride seemed like an enactment of a utopian vision. I likened our action to the civil rights movement tactic of blacks joining whites at segregated Woolworth's lunch counters. We were going to assert a positive vision of how things should be in order to expose the current injustice of car dominated public space and let the powers-that-be respond. Though the police might react violently, we felt that our righteous assertion of our rights to the road, demonstrating a simple solution to the pavement and pollution that plagued our city, was worth the risk.

But civil rights activists had been trained in nonviolent civil disobedience tactics and had strategized extensively on their actions and possible outcomes. Could a group as amorphous and individualistic as urban cyclists come together to express a common message on their right to public space without it exploding into chaos and violence?

As we circulated hundreds of fliers and the date of the first Chicago Daley Plaza Critical Mass finally arrived, many of us were full of nervous anticipation. Josh and I brought cardboard signs to wear on our backs with innocuous messages like "Share the Road" and "Peace in the Streets," hoping to perhaps preempt any conflicts with police or drivers. Jim passed around the route map and streamers to give our bikes a festive appearance.

The cyclists gathered at the base of the Picasso statue. The number of cyclists quickly surpassed the two dozen police awkwardly lining the periphery of Daley Plaza. One of them asked me, "Why are you doing this?" in an irritated, sarcastic tone.

I told him because the city streets were unsafe for cyclists. I motioned to a nearby bicycle cop and said, "Ask him, he'll tell you." The bicycle cop nodded to us, knowingly.

"Can I have one of those?" asked the ill-tempered cop, pointing towards the stack of route maps in my hand. I wasn't sure what to do, but I felt an urge to keep within the good graces of the cops in order to keep the peace. I handed over a map and I shuffled back towards the swelling group of cyclists, that now numbered well beyond our hoped-for 100 riders. My giddy feelings over our good turnout were soon tempered by one of the A-Zone anarchists.

"You gave the cops a map? What were you thinking?!"

I pleaded inexperience, not sure if I had actually done anything wrong. But there was little time to brood over my action as the cyclists began to swarm around the Picasso and then pour out onto Dearborn Street. As we took all three lanes, a feeling of euphoria overtook me amidst honking horns, ringing bells and hooting cyclists.

The mass was far too large for the police to do anything but facilitate our movement. We slowly wheeled northwest, waving to surprised pedestrians, giving fliers to idling motorists, and most of all, sharing conspiratorial smiles with each other at our creation of a beautiful social space in the usually cold, congested city streets.

The ride ended at a backyard party in the Wicker Park neighborhood, with our social intoxication from finding each other supplemented by a keg of cheap

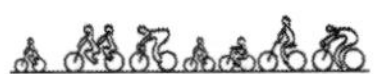

beer. A yellow legal pad was circulated and filled with dozens of names, phone numbers, and e-mail addresses. That night a new community was born.

Just as Critical Mass has helped countless Chicagoans become urban cyclists by providing a safe biking space during the rides, the Critical Mass community has provided inspiration and a nurturing space for countless rugged individualists. The wide variety of creative projects, campaigns and splinter groups that emerged from the Chicago Critical Mass stand testament to the richness and depth of our community.

But the real ties that bind us are the many personal relations we've developed while working and playing together. Jim and I lived across the street from each other for years before Critical Mass brought us together. Besides goading each other on numerous crazy cycling projects, we bought a sailboat together, recently traveled to Ecuador and count each other as cherished friends. And I still vividly remember the day in 1998 when Gin Kilgore walked down the stairs to join in her first CM activity, a banner making party. In August, she and I will be married and we'll lead a CM style bike parade to our wedding reception.

I still love the Wild West elements of my daily bicycle commute, the physical exertion and the opportunity for quiet contemplation. But now I also enjoy waving to my many two-wheeled friends. Chicago feels warmer and less lonely. And through the collective will of many individuals, Critical Mass has changed the streets of the city.

Rugged Individualists Unite to Change Chicago

Are you artistic? Submit your work to the CM art show. Is street theater more your style? Come on out to the annual Santa Rampage or St. Patrick's day ride. Feel like protesting car culture? Join us for the yearly shutdown of the Chicago Auto Show. Pissed about the elimination of Bike Lanes on Halsted Street? Work with the Bike Lanes for Boys Town Campaign. Feel more like helping educate lukewarm riders to stay in the saddle year round? Get involved with the Bike Winter classes. How about promoting gender equity in cycling? The Cycling Sisters may be for you. Or perhaps you'd like to promote walking and public transit as well as urban cycling? Check out Break the Gridlock. Or maybe you're sad that Chicago's lakefront is saddled with an 8-lane superhighway. Have you heard about our campaign to depave Lake Shore Drive? Do you have a penchant for choppers and alley scavenging? Join the Rat Patrol for a wild ride. Or how about long distance riding— join us for our annual trip to Starved Rock. Enjoy writing? Edit the *Derailleur* next month. HTML more your bag? The CCM website could use your talents. Or how about curling up with a good book? Travis Culley's *The Immortal Class* should be at the top of your reading list. Just feel like riding? The list goes on and on. And if none of these activities strikes your fancy, pitch a new idea to the community and you'll no doubt quickly find a few active co-conspirators. And don't forget: the last Friday of the month, 5:30pm, Daley Plaza. See you there!

Montréal, Québec, Canada

SPRAYPAINT SLINGERS, CELEBRATION, AND A TIDAL WAVE OF OUTRAGE

BY SARAH BOOTHROYD

Critical Mass is a many-splendored beast. The next few pages are an attempt to sketch its nature through exploring its parallels to and distinctions from three other forms of creative dissent. Graffiti, 'Reclaim the Street' Parties, and the Protest March will each be compared with the Canadian species of Critical Mass; thus shaping a portrait of Critical Mass—its dimensions, definition, foibles and future.

Colourful Mutiny

"La forét précède l'homme, le désert le suit"
Forest preceded man, desert follows him.
—Graffiti scribbled in Sorbonne, Paris, May 1968

What does the pictorial lingo of subway walls and bathroom stalls have in common with Critical Mass? Surprisingly, the two genres of creative dissent are symmetrical in several respects. To begin with, graffitists write their discord across perpendicular cement space, while Critical Mass cyclists ride their insurgence across horizontal cement space; and both employ a form used worldwide—a mode *du monde [of the world]*, hanging their missive to the masses between the ocher-sky and slate-ground of urban public space.

Graffitic din veers across the denizen's den—it is a painted expression of artistic dissent and creative nonconformity, and it is sprayed into the mallified public zone of dominant culture. In like fashion, the merry band of Critical Mass vélorutionaries are also subversives, interrupting the "consumption-oriented theme park"[1] of downtown with their no-motor mottoes. They move in harmony with Wolfgang Sach's notion that "those who wish to control their own lives and move beyond existence as mere clients and consumers—those people ride a bike."[2]

Modern scribes litter letters across walls, thus making their marginalized voices visible; similarly, when city cyclists morph into Critical Mass'ers, they emerge from the skinny margin of the street to bask in the middle of the traffic lane, thus making the auto-alternative visible. Both of these images, the one on the concrete canvas and the one on the paved landscape, are revolutionary in form since the very mechanism of communication in each case embodies a skepticism toward the status quo.

Assorted slingers of graphic slang may use the same form, each arranging some combination of line, shape, and colour; however, the content of such cursive discourse varies from writer to writer. From rider to rider, the intent of Critical Mass participants is equally varied, as are the participants themselves. In 1994, the *Toronto Star* described the San Francisco massers as "A hodgepodge of hard-core

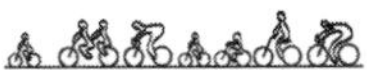

bike messengers, suited business people, body-pierced rockers, environmentalists, parents with kids in tow, and just about everyone in between."[3] Critical Mass is a communal forum for sundry partakers who wish to peddle divergent ideas, just as the primal scrawl is penned and painted by myriad messengers of disparate purpose. Said messengers are often stigmatized as delinquents, as derelicts smearing the stucco skin of the city with crude vulgarities. Their dialect is read as rebel babble, just as the dialectic of Critical Mass is often read as the rabble rousing of anti-traffic riff raff. In August 1998, the *Calgary Herald* ran a story entitled "Bike Messengers Defend Road Rights," in which the Deputy Chief License Inspector described Calgary's June Critical Mass ride: "They cut people off, they kick car doors. They swear and curse at people. They almost run people over on sidewalks."[4]

When Scott Martin wrote a favourable article on Critical Mass in *Bicycling* magazine's January 1994 issue, several reader retorts ensued; including "I'm disappointed to see Martin supporting this perverted brand of Street Justice," and "Your glorification of juvenile delinquents blocking traffic and assaulting motorists upsets me."[5] In the public eye and mind, Critical Mass is opposed, glorified, and defined in numerous ways. Analogously, 'graffiti' is simultaneously a synonym to both 'vandalism' and 'street art,' while it denotes both the ancient cave scenarists at Lascaux and Pompeii, as well as the idiom of so-called idiots who demur *sur le mur [on the wall]*.

There exists the ball-point-pen variety of graffiti—generally decipherable, more textual than visual, oft-sighted in lavatories; flipside, there exists the abstruse-spray-paint variety—requiring a graffiti glossary, more cryptic than clear, oft-sited in subterranean tunnels. Critical Mass may differ from graffiti in that the former is formed in the broadest of daylight by a plurality of persons, while the latter is commonly the nocturnal creation of an anonymous individual. I wonder, however, whether there is a difference between the legibility of these two acts of dissent.

From Victoria, British Columbia to St.John's, Newfoundland, witnesses frequently respond to the massing flock of two-wheelers with "What is this *for* anyway?" (insert wrinkled forehead, pointed finger, bewildered expression here). Delivering an answer vocally and/or handing over a flyer offers a translation to those in the direct proximity of the mass. Unfortunately, the majority of the thronging traffic who witness the Critical Mass only glimpse the blur of spokes and signs, or catch a wisp of chant amid rush-hour carcophony. Perhaps this zesty taste of Critical Mass prompts such spectators to peruse their local newspaper in search of an article to explain the nexus of pedal power and politics happening in their neighbourhood. It is unlikely, however, that such spectators would find a paraphrase of Critical Mass purpose inked in their daily rag, since Canadian newspapers have provided little information on Critical Mass of late. Major print media in Canada most recently ran articles on Critical Mass in 2001 in Victoria, 1998 in Toronto, Calgary and Hamilton, 1996 in Montréal, 1995 in Vancouver, and 1994 in Edmonton.

The question of legibility rephrased: What does a roaming heap of cyclists signify to those who are behind the caboose of the mass—is the intent clear to the average spectator, who is unequipped with media coverage of the event?

Furthermore, if riders participate in Critical Mass for various reasons, does there even exist a common answer to the question of what Critical Mass signifies? And finally, if Critical Mass's are held *for* different purposes—to protest the G8, to recognize a cyclists' death, to protest the war in Afghanistan—does Critical Mass signify anything in itself, or is its meaning dependant upon a chosen issue?

The CMovement, including its foibles and its future, is as complex as the elaborate tangle of aerosol and hue that tattoos the cracked and sweating surfaces of urbanity. These two different designs of dissent each find their place in the cementscape, where both marginalized voices speak out against the cartography of the city; one in a vehicle without walls, the other using walls as its vehicle.

Camelot Monthly

> *"The meaning of the Street in all ways and at all times is the need for sharing life with others and the search for community."*
>
> —Virginia Hamilton (b. 1936),
> African American writer of children's books.

Critical Mass and "Reclaim the Street" Parties each reach into the same bag of carnivalesque antics, drawing out a handful of song, a pitcher of costume, and a bucket of ethos with which to compose their playful display of creative dissent. For both forms, center-street is stage to a car(e)free spree: smiles boomerang between strangers, and celebration is the main sensation from curb to curb.

The urban street is a sun-up to moon-down perpetuum of people fastforwarding through The Inbetween; and in this way, the boulevard more closely resembles the conveyor belt than it resembles its sibling, the village green. Critical Mass and Street Parties alike recognize the modern road, with its ashen complexion and car-clots, as a sullied version of its former self. Long before the sky began to fade, the street spent several centuries as the stage for weddings, funerals, education, public debate, prayer, processions, commerce, theatre, music and the "triumphal entry of kings and queens."[6]

Street Protest and Critical Mass relive those days of yore by reviving the concept that public space is not just the gap between departure and arrival; rather, it is a gallery for public expression. Street Protesters and Critical Mass'ers dare to venture beyond the privacy of the living room—both the stationary salon and its four-wheeled cousin—to disclose themselves within the (c)architecture of the public zone. Both movements hold the conviction that the avenue is an ideal venue for communication and communion. They embody this view by displaying their beliefs on its white- and yellow- lined surface; thus replacing the thoroughscare of the thoroughfare with a sharing of ideas.

Much like Street Protest, the idea of Critical Mass is concretized by the carnivalesque crowd, and soundtracked by the melee of bells, horns, and voices that swerve through the smogsong of rushhour. The Critical Mass scene welcomes unusual accoutrements to both ride and rider, from superhero garb and cardboard bicycle-adornments to body paint and animal-inspired helmet ornaments. Amid the wink of reflective gear and the intimacy of collective purpose, the ebullience is palpable: "The point is to make a statement, but at the end of the day, it's a parade on two wheels. It's a fun and festive thing. It's not anti-car, it's a celebration of alternatives," explained Hamilton Critical Mass organizer Neil Croft in 1998.[7]

This rather cordial portrait of Critical Mass as a frolic of beatitude with a pro-pedal+person–power subtext, implies that Critical Mass's intention is to illustrate a Bravo! to the vehicle credited with putting the gaiety into 'the gay 1890's.' On this view, when the legs of the CM bicycle-bevy go round and round—tracing '0's with their pedals, this is Whoopla! for the zero injury this vehicle causes to the environment, the flora and the fauna. Critical Mass, in this light, is a Hooray! for the vehicle that costs approximately 2% of the capital needed to maintain a car,[8] and travels up to 9.5 kilometers faster than the car during rush hour.[9] Into the wheel-spun air Critical Mass projects a Whoopee! for the vehicle commonly considered the first democratic means of transportation, a Hurrah! to the mobility-booster and corset-alleviator of women: in 1896 Susan B. Anthony declared that "The bicycle has done more for the emancipation of woman than anything else in the world."[10]

Although this depiction of Critical Mass as a moving exhibition of ecstatic saturnalia and bikephilia is certainly an alluring advertisement to potential-CM'ers, I wonder whether fun-lust alone is enough to motivate returnees. Can the Critical Mass -verve and -vim keep riders recycling the event month after month, especially when the weather delivers a whammy? Will a veritable 'mass' of people choose to experience Critical Mass-as-watersport on a sodden afternoon in the Lower Rainland of British Columbia just for the fun of it? And when Decembrrr descends on Montréal, will many fancy r/gl iding their bicicle around the city's glacial corners for the jollity-quotient alone?

"The major problem [with CMontréal] is the difficult climate," concurs Robert Silverman, co-founder of Le Monde à Bicyclette/Citizens on Cycles, a Montréal bicycle-rights group that has been tremendously successful in its lobby for bicycle rights and parking, a network of safe bikepaths, bike access to bridges and public transit.[11] He also surmises that fury is perhaps a more effective impetus than fun: "It's almost as if you can get more people out to a protest than to a celebration;" this is true for both riders and media, according to Michael Thibault, a CM'er during the fledgling CMontréal movement of the early 90's.[12]

Le Monde à Bicyclette's debut event was the Great Bicyclist's Parade in May 1975. Silverman explains that it was composed of a duo of cyclists carrying a banner between them which read 'Pedal for a Better Planet' followed by 3000 cyclists—their wheels pirouetting down Montréal's Ste. Catherine's Street, a boulevard often opaque with traffic. Annually, this carless cavalcade would take to the street, resembling Critical Mass in its form and its repetitive nature; however, the content of "[LeMàB's parade] was strictly militant and the demands were clear—clearer than with the Critical Mass rides, which are mainly a social thing," Silverman remarks.

Chris Carlsson, a founding participant of Critical Mass in San Francisco, in conversation with the *Toronto Star* in 1994, described Critical Mass in like fashion: "This is really a very amorphous social movement. Achieving specific changes is not what it's about. The social experience makes it worthwhile."[13] In sharp contrast to LeMàB's specific proposals, Critical Mass'ers do the legwork for assorted causes, and are armed with diverse agendas. Critical Mass's multi-focal rather than uni-vocal personality has roused a rash of criticism, the tenor of which is represented by a reader's letter to *Bicycling* magazine in April 1994: "[CM-riders] don't have a bicycle agenda. While some mention their frustration with motorists, most espouse anti-car rhetoric or a 'Save Mother Earth' message. They are only coincidentally cyclists. They could just as easily be rollerbladers."[14]

Due to the fact that Critical Mass does not espouse a rigid set of tangible goals, it is very difficult to accurately judge the effectiveness of the CMovement. One cannot count the kilometers of bike paths, tally up the bicycle parking spots, and finally factor in the expansion in bicycle-awareness to produce a calculus of Critical Mass efficacy. Perhaps Critical Mass should be regarded as a party, with only the roadway as its platform; it's success evident in the sum of smiles and transported spectators.

Carsick & Miffed

> *"Protest, evasion, merry distrust, and a delight in mockery are symptoms of health: everything unconditional belongs in pathology"*
>
> —Friedrich Nietzsche (1844–1900), German philosopher

An aggregate of individuals forming a highly visible unit which roams the paved floor between skyscrapers = a textual sketch of both Critical Mass and the Protest March. Moreover, both species of creative dissent are "movements" that manifest this designation literally, and both breeds of public objection are at least partially motivated by ire.

Protest Marches are epitomized by the image of an unyielding, sign-wielding coterie of bipeds marching across the thunder-cloud-grey ground. Analogously, the postcard picture of Critical Mass shows a speedway deluged with chanting bipedlars, plugging the Friday afternoon flood of autos with tsunami-sized enthusiasm; a post-car utopia.

To protest is to complain about _____; hence,

A Critical Mass

In recognition of the recent tragedy and in opposition to further violence and militarism.

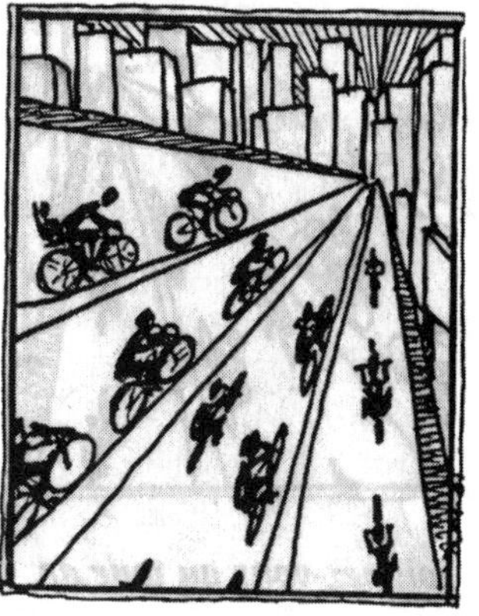

Come on a bike ride to spread information and encourage critical thinking about the threat of war.

5:30 pm
Wednesday
September 19
Meet at Phillips Sq.,
Rue St. Catherine
(across from the Bay)

A non-affiliated, non-confrontational, unorganized coincidence.

each Protest March is imbued with anti-______-sentiment. Critical Mass commonly fills in this blank with the rapscallion named 'motorized transport,' as the Critical Mass custom of slogan-saturation evinces. The Canadian Critical Mass repertoire includes such classics as the instructional "Get Out of Your Car, It's Not that Far!" the chiding "Get Off Your Ass, Save Some Gas!" the prophesying "*Auto à la Poubelle!*" *[car in the garbage can]* and the striking "Cars Kill, Bikes Save!"

There exists a melange of motives to spark one's joining a PM; equally, there are myriad reasons to join the sentience-engined Etcetera of the roadway as they become the content of the street through Critical Mass. Many riders participate in Critical Mass because of their unflickering vexation with auto-culture, its unconscious machinations, and its dire consequences. Some ride to protest that their kids can only trot *sur les trottoirs [on the sidewalks]* because it's a zoo *dans la rue [in the street]*; they are frustrated because the road has become a moat filled to the brim with hollow-tailed serpents. Others are fed-up with riding the tight rope of road between swinging car doors and gas-guzzling-hubbub. Others are irate because they do not have the freedom to practice what they believe is ethical without being (dis)regarded as penniless paratraffic. Many are pushed to pedal by the rueful fact that over 17 million people have died worldwide because of the car, since the first cockcrow of the automobile age.[15]

A tidal wave of outrage is sometimes the force necessary to carry a huge drift of CM'ers into the autopolis. According to Robert Silverman, the largest Critical Mass in Montréal to date included a "die-in" as protest against the death of a cyclist. Michael Thibault recalls this early '90s Critical Mass:

> *The route chosen ended at a point on Avenue du Parc, just above Sherbrooke, at the site of a recent cyclist's death. The ride occupied half the street, and people were flyering motorists who had slowed to beetle their way around the massing of cyclists and bicycles that had stretched across two lanes. The politicos and media in attendance did their thing. People watched dutifully. Bob dropped his bicycle and lay down. I caught on, and lay down too. The mass followed suit. In seconds, we had a die-in.*

This tale suggests a ratio betwixt Critical Mass size and the degree of fervor in the community, as Silverman recounts: "To my knowledge, Critical Masses have been biggest where the cycling conditions are the worst and where the people imagine how it could be." In Québec, where over 3000 kilometers of bicycle paths are either built or planned,[16] complacency has largely displaced the furor necessary to amass criticism via Critical Mass. "The general level of what Bob Silverman calls 'cyclo-frustration' is low among Montréalers—ironically, thanks to the many years of cycling advocacy by Le Monde à Bicyclette itself, an organization co-founded by Claire Morissette, Bob Silverman, and others," notes Thibault.

Despite a measure of post-success apathy, Critical Mass's in Montréal have continued to swell > shrivel < surge > shrink and to survive throughout this metamorphosis for over a dozen years. Thibault has had rendezvous with a few of the recent incarnations of CMontréal, and "didn't come away with the desire to return," having found the current CMontréal rendition just "a little too yahoo and confrontational."

Michael MacDonald, an organizer for CMontréal, comments that many riders did not reride following the October 2001 mass.[17] This particular bike-in, like most in recent CMontréal history, reached its finale at the main gates of McGill University, where the (de)riders began circling the intersection of Sherbrooke and McGill College as a denouement to their spin around town. The loop of cyclists continued to orbit the major intersection as the traffic lights turned yellow, then red, then green, then yellow, then red, then green, then yellow, then red, then green, then drivers began to inch through the rotating ring of rubber, and metal, and skin.

CMontréal's human twister, as described above, may be evidence of enough 'cyclo-frustration' to keep Critical Mass attendance *dans La Belle Province [in the Beautiful Province]* at least double-digited; however, it may also signify a rumbling of vitriol sizable enough to ignite civil disobedience and kindle a showdown. Speaking on this Critical Mass issue, the executive director of Cycling B.C. informed the *Vancouver Sun* in June 1995: "Our association does not hold with civil disobedience. Over all it hurts us more than it helps us. But I understand the frustration of cyclists when you see how long it takes to implement change."[18]

This comment implies that the firebrand's march on wheels blocks both traffic and progress; however, what the bystander reads as tempestuousness and commotion may be more accurately translated as vivacity and co-motion—as is the verity from the vantage point behind handlebars. The vocabulary of Critical Mass is replete with double entendres, with gestures legible as both protest and celebration. Perhaps we should spin our wheels toward evolving our coordination between dissent and creativity as we monthly sign the concrete crust of our cities with Critical Mass' colourful lexicon of movement, jubilation, and pique.

Footnotes

1. Gust (Ghent Urban Studies Team). *The Urban Condition: Space, Community, and Self in the Contemporary Metropolis*. Rotterdam: 010 Publishers, 1999.
2. Sachs, Wolfgang. *For Love of the Automobile: Looking Back into the History of Our Desires*. trans. Don Reneau. California: University of California Press, 1992.
3. Heft, Richard. " Pedal Power Seizes San Francisco." *Toronto Star* 3 Dec. 1994: E6.
4. Lunman, Kim. "Bike Messengers Defend Road Rights." *Calgary Herald* 5 Aug. 1998: B4.
5. Macgregor, Cairn. "Cycling for the Urban Masses; Critical-Mass Rides a Statement for Riders' Rights in the City." *Montreal Gazette* 20 May. 1994: D4.
6. Engwicht, David. *Reclaiming Our Cities and Towns: Better Living with Less Traffic*. Philadelphia: New Society Publishers, 1993.
7. Hughes, Rick. "Cyclist' Protest Ride Shouldn't Tie Up Traffic." *Hamilton Spectator* 28 May. 1998: A5.
8. Spokes Info: Benefits of Cycling, Ministry of Transportation, 5/10/93.
9. *Ibid.*
10. "A Quick History of Bicycles." http://www.pedalinghistory.com/PHbikbio.htm.
11. Silverman, Robert. Personal interview. 2 April. 2002. All subsequent quotes from Robert Silverman are gleaned from this interview.
12. Thibault, Michael. Personal e-mail. 4 April. 2002. All subsequent quotes from Michael Thibault are garnered from this e-mail.

13. Heft, Richard. *op. cit.*
14. Macgregor, Cairn. *op. cit.*
15. Engwicht, David. 2040: A Message from the Future. Video recording. Australia,1993.
16. Weisbord, Merrily. "The Don Quixote of the Bicycle." http://www.cam.org/~rsilver/don-quixote.htm.
17 MacDonald, Michael. Personal e-mail. 9 April. 2002.
18 Ward, Doug. "Bike-Car Wars Have Some Road Warriors." *Vancouver Sun* 1 June. 1995: B11.

Climate Change Caravan—CANADA

by Jeremy Murphy

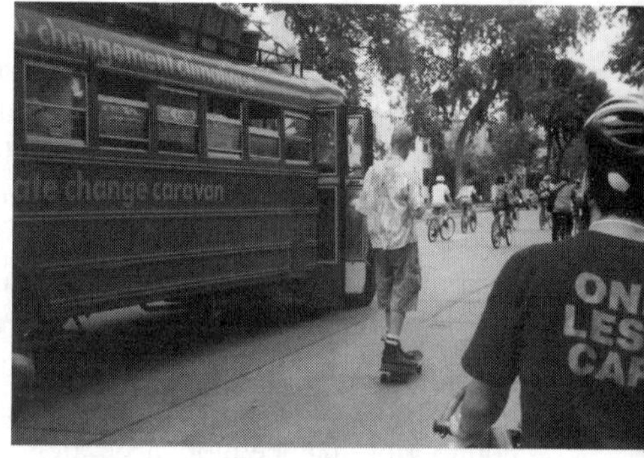

I am a cyclist who has recently biked across Canada on an environmental campaign called The Climate Change Caravan (www.theBET.ca). One of the ways we brought attention to ourselves was by holding Critical Masses in the towns we passed through. I was a little skeptical at first when we were presented with the idea of instigating a Critical Mass in Calgary, Alberta, let alone in every major centre across the rest of the country. We cycled from Tofino, British Colombia to Halifax, Nova Scotia; we treaded on every provice in the nation, some 10,000 km. We had an environmental challenge to Canadians: to reduce their personal greenhouse gas emissions. We made several suggestions, the most important being to drive less, much less. Holding press conferences, giving public presentations, and handing out pamphlets was pretty standard fare. But a Critical Mass?! I didn't think that the best way to get our message out there was to purposely rile motorists by slowing them down or stopping them entirely and then going to their windows to ask, "Excuse me, are you concered about climate change?" It didn't seem effective, or safe either.

Despite my reservations, we decided to give the Critical Mass a shot. Not just anywhere, though, not in a small town nor in a town where cycling was a popular mode of transportation to begin with. We would hold our first Critical Mass in Calgary. Here were people born with divine rights to have a full ton truck or SUV. The fervor for speed and asphalt is in their genes. These people had bypassed bicycles and gone straight to diesel power. With this in mind we set to the streets and were joined by about 15 other enthusiastic Calgarians. So, 35 cyclists strong, we nervously set a pace of about 5 kilometers per hour and tried our luck at this new tactic.

Motorists weren't pleased, to be sure. But, surprisingly, they weren't as rude or as impatient as we had anticipated. Also, most were open to hearing about our campaign and why we would do something as odd as bike around in a huge group, purposely getting in the way. I found we were quite good at keeping together and thus were quite safe. The people pulling up the rear brazenly slowed the traffic immediately behind us while people up front plugged traffic at the intersections allowing us safe passage, even if the lights turned. My friend Tim was particularly good at this; Tim raced ahead of us all into an intersection where the light was already stale amber against us. He hit his brakes and stopped dead in front of two lanes of traffic coming into the intersection from our right. The light turned red but Tim held up his arms, palms towards the drivers and confidently yelled, "STOP!" It was then that I realised what a great event this was. The cars were immobile, held static by Tim's commanding stance. I raced up to help him block and we laughed at how absurd the situation seemed. It was an amazing experience. For a brief period, we took over the streets.

DILDO MAN

BY R. WILEY EVANS

27 Aug 1997 IMPORTANT PRESS RELEASE

Look, over there, stuck in traffic...is it a dick, a weenie, a bicyclist?

No, ITS DILDO MAN. He is asking everyone, "Don't Be A Dick" (or a weenie).

The infamous Super Hero Dildo Man, a pillar of safety and enjoyment, has been summoned to bring peace and happiness to the streets of San Francisco during this Friday's rush hour. Dildo Man will be riding a public bike to promote friendliness and general good feelings during Critical Mass. Being somewhat a critical mass himself, Dildo Man feels it was time to show his solidarity with the people-powered transport of San Francisco. In closing Dildo Man says, "There will be lots of people stuffed into a very small space Friday evening, please don't push too hard, it can cause Road Rage and Rug Burn."

Dildo Man obeys all laws, both traffic laws and the laws of physics.

Dildo Man is not a leader, but a symbol of safety and enjoyment.

Attendance was high for the August 1997 ride. The media vans had circled all around Justin Herman Plaza. The Embarcadero was congested as helicopters hovered above. Traffic radio reported on the movements of a pack of thousands of bicyclists. It felt like a face off. The police were given public orders to ticket any and all cyclists for breaking the law. Cyclists jokingly pointed out that the police had riot gear and plastic handcuffs for bicycling red light runners, and blinders for automobile red-light runners.

The media attention was astounding. Critical Mass was live on TV. There had been the occasional TV reports and newspaper reporters, but this time there

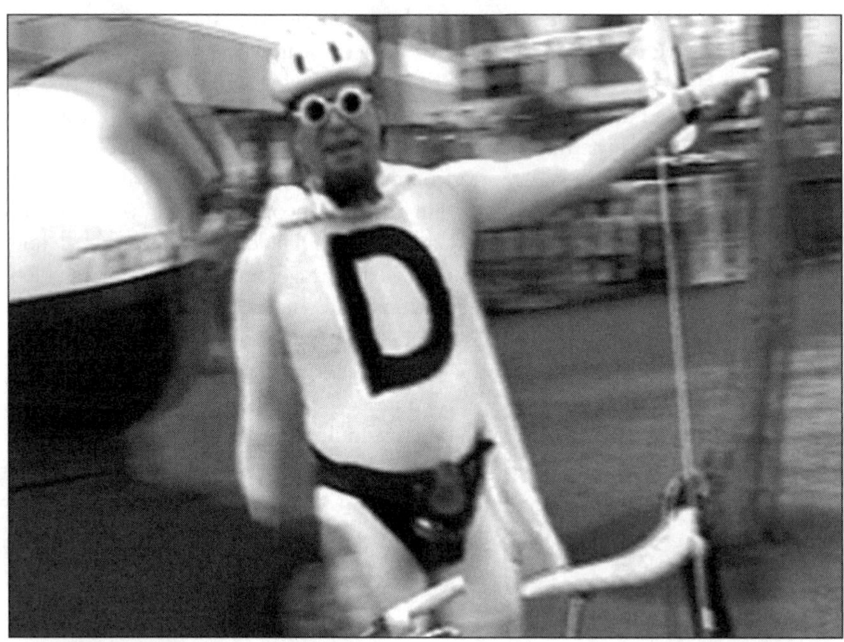

were TV cameras everywhere. Tag team reports seemed intent on finding the story right then and there, while everyone was standing around. You could sense that the media was also pissed off that there was no one in charge, nor any underlying statement to characterize the protest's purpose. Even the route of the ride was a mystery. The most popular question was, "where are you going?" Each person answered differently, unsure of destination but well versed in the near death experiences of riding the streets of San Francisco.

I knew from running in the Bay to Breakers that there would be a wide variety of rude and derogatory comments directed at Dildo Man, so I decided to make the identity switch near Justin Herman Plaza. The initial response from the cyclists was to give Dildo Man a wide berth. But after several fliers were handed out, the joke started to spread. It was good to get support from fellow cyclists. As we rode out of the plaza through the gauntlet of reporters, police and angry bystanders, Dildo Man received a vocal reception of praise and disdain. Some clever, most were predictable; "Hey, Dick Head!" Dildo Man was used to it. They didn't understand the throbbing intensity of a sex toy super hero.

From out of nowhere, a retort was shot back into the crowd from the cyclists, "That's not a dick head, that's Dildo Man, you asshole!" And with that spark of intellectual discourse, the anger was dissipated.

At first there was confusion about stopping at red lights. But with police guarding intersections, few had the nerve to tempt the police into a skirmish. Stopping at intersections caused the Mass to split up into several massive crowds of cyclists spread all over the downtown area. It got to the point were hundreds of cyclists were waiting at a redlight while hundreds of other cyclists crossed through on the green. Banter and innuendo rolled through the streets along with Dildo Man. Dildo Man was being accepted into the community, taken on as a sort of mascot.

Once again, Critical Mass had quieted the downtown area. Having Critical Mass stop at all stoplights had backfired. This time downtown was not only tied up with car traffic, but bike traffic was so heavy that even bicyclists were having a hard time winding through the blocked streets. As Dildo Man approached an intersection he could see things were getting tense. It was amazing how people would drop their guard and anger when Dildo Man appeared. Dildo Man turned outrage and anger to the sudden realization that this was a once-in-a-lifetime San Francisco experience. More often than not, the parting quote was heard, "where else but San Francisco?" By the end of that ride, Dildo Man was standing tall on his pedals, waving to onlookers, spreading joy and love all through town.

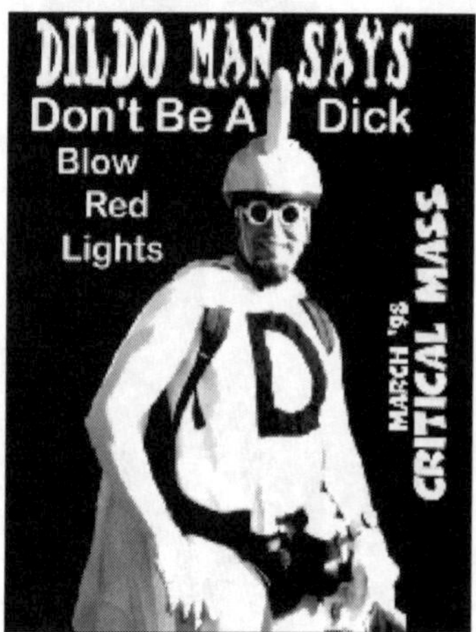

There was a lot of discussion on whether or not we (as a Mass) should return to the lawlessness of redlight running in order to keep the Mass together and on the same path. Dildo Man's notoriety began to swell over the next few months. He began flyering about "blowing red lights" for the March ride (1998). It was an ambigous flyer. (He still denies that it encouraged the blowing of red lights.)

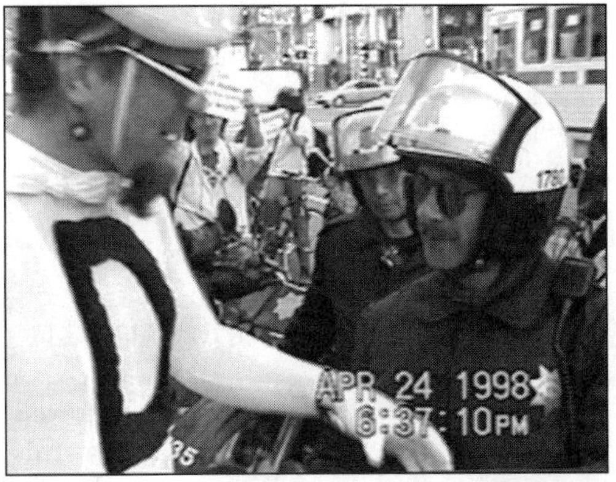

Like many of the rides following the big August 1997 ride, the Mass headed up Market, stopping at each light. People shouted "it's turning yellow," "we should go through it." Dildo Man's bicycle was a one-speeder, so stopping at stop lights was fairly easy. Anyway, he was only tipping the speedometer at 10 mph, tops!

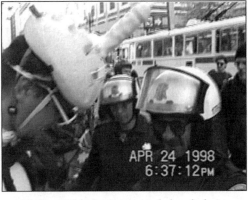

At Market and 5th streets, Dildo Man was riding alongside a motorcycle cop. Just as both of them entered the crosswalk, fellow cyclists alerted Dildo Man that he was about to blow a red light. Dildo Man noticed that light was a stale yellow and there was time to stop, but since the cop was going through, Dildo Man plowed right through, too

It was pretty obvious that Dildo Man had blown the red light. And there was a fairly large group of people shouting at the cop to pull Dildo Man over and ticket him. The Cop hesitated for a split second, but then snapped into action, closing in on Dildo Man. The Officer, asked Dildo Man to step off the bike and stand on the sidewalk. Dildo Man, suddenly felt so alone. In fact, Dildo Man had been cut off from the Mass by two motorcycle cops and a bus full of angry commuters shouting obscenities.

After both of the cops dismounted their motorsteads, Dildo Man began pointing out the uneven enforcement. Dildo Man blowing a red light is much less harmful and lethal than a 35 mph Detroit Bomb running red lights. They were embarassed. Not only did they have to be seen by a growing audience, but that this perp was going to be a dick too.

"Do you have any I.D.?" said the motorcycle cop #1780.

I then realized that I only had my keys and a twenty dollar bill on me. So I thought I would stay in character as long as I could.

"No, I don't have any ID," Dildo Man said. This did not go over very well with #1780, especially because the light was now green and a swarm of cyclists was approaching for the show.

"Do you have anything with your name on it?" raising his voice over the rumble of diesel buses.

"I have a 'D'—that's all I have."

"Huh?"

"I have a 'D', that's all I have," Dildo Man proclaimed again.

This initial exchange did not go over well with Officer 1780. He wasn't going to play this game, and reached the end of his rope. Here he was, a highly trained motorcycle cop with several years' service, in the middle of the tourist area writing a red light ticket to a freak in a white suit with a dick on his head! And the character was blathering about bicycle rights and asking "why aren't you ticketing cars that run red lights?"

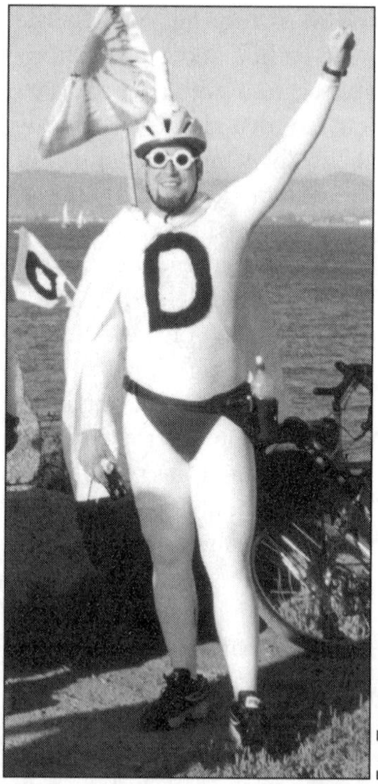

The cops looked at each other with a 'what are we going to do with this jokester' shrug and turned back to Dildo Man. "What is your legal name?" one asked with a ready pen, looking downward.

"I am Dildo Man!" Dildo Man exclaimed, "I'm a Super Hero."

Eric Zuckerman

Dildo Man salutes his admirers at the Wave Organ during Bikesummer 1999

In his best John Wayne walk, Officer 1780 waddled around from behind his motorcycle and stood close to Dildo Man. With a threatening voice, he said, "Y'know if you want to give me false information, I'll take you downtown and book ya, or you can give your real information and I'll just give you a ticket."

I instantly caved into the long arm of the law and started spewing my personal identification, but by this time an audience of about 20—30 cyclists had gathered and begun to shout at the officers. "You should be ashamed of yourself taking orders from the Mayor, having to hand out traffic tickets that won't stick in traffic court." They were right, of course. These guys were being used as political pawns. They were angry and humiliated at having to write Dildo Man a ticket for Blowing a Red Light. But they did.

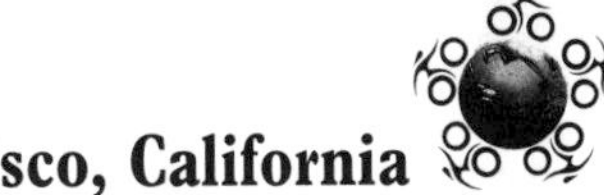

HALLOWEEN

San Francisco 1998 Report

BY JYM DYER

I had a great ride! I dressed as Akbar (or maybe Jeff) from from Matt Groening's *Life in Hell* comic strip. Basically it's a Charlie Brown shirt and a red fez, which was way oversized because I built it around my bike helmet. Most people seemed to think I was Charlie Brown with a lampshade on his head.

My favorite ensemble at Pee-Wee Plaza was a group with big white birds flying overhead, with "Reclaim The Streets" written on their bird bellies. They identified themselves as a local RTS collective. Right on! Other great stuff:

• A bike/wheelchair musician setup with an accordion player sitting in the chair. I saw a number of wheelchaired folks on Market, and their faces totally lit up when this went by. • A grumpy skinny Santa (he'd downsized the reindeer, the elves, and his belly) who told me I wasn't getting anything for Christmas. • A very convincing Krusty the Clown (he had the voice and the patter down perfect!) on a folding bike. He was the only other Matt Groening character I came across, and *he* was getting the same treatment (people thought he was Bozo). • A shriner with a little bike instead of a little car. (He told me that I gave him "fez envy.") • Speaking of size envy, Wonderbrawoman was there. Bikehilda was there with a horned helmet, "Flight of the Valkyries" on tape, and a breastplate that figured in a TV cameraman's extreme close-up. • Did somebody mention size envy? Dildo Man joined the party, disguised as a mild-mannered alter ego. Other superheroes there were Transit Man and Patch Man (with Schrader *and* Presta valves). Also, an action-packed Captain America/Spiderman crossover! • A priest with an alarming voice-

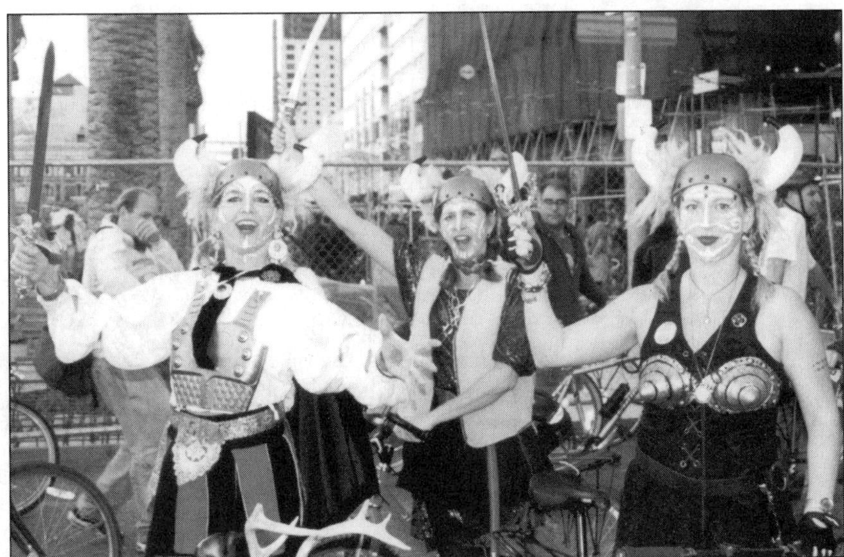

CHRIS CARLSSON

Super Heroines from Valhalla

of-authority megaphone. He made me feel like confessing, but I didn't know whether I should confess my sins or Akbar's (or Jeff's) (or Charlie Brown's, I guess). • A devil/angel tandem. • A Muni tandem with an orange-hat construction worker and an orange traffic-diverter cone. • A "cigarette girl" peddling worms and chicken feet (eeuw!) and pubic hair and roaches and candy corn. • A candy corn. • Mona (the mural artiste) [and cover artist for this book—ed.] had this beautiful elaborate winged insect outfit. • A big chicken with convincing birdlike eye movement; very unsettling. • A big fuzzy dog who said "Ruff!" but didn't recognize the old "rough/roof/Ruth/DiMaggio" joke. • Two Y2K bugs, replete with insect wings and nerdy slogans such as "COBOL Rules!" Scary.

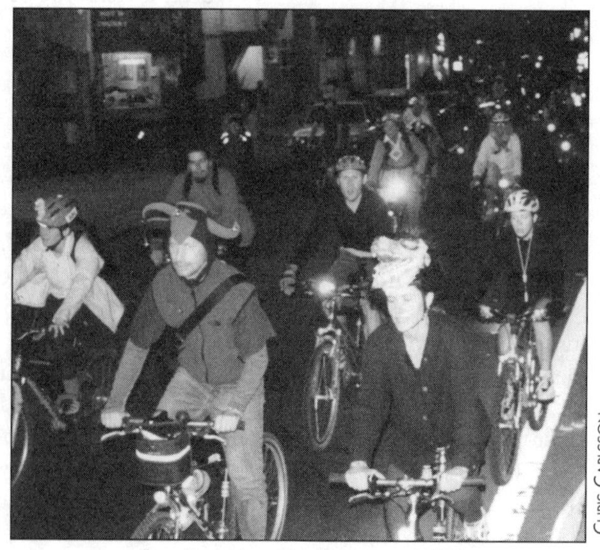
CHRIS CARLSSON

San Francisco Halloween 1999

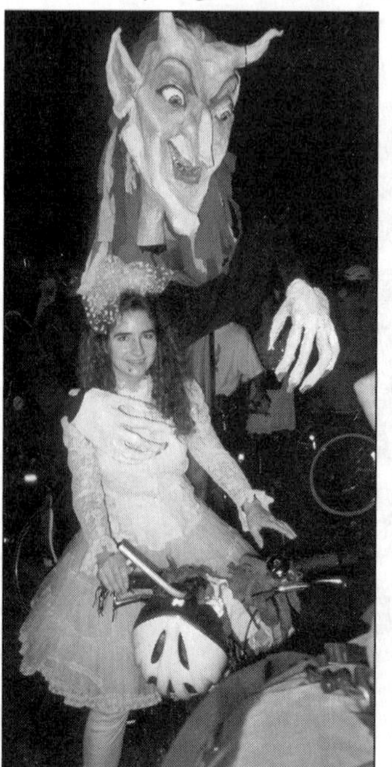

Dare I say it? I think we had better costumes going than at last night's Halloween party in the Castro. We started going up Market, which was boring, I thought, except that I'm really glad all those folks in wheelchairs got to enjoy the accordion player.

I was kind of hoping for a long ride (on a beautiful clear night before winter set in), and I got it: we went down Valencia (who needs bike lanes?) and into The Castro. Akbar (or is it Jeff?) was duly recognized in The Castro, by the way. We swung up Divisadero to Geary, and there was a loop through the little Geary underpass. Then we headed down to The Haight, then to the lower Haight, then to the Bike Mural. I loved partying by the Mural, because we got to see all the excellent little details, like the traffic jam on Market. We also had fun waving and and dancing for the Muni passengers. ("If you rode a bike, you could be here with us now.") Great ride! Great party!

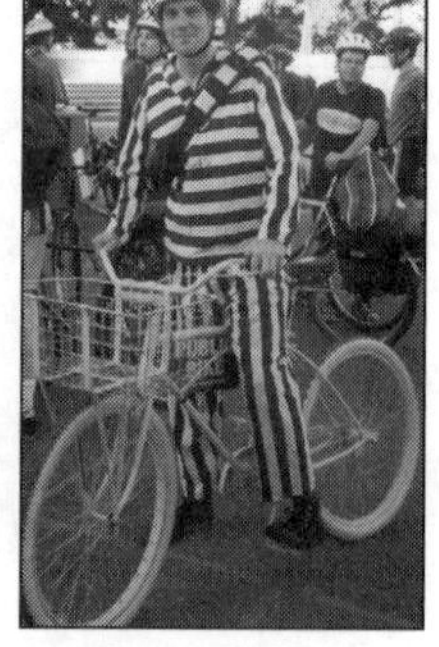

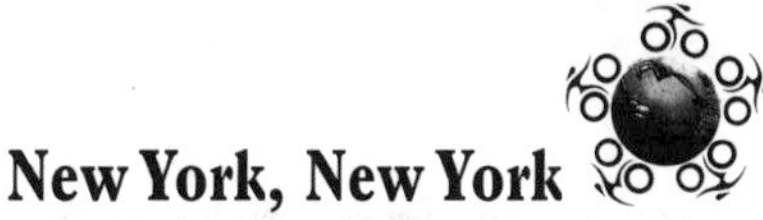

New York, New York

PHANTASMAGORIA.. .ON WHEELS

BY MARILYN HORAN
FRIDAY NIGHT, OCTOBER 26, 2001 / UNION SQUARE, NEW YORK / 7:35 P.M

The wind blustered but the atmosphere was electrifying as, with a roar, hundreds of costumed Halloween revelers hopped on their bicycles and flooded 14th St. to begin Manhattan's 3rd Annual Critical Mass Halloween Ride.

The spectacle they presented, spanning four or five city blocks, was truly dazzling. Amidst the pantheon of skulls, ghouls, and demons were several masked marvels, a hiphop witch in high-heeled sneakers, a rockabilly heartthrob wearing a suit that twinkled all over in yellow lights, a Mother Goose who was really something else, and a fat cellulite-riddled stripper in tassels and g-string (whom I tried not to ride behind). Towering over the rest on an old-fashioned bicycle with a front wheel four feet high was someone in mask and standard issue anthrax-resistant, anti-contaminate white jumpsuit, just in case anyone forgot who or where we were. There was also a woman with almost nothing on except some sweatery stuff around her elbows. I have no idea who she was supposed to be, or how she didn't catch pneumonia.

There would be no jockeying for lanes this time round. From the start our jolly crew of vampires, strippers, saints, and sinners filled the entire street pedaling up Sixth Avenue. Granted, crossing 42nd Street was a dicey affair, but we weren't about to let a horde of dirty stinky noisy polluters—going nowhere fast—slow us down. And since they were going nowhere fast, the polluters got to feast their eyes on a gala performance better than anything Broadway or Fellini had to offer, as they sat gaping at the bewitching apparitions rolling by, so resplendent in their All Hallow's finery.

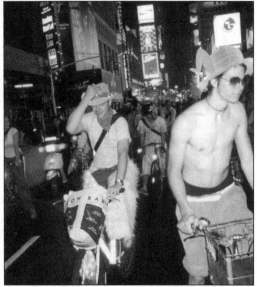

ALISA CLARK

Halloween Critical Mass, NYC 2001

As the first wave of riders turned north on Eighth Avenue there was a traffic policeman and something happened. The absence of lurid testosterone posturing indicated it was nothing serious, but a small group of cyclists near the cop had stopped, or been stopped, in the street. With barely a moment's hesitation the rest of the gang boldly launched themselves up Eighth Avenue. It's times like this when having no fearless leader really comes in handy.

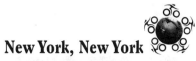

By the time we reached 47th Street, at least one costumed charac-

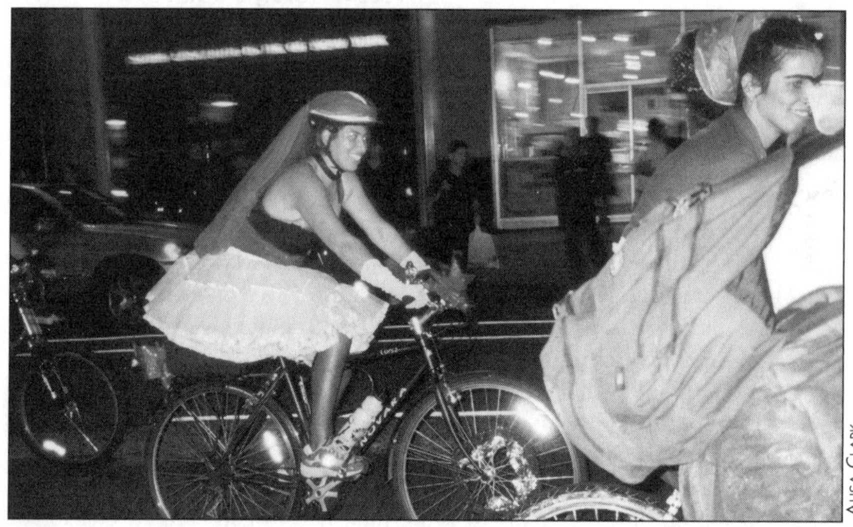

Alisa Clark

ter—who made a big mistake when she assumed pedaling would keep her bare legs warm—was ready to head over to Broadway and cruise on down the strip. But that was not to be. It was up to Columbus Circle and four times round the loop, three too many for the same shivering malcontent who scowled at the lot of them while she waited on Broadway.

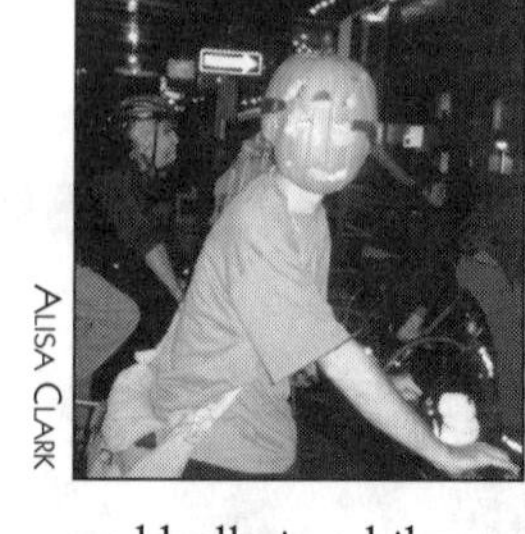

Alisa Clark

And then it was all downhill, rolling through the glittering canyon of dreams and desire—well, lights anyway. The crowning triumph came at 42nd and Broadway. For five glorious moments cyclists RULED Times Square. It was ecstasy, delirium, pandemonium. Amidst the hooping and hollering, bikes were hoisted triumphantly to the heavens. Even the 42nd St. traffic cop was having a ball. Cameras flashed, videocameras suddenly appeared, and some of the stars on wheels graciously allowed themselves to be photographed with the clamoring throngs.

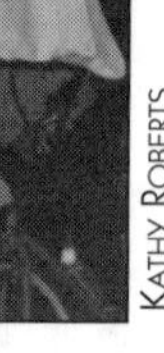

Kathy Roberts

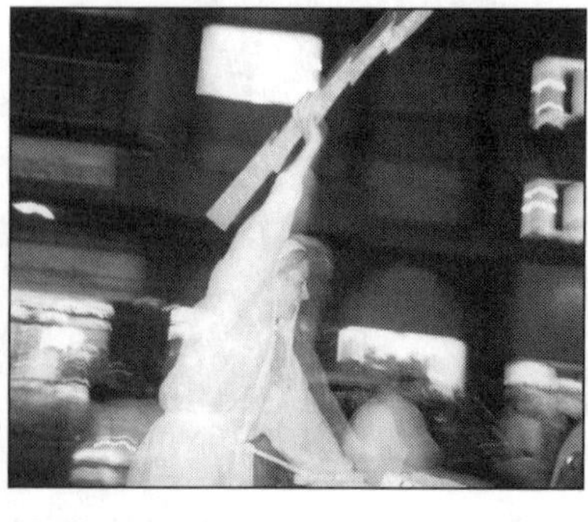

Alisa Clark

On my way out of Charas later that night, I ran into a fellow rumored to have something to do with the evening's events. Going by he muttered, "It went well." Recognizing a burst of enthusiasm when I saw it, I took this to mean the night was a rip-roaring success. I know it was for me.

Toronto, Ontario, Canada

CRITICAL MASS TORONTO

BY GUIDO BRUIDOCLARKE

Toronto's Critical Mass started in the crazy days of 1995. Revolution was in the air, the Cycle Messenger World Championships were coming to town and the city was ripe for change, bicycling style. It was a time of innocence in Toronto, a time when it seemed possible that the tide of the automobile could be turned back to the suburbs. It was during this time that bicycle messenger Dave DeYong returned from Washington DC. He brought with him the idea of cyclists getting together and riding around in a peaceful group. It was called Critical Mass.

Who knew where Dave got the idea to carry on a simple idea of getting cyclists to ride together in downtown traffic. It might have been from the messengers in DC, or San Francisco or perhaps from Mexico City where rumour has it that Critical Mass was originally conceived.

Dave wanted to have Critical Mass in Toronto. So with the help of other messengers, they made up some simple leaflets and flyered the neighbourhood. The last Friday of every month has never been the same. Bicycling in the city was different. People would run down cyclists and think it was normal. And although back in those crazy days the police seemed to care a little bit more, there was still something unwritten about bicycles not belonging on the road.

In comparison with today, the early Critical Mass's were crazy. There were definitely more confrontations with drivers, fistfights and property damage. One Critical Mass had a messenger bouncing his back tire off the front of a bumper of a car, while other participants rocked the unfortunate car back and forth in an attempt to tip it over. But over the years CM matured and changed and became a little more peaceful, but still confrontational.

It was from one of these confrontations that Advocacy for Respect for Cyclists was born. A police cruiser was responding to a call about dangerous cyclists holding their bicycles over their heads in an intersection. By the time the police showed up, sirens howling, the ride had moved down Yonge St. The cruiser struck a rider from behind and then the police promptly arrested him. The resulting confabulation shut down Yonge St for an

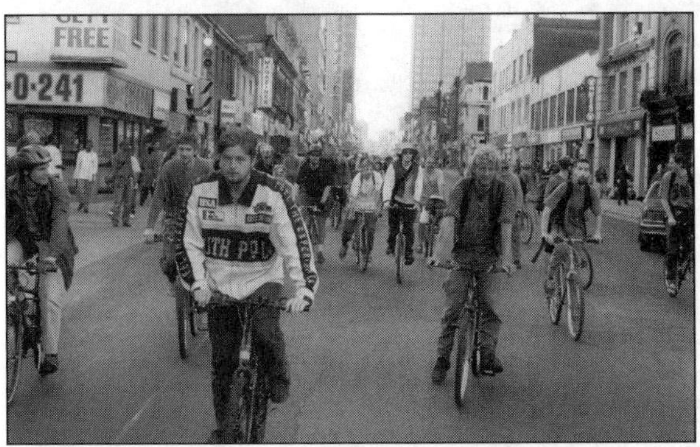

CM heads south on Yonge St. Yonge St. is the longest street in the world (no bike lanes) and one of Toronto's major streets.

hour. This arrest and a separate incident of a woman being run down by a dump truck at Queen and Bathurst made many a cyclist realize that the only people who would be looking out for cyclists' well-being were cyclists.

This was the first of many times that Critical Mass caught the media's attention. After a columnist for the *Toronto Star* said it would be all right to start shooting cyclists, perhaps in response to a certain cycling 'zine that suggested a bullet should be given to every driver, with the appropriate delivery device. Critical Mass went to the offices of the *Star* to get some answers. The columnist was not there, but the police were.

It was not long before ARC members quietly took the lead in making the ride more accessible to those who just wanted to go for a ride. Some of the tactics changed. Instead of everyone hanging around while the police dealt out tickets, the ride would continue on, but a few ARC members would stay behind to help the unlucky cyclist. Instead of staying for a long period of time on a major artery, the ride would stay just long enough to make a point and turn off before the police could be alerted to its presence.

In the early days of CM the police had no idea that Critical Mass even existed. Once in a while they would stumble upon the ride. Their reaction would never be the same. Sometimes they would arrest people straight out, pulling over the ride and ticketing everyone. Other times they would cork intersections for the ride. At those times it seemed like it was all of us against the car drivers. As the ride grew in numbers, the local authorities began to take notice. They knew the rides happened at regular intervals, but could never pin down the date.

They would sometimes show up at the beginning of the ride demanding a route map or wanting to talk to the leader. Both of these requests were met with blank stares. Toronto Critical Mass has always been adamant that there is no pre-

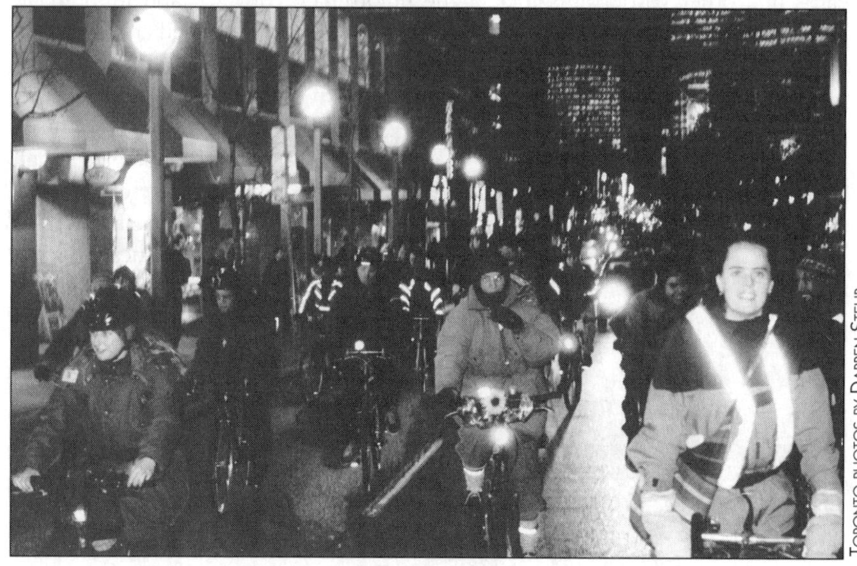

Toronto photos by Darren Stehr

A cold Critical Mass in February 2000 in Toronto.

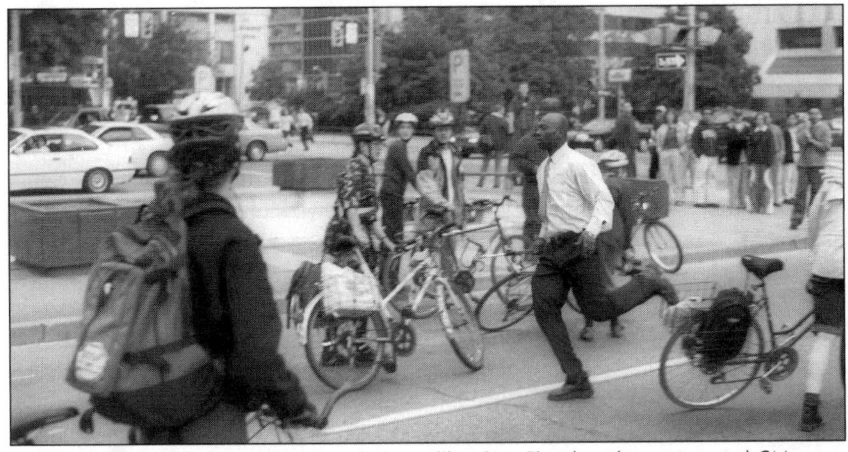

This motorist decided that he did not like CM. First he drove around CM on the sidewalk and through a group of pedestrians then he tried to 'brain' a few CM'ers with his CLUB (anti-theft locking device for car steering wheel).

determined route and there is no hierarchy. Whoever is in front is the person who leads the ride wherever they want to go.

The police could never understand this kind of structure. They eventually thought it was best to leave the ride to itself. That was until Officer Rodriquez made it his life mission to harass cyclists all over Toronto. Rodriquez was an officer out of 52 Division, the division that keeps a lazy eye on downtown Toronto. Rodriquez announced to one ride that he was the new sheriff in town and that he was going to tame Critical Mass.

For a while Rodriquez became Critical Mass's boogeyman. His name was whispered when his car would suddenly show up in the middle of the ride. He would harass participants in the vain hope that they would stop attending the rides. Some people stopped going to the rides, but new people kept showing up. He was a constant thorn in the side of the ride and then he disappeared. Rumor had it that he was sent to Ottawa to be turned into a special Critical-Mass-destroying-cyborg. He eventually returned, but not with the same gusto and only occasionally appeared to harass the ride.

The last the ride saw Señor Rodriquez was on College Street, when he did everything in his power to disrupt the ride. He would drive into oncoming traffic to get to the front, like a lunatic. He finally stopped one participant and tried to ticket him. The ride took up a chant of his name until the noise was unbearable to the officer. He finally jumped into his car and squealed away. We hoped that with our strange garlic and mystic chants that we have finally seen the last of this peace officer.

Over the years CM has changed from a ride of confrontation to that of a social ride with teeth. Most drivers either avoid the ride, or treat it like a parade that will eventually go away. There are still problems like the driver who chased a rider with a tire iron, or when the police stopped the ride on University and then got crap from his superior officer for tying up all four lanes of traffic. But these moments have become fewer and farther between.

During the earlier rides Critical Mass put the word out through flyers and word of mouth. The few times that announcements were put in the weekly free paper was met with confusion. The paper never really got the date right, or the time or the location. So the attempt to alert the general populace of the upcoming rides was left to such devices as word of mouth and the occasional flyering.

Over the years the number of people who showed for Critical Mass changed like the seasons. From the twenty-five people who showed up in December to the two hundred plus who would show up in the summer, it all depended on the weather. But one of the amazing things about Mass in Toronto is that it rarely has bad weather. After seven years of mass rides, it has only rained on the ride once and that was at the end of the ride. One memorable ride had the rain coming down hard all day, the ride started, the rain stopped, the ride rode until it was over and then the rain started *[EDITOR'S NOTE: this same magical weather pattern prevailed in San Francisco for the first eight years!]*.

Although Critical Mass has been about riding your bike in Toronto, other groups have piggybacked to get the word out about their own event. The largest mass ever was during the Days of Action. This was a time when government workers went out on a province wide strike. The streets were shut down and Critical

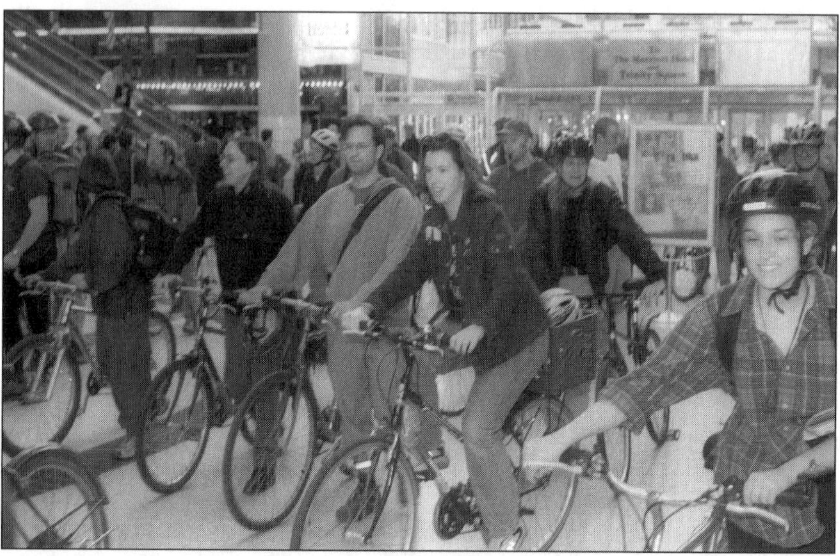

Critical Mass enters Eaton Centre, Toronto's largest shopping mall.
"My favourite Toronto CM moment was when we went through the biggest mall in town, 200 riders walking our bikes, and came across a bunch of contestants for a free SUV inside the mall. They were all dressed in stupid T-shirts from the car company each one touching the car with one hand (last still touching wins). One of them thought we were part of the contest! Hardly!"
—Martino Reis

Mass had an astonishing turnout of over 300 participants. Others have tried to turn the ride into a political movement, but it rarely ever works. Critical Mass is non-political no matter how some people and the media would like to change that.

Unfortunately not all cyclists see the good in Critical Mass. Many early participants dropped out because they considered the rides too dangerous. For a while some city councilors would ride, as did some members of the City Cycling Committee. But when the police began to show up at the rides, these officials quickly disappeared.

Toronto has changed a lot in the last seven years. What used to be a forward thinking council looking after the disadvantaged has changed to right wing advocates of the automobile and sprawl. The almighty dollar rules now and if you don't drive a car you are just something else that gets in the way of the smooth flow of traffic.

Critical Mass will continue in these darkening times. As Ontario and the city of Toronto continue to move towards a police state, CM will ride on and hopefully in the end make a difference for those who want to make a difference.

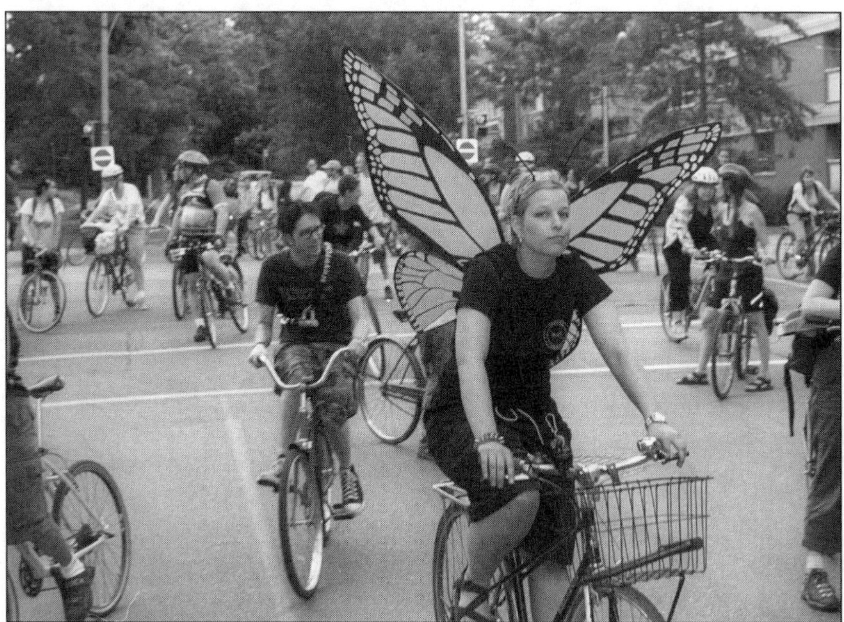

Lisa Butterfly, Toronto. *PHOTOGRAPHER'S NOTE ON CAPTIONS:* Critical Mass attracts a lot of people that help the poor. This attracts the police who use CM as a fishing pond. Less and less traffic tickets and more and more information gatherng. Traffic tickets require that you identify yourself. . . taking of info with no ticket usually means that they will ask your life story and file that info. I got threatened by a cop once and filed a complaint. During every interview they were more interested in my identifying members of the Ontario Coalition Against Poverty (I am not a member) than my complaint. No one in CM Has ever complained that I am posting pics (to the web). Many have asked that their names not be posted.

Stuttgart, Germany

I AM A CRITICAL MASS

BY MICHAEL HUMPHRIES

The first Critical Mass in Germany took place on a cold September 26, 1997 five years after the first Critical Mass took place in San Francisco. Then things slowed down a little. CM took place in Stuttgart in April 1999 and was followed by further Critical Mass events in Heidelberg, Mannheim and Erfurt. On January 1, 2001, the high-tide of Critical Mass activity in Germany, some sixteen towns took part in a synchronous ride. Since then, some of the towns involved no longer stage Critical Mass events.

Taken as a pattern what you have here is not so much the chain reaction implicit in the CM idea as a series of sporadic brush fire protests that the authorities have managed to contain and in some cases snuff out completely.

This article is a brief account of two Critical Mass's that took place in Stuttgart. I was told about the first by one of the participating riders.

About thirty riders assembled at the designated starting point but found the place bristling with a heavy police presence. According to the German law a cycle ride constitutes a gathering and the police have no right to dissolve it since the right of assembly is fundamental. However, if you notify the police that you are gathering together for whatever reason you become subject to the controls they can impose under statutes relating to public order. Then, to forestall any trouble they think might flow as a consequence from your assembly, the police will specify or vet locations and prescribe routes. If you happen to swarm spontaneously the letter of the law is slightly different but the police will police you just the same once they get on to your case.

Once the Critical Mass riders had assembled the police issued them with route maps showing them exactly where their mass could be concentrated. The riders studied and discussed the maps and got hot under the collar because they felt they were being dictated to in a manner contrary to the nature of CM as they understood it.

They considered themselves to be free spirits and would not be poured down a conduit chosen by the cops for their convenience. By way of protest they improvised a plan to escape from the constraints imposed on them. They set off, apparently in obedience to police instructions, but then quickly dispersed in all directions and reconvened at a prearranged spot. This tactical maneuver reduced their number by half as some riders probably took the opportunity to review the gathering in the ominous light of the large police presence. Those that remained now, minus their police escort were able to advance at least for a short distance along on their preferred route. The police caught up with them in one of the many tunnels that pierce the hills of Stuttgart (Stuttgart is similar to San Francisco in its hilliness and that has been one of the more feeble reasons put forward by town planners for the paucity of cycle paths.) The CM'ers were intercepted at some traffic lights and the demonstration stopped dead and the police went to work on the Critical Mass concept.

The riders' bikes were confiscated to be picked up later but at a time and place guaranteed to cause the maximum inconvenience. The riders' personal details were recorded for undisclosed future purposes. The whiff of anarchy explicit in the Critical Mass agenda and as clearly manifested in the riders' refusal to obey orders (and also by the fact that they had been fooled by a bunch of cyclists) had triggered a snarling nastiness in the cops. The riders were made to feel uncomfortable. My informant, a sprightly character of about sixty, managed to slip away as the cordon closed. He then changed out of his distinctive red trousers and sat sipping a beer in a nearby park watching with some amusement while the police hunted for him along the thoroughfares. Apart from the uplifting story of The One That Got Away, the CM was a debacle with few encouraging signs to be read from the ashes. To understand the shock the police delivered it must be understood that the majority of German cyclists are middle-class, peaceful, and with Green or Green-tinged politics.

They are also deeply law-abiding—as are most Germans. Jerome K. Jerome, writing in 1900, described a cycling tour through Germany in a book entitled *Three Men on a Bummel*—a 'Bummel' being a sort of meandering trip with no fixed objective such as the Critical Mass'ers had been forbidden to follow in Stuttgart—and observed then that the Germans were not merely law-abiding but sometimes dangerously so. A hundred years and two world wars have done little to put even a small dent in this national characteristic. So, for a law-venerating cyclist to be tongue-lashed and intimidated by the police is a significant matter—an almost schizophrenic experience because the offending cyclist is instinctively on the side of the law. Also, because these cyclists are perfectly respectable, they have orderly lives and established routines and good quality bikes that they value and take good care of. To be jarred out of their routines, stigmatised by having their names entered into police files and having their bikes confiscated was traumatic. And for what?

Reporting the event the Stuttgart press was uniformly hostile and scathing. *Bild* (*The Sun*) wailed about cycle anarchists holding up commuter traffic. A follow-up piece in the same paper screamed, 'When is this madness going to stop?' There was a quote from the Police Commissioner who described Critical Mass as a contravention of Paragraph 1 which forbids any traffic participant from impeding another—which seemed to imply that anyone stuck in a traffic jam was breaking the law. Then there were more column centimetres designed to reassure an alarmed populace, detailing the counter-measures the police were adopting, getting tooled up with video cameras to catch the Critical Mass cycle anarchists in the act of perpetrating their nastiness. The point of the Critical Mass evaporated in the heat of the denunciations. The voices of the individual riders were not heard. None were invited to articulate their individual motives in any of the available media. The overall result was that opposition to the cycle lobby, which is already strong in Stuttgart, now inoculated with a particularly mild strain of the CM virus, grew even stronger.

Of course, this event did not happen within a vacuum but inside a series of contexts, political, geographical and historical. It happened in a particular city in Germany within Europe and at time when the bicycle agenda is being pushed often with conspicuous success by a variety of pressure groups. Germany also has the Danes as irritatingly good model neighbours in this respect. Provision for cycling in Denmark is probably the best in the world so German politicians frequently get pestered by the question—Why can't we do it like the Danes?

One factor probably contributing to the limited effect of Critical Mass in Germany so far has been the lack of overt support from ADFC (the Allgemeiner Deutscher Fahrrad Club, a national association that lobbies for cycle-friendly roads and transport planning). While ADFC has given column inches to Critical Mass in its magazine *RAD-Welt* and some ADFC members have moonlighted on CM demos, there is a clear difference in approach to the same problem by the two movements. One is evolutionary and the other appears to be revolutionary.

It is also possible that the amorphous nature of Critical Mass—no organiser, no organisation, no single message, anyone can decide to lead everyone anywhere—is anathema to the orderly German mind. The ADFC, a large powerful organisation, is also well-connected and has some high profile members. One such is the German Transport Minister Kurt Bodewig, a keen cyclist and a key figure in the National Cycling Policy now under development. The ADFC promotes and organises huge pro-cycle rallies within the law—an annual 50,000 rider bike event in Berlin is one example of this. ADFC would thus have much to lose and nothing very much to gain by aligning itself too closely with an apparently reactionary and confrontational organisation that not only moved at a different and unpredictable tempo but also lacked rigorously defined objectives. ADFC might easily upset its network of relationships with the ruling powers and so endanger its own agenda. The ADFC could also claim with some justification that its policies are working well if a little slowly in some places. So who needs Critical Mass?

The trouble is that some cities, for various reasons, are tough nuts for the cycle lobby to crack and the ADFC "softly-softly" approach can seem a painfully slow way of effecting urgently needed change. Stuttgart is one such city. Chief among the reasons here is that Stuttgart is a base for Daimler Chrysler which is a significant employer and has a loud voice in local government. There is a powerful and sometimes irrational lobby not just *for* cars but *against* cycles. Some go so far as to fear and predict that a proliferation of cycle-paths would lead to a downturn in auto production which would in turn lead to layoffs and mass unemployment and famine stalking the streets. However unfounded and intemperate these beliefs may be they have to be recog-

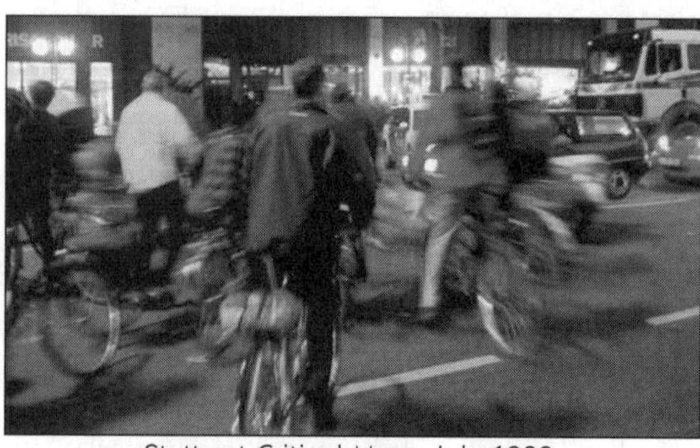

Stuttgart Critical Mass, July 1999

City 100 Radfahrer-Chaoten stoppten Berufsverkehr

Von ROBIN MÜHLEBACH

Gestern 17 Uhr: Alarm beim Verkehrs-Dienst der Polizei. Hundert irre Radfahrer legten in der Stuttgarter City den Berufsverkehr lahm.

★★★

Öko-Demonstranten! Eine Organisation mit dem Namen *„Kritische Masse"*, nach Vorbild der amerikanischen Anti-Auto-Bewegung *Critical Mass*. Die Kriegserklärung an Stuttgarts Autofahrer: „Wir sind Radfahrer, die Spaß am Stau haben."

Die Rad-Blockade begann auf der Willy-Brandt-Straße (B 14) beim Schloßgarten. Die Radfahrer versperrten beide Fahrspuren, lachten hupende Autofahrer aus. Rund 5 Kilometer Stau (ab Leuze-Tunnel und rund um den City-Ring). Hauptkommissar Raymond Schmidberger (34): „Über Notruf 110 bekamen wir ständig Anrufe von wütenden Autofahrern."

Am Rotebühlplatz griff die Polizei endlich durch. Etwa 50 Beamte mit Schlagstöcken kesselten die Demonstranten ein, beschlagnahmten die Räder. Ein Aktivist hämisch: „Ihr könnt uns gar nichts."

Schlimm: Die Polizei gab die Räder wieder zurück, schrieb keine Anzeigen wegen Nötigung. Ein Beamter: „Die Beweislage war zu schwach."

Warum die Polizei nicht ihre Video-Kameras einsetzte – unbegreiflich! In Flugblättern kündigen die Radler jetzt regelmäßige Störaktionen an – den ganzen Sommer über.

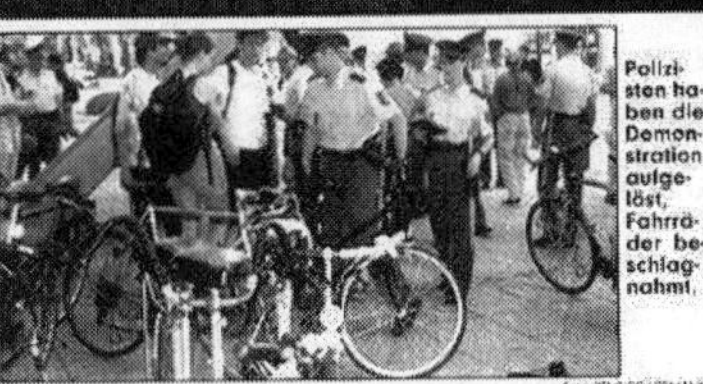

Polizisten haben die Demonstration aufgelöst, Fahrräder beschlagnahmt.

Foto JENS OELLERMANN

Natalie (4) aus Weilimdorf: „Danke, liebe Polizei..."

Großes Lob von einer kleinen Stuttgarterin an die Polizei. Natalie (4) aus S-Weilimdorf in einem Brief an die BILD-Redaktion: „Mein schönes Fahrrad war verschwunden. Die Polizeimeister Thorsten Bertsch (24) und Michael Dietmann (24) sahen mich weinen, fanden das Rad im Gebüsch. Ich hab' die Polizei ganz arg lieb..."

West

Neue Lastwagen für Hilfsdienste

Im Katastrophen-Schutz-Zentrum (Im Vogelsang

Neuer ICE T in Stuttgart

Heute testen

Der neue Super-ICE T der Deutschen Bahn – heute können Sie ihn im Stuttgarter Hauptbahnhof schon testen. Beim Bahnhofsfest ... herige D-Zug. Dafür sorgt die „Pendelino-Technik" des modernsten Zuges der Bahn. Wie ein Motorradfahrer legt sich der ICE in

News headline in *Bild*: "100 Cycle Rowdies Stop Commuter Traffic"

nised before any dialogue can take place.

My own attitude, after some twenty years riding and campaigning for cyclists' rights by every means I know of, is that anything that might influence events by even so much as another metre of cycle path is worth trying. So, when I learned through a web-page that there would be another Critical Mass in Stuttgart I thought I should attend. I had no preconceived idea of exactly what I would do but a clear agenda about what I wanted to achieve. The event was set to take place in the centre of Stuttgart on Friday at 5pm 29th June 2001. When I arrived at the designated starting point outside an adult education college there were no other cyclists around. There were a few bikes chained to the railings but no owners, no CM'ers. There were though, eight motorcycle cops waiting on their machines.

After some fifteen minutes the tally of those present remained at cops eight, cyclists one. At that point one of the cops came over and asked if I was there for the Critical Mass: *"Hallo—Sind Sie hier für die Kritische Masse?"*

I said I was. He asked if there were any other cyclists coming. I said I thought so. He went back to his machine and we waited a further ten minutes. It was a long ten minutes because it was beginning to dawn on me that no-one else was going to turn up.

I had a little time to reflect on what I was doing there and whether CM was such a hot idea after all. Perhaps it worked perfectly well for the Californian lifestylers, free-wheeling in the sunshine, but simply would not ignite at rush hour in a gritty, bike-hostile industrial German city.

There were also my doubts about the name itself with all its explosive and dangerous connotations and borrowed from the nuclear industry which I happened to loathe and fear. There is much to be said for stealing the enemy's signs but the process of converting them from one meaning to another is often a costly and bloody business.

Critical mass for Pete's sake!

I remembered reading about the very first critical mass which took place on 2nd December 1942 in a squash court at the University of Chicago. Enrico Fermi, who was supervising the start of the world's first nuclear bonfire had—necessarily—only a theoretical understanding of what would happen once it got going. One of his last line safety devices—just in case the nuclear conflagration ran amok—was a character armed with an axe to cut a rope which would release a cadmium rod which would fall into the centre of the pile and—theoretically—soak up all the fizzing uranium activity. History does not record if the name of this pioneer nuclear worker was Homer Simpson. However, when Fermi uttered his immortal words 'Zip in!' anyone might have been subject to sweaty palms knowing that one inefficient stroke of the axe could mean the cremation of Chicago. And the development of that critical mass has thrown a spotlight onto a number of places hitherto only vaguely known—Hiroshima, Nagasaki, Chernobyl, Three Mile Island ... I had to do my own renegotiating about the value of Critical Mass.

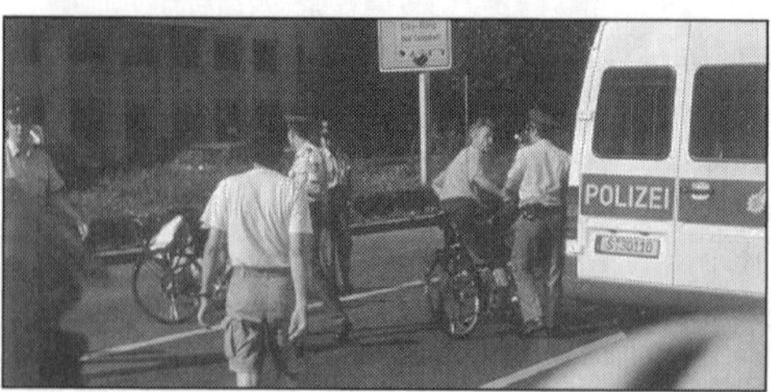

Again, while I understood that on a Critical Mass anyone could be part of it for any reason, my own reasons were clear cut and urgent. Cyclists in Stuttgart were not getting a fair slice of commuter space. Their health and their lives were being constantly put in danger by motorised traffic.

That to me was a situation to be challenged and changed. And what exactly was a critical mass of cyclists? Most of the cyclists I knew were distinctly amiable and non-fissile material. The only really two-wheeled critical ball of fire I had seen in action was the sometimes drug-fuelled peleton that rockets around France when the Tour is on. And where was that when I needed it?

In his masterpiece, *Crowds and Power*, the Nobel Prize Winner Elias Canetti defined crowds according to their prevailing emotion and showed that it is possible to predict fairly accurately how any given crowd will behave once its purpose is

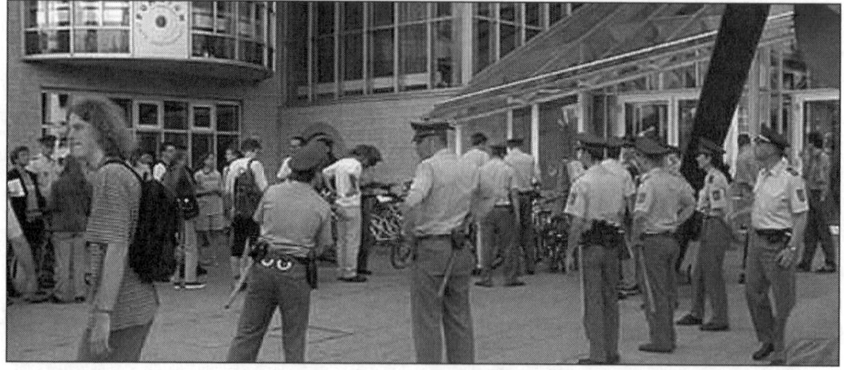

defined. Among these crowd types he identifies the Baiting Crowd, The Flight Crowd and the Prohibition Crowd. According to Canetti's taxonomy CM would fall into the latter category. I quote:

> "*A special type of crowd is created by a refusal: a large number of people together refuse to continue to do what, till then, they had done singly.*"

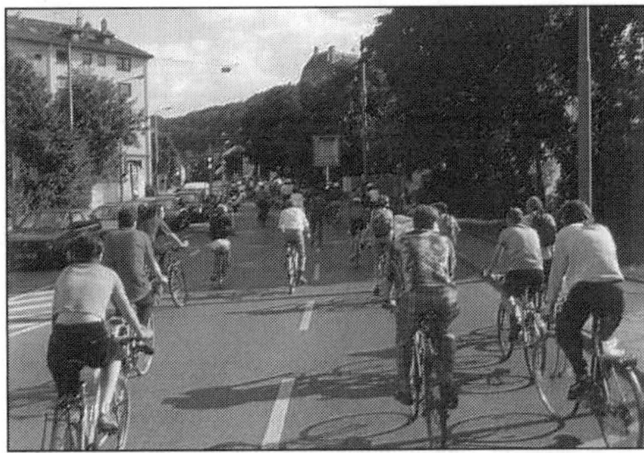

Stuttgart Critical Mass, July 1999

He then goes on to explain the dynamics of such a crowd but the main point is, these people are on strike. In Critical Mass the cyclists who have individually tolerated the injurious and adverse conditions imposed on them by their commuting brethren bare their teeth and say, "Up with this I will no longer put." And they hit the streets aiming to kick the chips into the air so when they next fall they will be more equitably distributed. At least, that was my take on CM at that point in time.

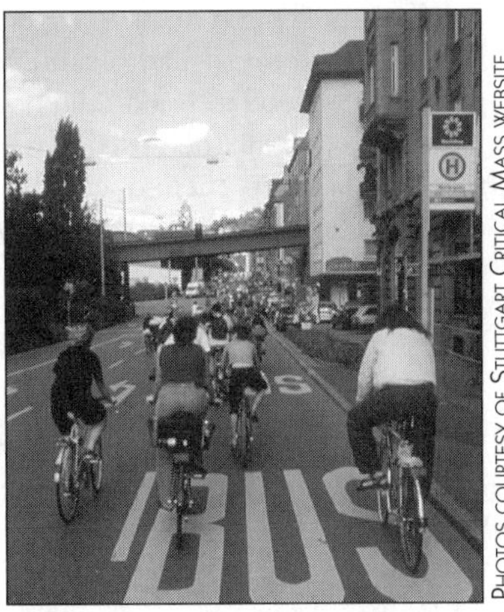

PHOTOS COURTESY OF STUTTGART CRITICAL MASS WEBSITE

The spokes-cop came over and asked how much longer I intended to wait. I said ten minutes. And if no one else comes?

To me this sounded a strange question because the obvious answer was that nothing would happen because the way they had dealt with the first CM had killed it off. And if no-one else turned up I would have to disperse. They had steamrollered the thing flat before it even began. But on the other hand ... I suddenly realised that they were stuck in their groove of needing to control the event down to the last individual.

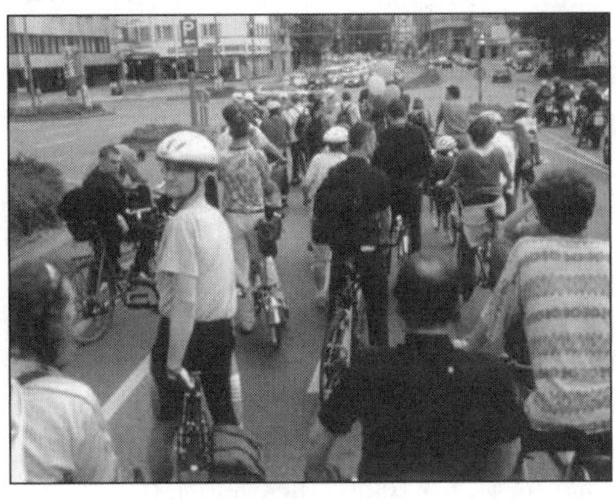

Like conscientious social firefighters they believed that until they had extinguished the last spark of Critical Mass cycling anarchy the danger to the public remained—so the fire was not out until I had gone. It was a critical moment. Luckily two diverse but useful historical examples came to mind. One is perhaps better known than the other but they had a lot in common. The first was King Christian X of Denmark who during the German occupation of his country rode alone around the streets of Copenhagen each day on a white horse (in defiance of German orders) to show the people in the only way he could that the soul of Denmark had not been snuffed out. The other was President Kennedy's well-intentioned verbal gaffe when he stood on a podium in Berlin near the Berlin Wall and the Brandenburg Gate and declared '*Ich bin ein Berliner*' to show solidarity with the Berliners in the face of the Soviet menace (the words can be understood as Kennedy saying 'I am a donut'). I was in no way comparing myself to either but if someone sets an example ...

I told the cop I would do it myself.

—*Meinen Sie das ernst?* (Are you serious?)

—*Ja—ich bin eine kritische Masse* (Perfectly. I am a Critical Mass.)

The spokes-cop had not expected that and went away to confer. When he came back he said I had misinterpreted the idea of Critical Mass as they the police understood it. I said I did not think so. I said I had interpreted the idea as I understood it. He then tried to reason with me. He told me I should understand that the cops were there to enforce the law and to protect the cyclists. He related an incident in which a motorist, obstructed by a cyclist, had jumped out of his car and beaten the cyclist to a pulp. He said he was telling me the story for my own good so I knew what I was getting into. If you went around upsetting people bad things could happen. So, did I really intend to go?

When I said 'yes' he looked disappointed and handed me a sheet of paper that showed the route I had to follow.

He reminded me I had to abide by the highway code and must at all times obey instructions issued by the police.

We set off in formation with the motorcycle cops, blue lights flashing, forming the corners of a lead box that contained me, the Critical Mass. They may have worried about me giving them the slip and recovening with myself anarchistically elsewhere but that would have been simply surreal.

To begin with there was an immediate chain reaction of sorts that sucked in four other cyclists—but all veteran cycle-rights campaigners as I found out afterwards so there were no immediate converts—and a kid on roller skates. With the cops as outriders and with cops behind we ploughed effortlessly through the homebound traffic of Stuttgart jamming the streets and drawing a good, if uncomprehending crowd. I remembered to smile and wave because body language is important on these occasions and I wanted to create a good impression for the future of Critical Mass. Motorists pounded on their horns and wound down their windows and wanted to know what the hell as going on so it was good that the cops were there to protect us.

But the presidential treatment they were unintentionally giving us evidently embarrassed the cops into wanting to get the thing over with. With their help we swept through red lights and stopped all contrary vehicular movement dead in its tracks until we reached the finishing point. When we dispersed the spokes-cop made a point of telling me again about the motorist who had jumped out of his car

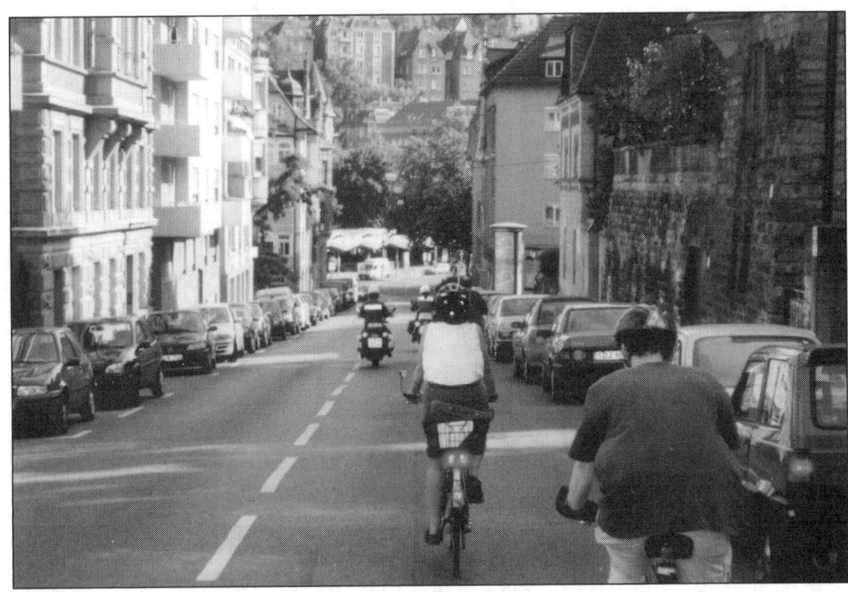

I am a Critical Mass!, Stuttgart, Germany

and pulverised a cyclist just in case I had not gotten the point the first time or because the story was uppermost in his mind during the ride. On the plus side he was by no means angry and from the police perspective the Critical Mass menace had been contained according to the letter of the law.

Conclusion? It had only taken a handful of cyclists and a kid on a skateboard to keep the Critical Mass counter in play in Stuttgart and to repair some of the PR damage the car lobby managed to inflict after the first Critical Mass.

For all its conceptual slipperiness—or perhaps because of it—I am persuaded that Critical Mass is a useful tool in the cyclist's kit for getting a fair deal on the roads. Also if I had not gone on the Critical Mass I probably would not have realised quite so clearly that I am a Critical Mass—*ich bin eine kritische Masse*. And so is every other individual.

Duisburg, Germany

BY ULRIKE GÖRTZ

I am 50 years old, married and mother of three daughters. My hobby is my bicycle, I am member of a cycling organisation (ADFC) and in 1999 I took part in a protest cycling tour. The protest was against a highway along the Eastern Sea, we rode 13 days about 800 kilometers. This was the first time I heard about Critical Mass and decided to initiate this in Duisburg. Duisburg is an industrial town of about 500.000 people. It took some time for me to organize this and we started first time in August 2001 (3 people)

September 2001 (12 people)
October 2001 (1 man)
November (1 woman)
December (me)
January 2002 (13 people, I am happy)

We meet on every last Friday of a month in the Duisburg City at the Lifesaver.

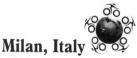

Milan, Italy

AN AESTHETIC REBELLION

BY GIOVANNI PESCE

Critical Mass in Italy grew out of an aesthetic rebellion. Contrary to common cliché, outside of some very beautiful but limited enclaves, Italy can be a hell of a country. Most of the country's environmental problems arise from hyper-motorization: Fiat-land counts among the highest rate of per capita car ownership in the world, the highest in the European Union. In Milan there are 66 cars for every 100 inhabitants. The problem is that Italian cities are not built for cars. Densities are too high, city centres are made of narrow streets with medieval structures and outside the urban centres, in the post-WWII era, cities grew in an unplanned manner, in what we could call a Taiwanese pattern, with a maze of roundabaouts and highways embedded together with factories and houses.

In Italy groups of two-wheeled urban rebels can be traced back to the '70s, mostly inspired by radical anti-consumerism and environmentalism. The aim of these groups has always been to revive the big Italian urban cycling tradition. In fact, before the 1960s and the motorization boom, bicycles were a very popular means of transportation in Italy, especially in the Northern continental part of the peninsula. In some minor cities of the North bicycles still retain an honorable position. Such is the case in Ferrara, near Bologna, where more than 30% of trips are made by bicycle. But in the big cities the trips made by bike are only 2% of the total, cars accounting for more than 70%, and public transport for the rest.

In recent years there has been a public upheaval about traffic. Frequent winter drought has caused very high levels of air pollution. In the most densely populated

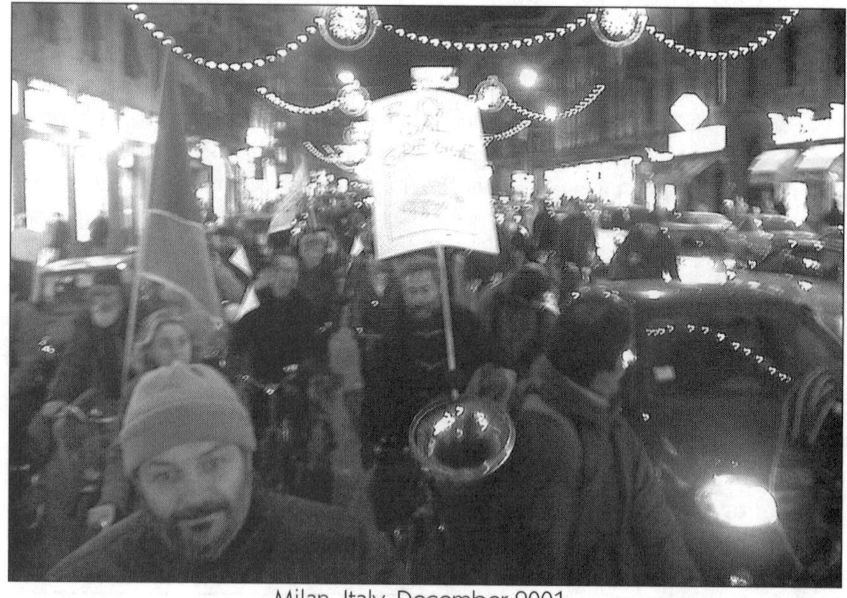

MILAN PHOTOS BY GIOVANNI PESCE

Milan, Italy, December 2001.

areas of the industrial North, mayors often had to order traffic blocks in order to tackle pollution. The surge of attention to traffic has given more energy to the urban cyclist movement. In winter 2001-2 Milan has taken the lead, with traditional environmental associations strongly calling urban cyclists to action.

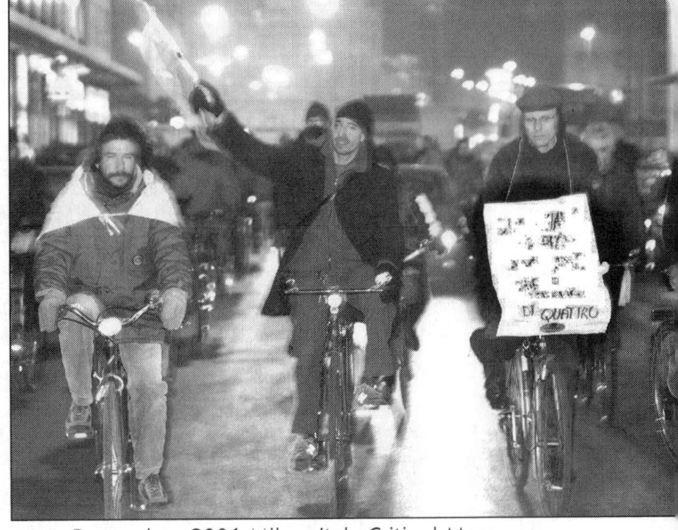

December 2001 Milan, Italy Critical Mass

A big parade was organized on December 6, 2001, urging motorists to "get out of the herd." Considering the cold season (temperature being around 5-10° C in Milan winters) this parade was quite successful, gathering about 400 cyclists.

But this was an authorized bicycle rally, nothing to do with the "organized coincidence" we are all so fond of. Some of the cyclo-activists gathered by that rally wanted something more. In February 2002 we had an evening meeting where a few of us discussed how to start a Critical Mass in Milan. At the end of the meeting we all hit the road to get a beer, and found out there was nothing to organize, we just had to cycle in the middle of the road to make it a CM. We arranged a new meeting for the next week. It was still winter time, still cold, but the next week 30 of us hit the road. The e-mail and sms announcments had worked. The wave had started to grow.

A web site was soon created (www.inventati.org/criticalmass) thanks to some independent media providers close to Indymedia Italia. On the web site two mailing lists were activated, one for the crew and one for announcements only. In the chinese quarter of Milan, a cycle lab was founded hosted by a squat called Bulk, to be used to fix bicycles but also as a Critical Mass café and a gathering hub for urban cycling culture. The cyclo-lab started collecting images and books and soon produced a video on CM around the word. Among the group of "founders" there were also some people from BiciG8, the group of cyclists from all over the country who rode through Northern Italy to get to Genoa for the G8 summit demonstrations of July 2001.

By the fourth week we got about 100. Traditional media started to talk about us, not only the local newspapers and radio, but also some national. The idea started to spread to other cities. Turin was the first to respond, followed by

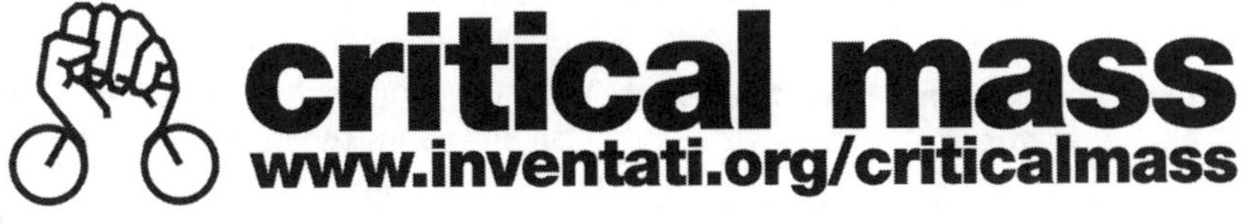

Bologna, Brescia, Roma and other minor towns. Throughout Italy rides are now held at the same time, every thursday starting at around 9.30 pm and going on until late. Rallies usually end with a glass of fresh beer, in squats, clubs or in suburban parks.

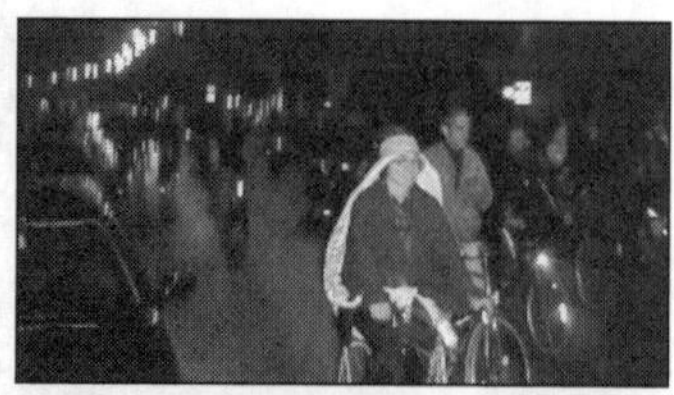

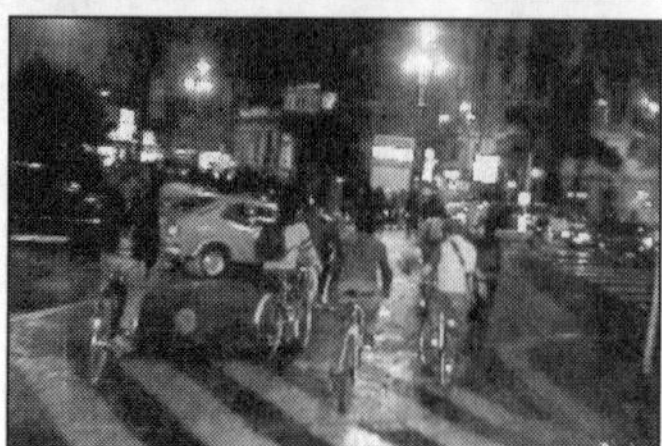

March 2002 Critical Mass

In Milan we still are the biggest crowd, a traffic bull dozer of 400 bicycles. So far we still haven't had big problems with the police. Sometimes they come and stay in the back of the group. Participants are mostly aged 25-35. We start from the city centre, through an area packed with motorized leisure hunters. There is no scheduled track. We like to confront crowded streets and traffic, because the sound of angry horns is music to us, but we also ride in silent park areas, in the train station halls, or in circles and swarms in the rounded piazzas, howling and whistling like crazy. A group of high-tech bicycle acrobats as also joined in, giving the group a spectacular touch.

Our communication with the press is kept very minimal: journalists who want to speak about us are just invited via mail to join in, watch and report. There are no official speakers, no explicit requests or political proposals: we decided to let the visual and audio impact speak for us. We seek no communication with the local government. We feel it's not our job. We just want to show everyone how fun and beautiful the city can get when bicycles take control of the streets. Anyone can create his own flyers and e-mails by downloading elements from the website. Texts tend to take a surreal tone, both light and hard, e.g. "Flabby bum? Feel like making the revolution? Come and join Critical Mass." There are texts drawning from diverse ideas such as situationism, psychogeography, ciclo-ufology, communication ciclo guerrilla, etc.

Problemi di fianchi flaccidi?
Voglia di fare la rivoluzione?

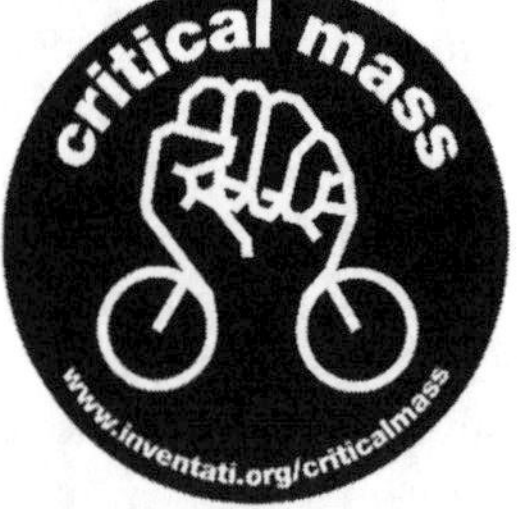

La lotta politica che fa puzzare le ascelle e fa tremare l'AUTOrità

Sciame di macchine a pedali
Ogni giovedì piazza mercanti alle 9 pm

"Noi non blocchiamo il traffico, noi SIAMO il traffico"

At the moment I am writing Critical Mass is growing very fast. The rain season has just finished, summer explosion just started. We have plenty of ideas, plans and enthusiasm. Probably when you'll read this, things will have changed dramatically. For fresh info stay tuned on www.inventati.org/criticalmass.

CRITICAL MASS I I I

BY MATTHEW ARNISON FRIDAY, 29TH SEPTEMBER 1995

The cop says, "Who organised this? Who's in charge here?" The guy they're hassling says "I don't know." He asks the guy next to him in a bike helmet, "Who's in charge?" The guy in the helmet doesn't know either.

Picture a police paddy wagon parked across three lanes, surrounded by 100 people on bikes, all shouting "Who's in charge? Who's in charge?"

"You've got no right to obstruct traffic like this," says the cop. Seems a bit ironic; it's the cop car that's blocking the road. They're leading the guy with white hair toward the back of the wagon... the crowd starts yelling "What's the charge?" Bikes have a right to the road, they've got nothing on him. The crowd decides to move on up along Oxford Street, where another wagon is parked in the way again. Pretty funny, this behaviour seems to stop the cars getting past, but the bikes just flow around it. Later, the cops find a role for themselves by escorting the Mass—but this mass doesn't need an escort, it's a Critical Mass.

It starts after work in Hyde Park, seems pretty low key, maybe 30 cyclists. Someone's playing pan pipes. One bike has a trailer you could fit a couple of kids in. There's a rollerblader, a tandem cycle, some bike couriers. As usual, there's a dog.

It doesn't seem quite together as we head down the middle of Hyde Park. At the first set of lights the mass splits apart. But by a few blocks it's all coming together, and we're shouting and whistling echoes off the buildings—it's a mob of cyclists half a city block long riding through the middle of Sydney! We stop for a red light, and there's a roar as it goes green. It's grown, there seem to be heaps of us.

Some agro motorist is honking at the back, just makes people ride

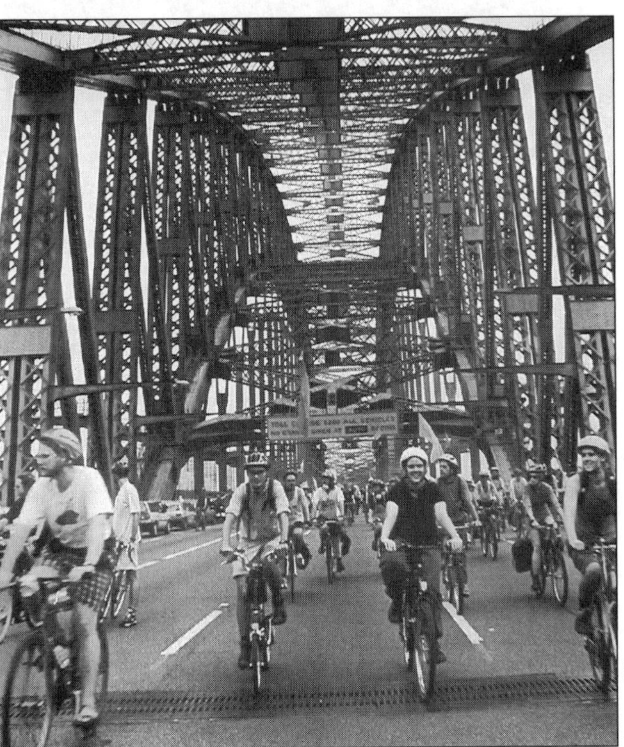

MATHEW WHITAKER

Sydney Harbour Bridge, November 1997.

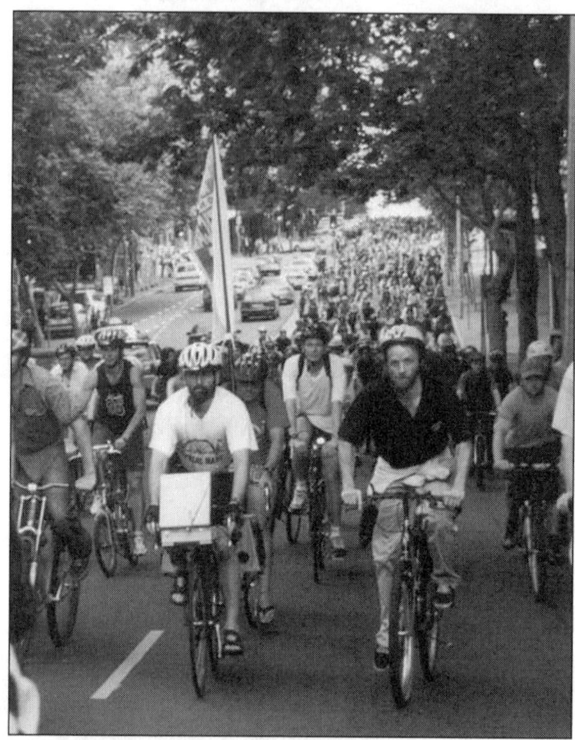

Miller Street, Sydney, November 2001

slower. The suit rams one of the bikes, squashes the bike's mudguard, but puts a huge dent in his own bonnet. "I pay taxes to use this road!" the red face screams. "So do we!"

At Town Hall, a dozen people are shooting across the intersection to join us. It's pretty big now, must be 200 at least. That's when the testy cop car turns up, gets to the front eventually, to triumphantly stop across our lanes. Gee, somehow the bikes get past and surround the car.

Later we're riding down William St, this mob has a mind of its own, the map said go down Bourke St. Some of the bikes have twin headlights blazing. From behind it's a mass of red lights twinking. Every intersection people go to the sides and cork the endless carflow from streaming into the mass of bikes. Someone flips over their bike, a flashy stack, at King. To finish in Pitt St. Mall, we're telling the cops where we wanna go—now you can go, we've finished (we didn't need you anyway).

"Tell 10 friends, to tell 10 friends for the next one, last Friday every month. It's happening in cities all over the world, burn fat, not oil."

"Two wheels good! Four wheels bad!"

With that cheer, sounds like we'll be back, and more.

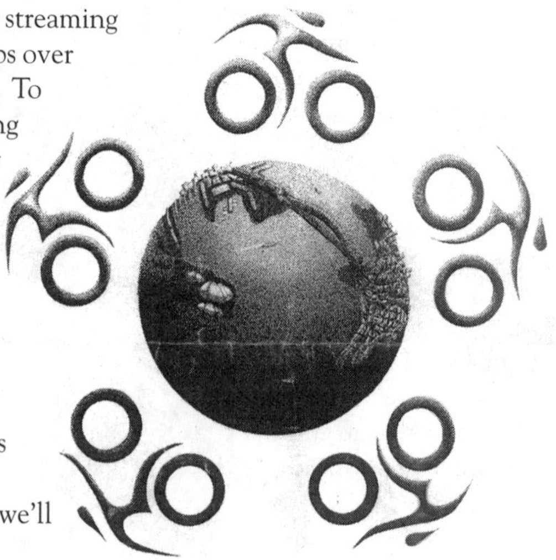

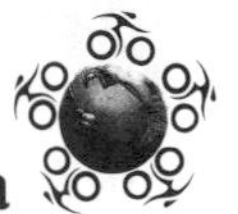

Melbourne, Australia

Herald Sun, Saturday, March 31, 2001 www.heraldsun.com.au 5

Protesting pedal power plugs tunnel

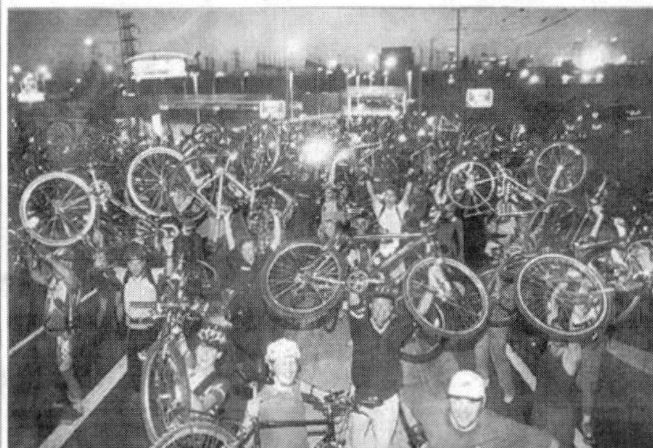

Wheely impressive: bike riders stopped traffic flowing through the Burnley tunnel last night. Picture: CRAIG WOOD

CITY traffic was thrown into chaos last night when protesting bike riders forced the closure of the Burnley tunnel for more than an hour.

Frustrated football fans travelling to the MCG and motorists heading in and out of the city endured long delays as cars banked up on main roads.

Police and CityLink closed the tunnel shortly before 6.30pm and it didn't reopen until after 7.30pm.

The protest, organised by Critical Mass, saw about 300 bike riders, skateboarders and roller-bladers travel through the tunnel for the first time.

Cyclist and regular Critical Mass participant Alex Carr said the group did not set out to antagonise motorists.

"We're just out to have fun," he said.

"We've got as much right to be on the roads as anyone else.

"We don't mean to stress out motorists."

CityLink spokeswoman Jeni Coutts said the toll road operator had no choice but to close the tunnel to ensure the safety of the protesters, who were given a police escort.

"There's nothing much we can do," she said.

By JASON FRENKEL

"It was aimed at causing maximum disruption and that's what it did."

The group began its journey at the State Library in Swanston St and travelled through the city before entering the tunnel at Power St.

Police immediately blocked the entrance behind the group and also closed off the South Eastern arterial, forcing the cyclists to exit at Burnley St.

A leaflet circulated by Critical Mass said the ride would encourage motorists to think about alternative means of transport.

"This is not a battle between motorists and cyclists, but a battle to save our city and the way we live from total car dependency," it read.

Critical Mass is an informal coalition of bike riders whose aim is to celebrate cycling.

The group's monthly bike rides has taken hundreds of cyclists twice over the Bolte Bridge and once through the Domain tunnel.

Melbourne Herald Sun, March 31, 2001

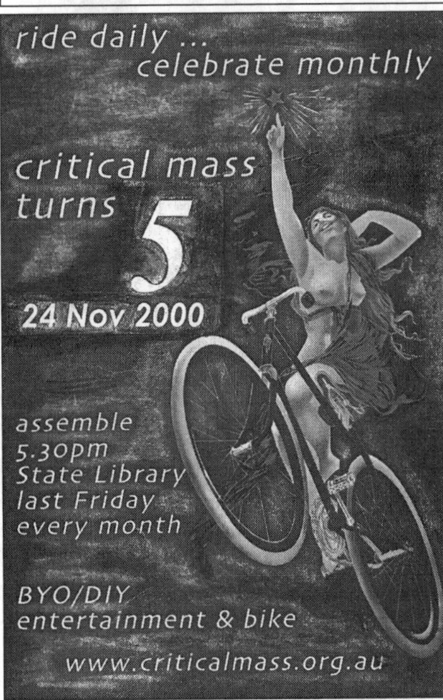

ride daily ...
celebrate monthly
critical mass
turns
5
24 Nov 2000
assemble
5.30pm
State Library
last Friday
every month
BYO/DIY
entertainment & bike
www.criticalmass.org.au

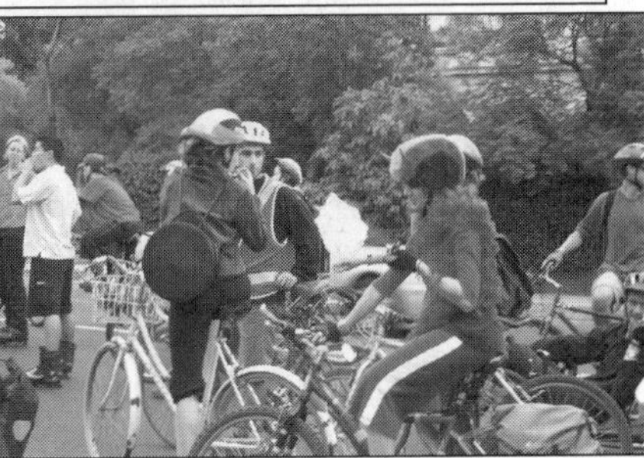

Devil Girl, Melbourne Australia

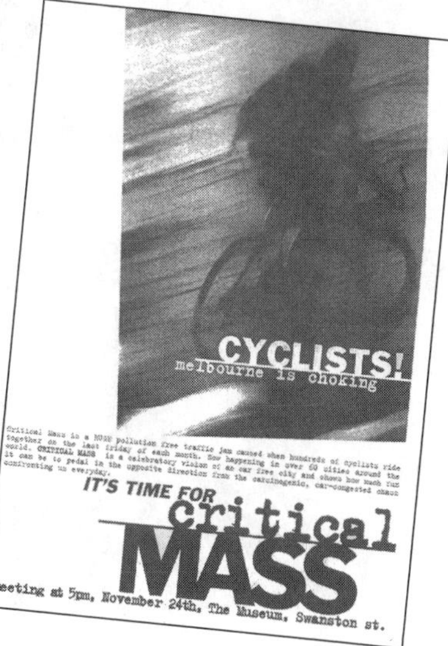

CYCLISTS!
melbourne is choking
Critical Mass is a HUGE pollution free traffic jam caused when hundreds of cyclists ride together on the last friday of each month. Now happening in over 60 cities around the world. CRITICAL MASS is a celebratory vision of an car free city and shows how much fun it can be to pedal in the opposite direction from the carcinogenic, car-congested chaos confronting us everyday.
IT'S TIME FOR
critical
MASS
meeting at 5pm, November 24th, The Museum, Swanston st.

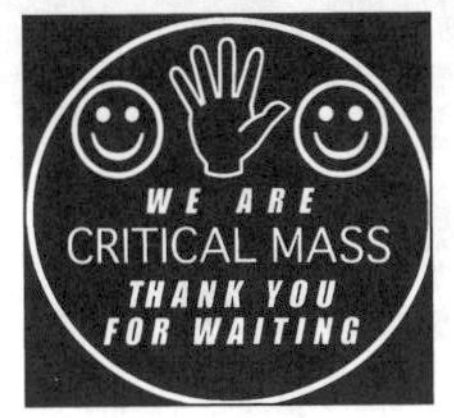

WE ARE
CRITICAL MASS
THANK YOU
FOR WAITING

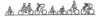

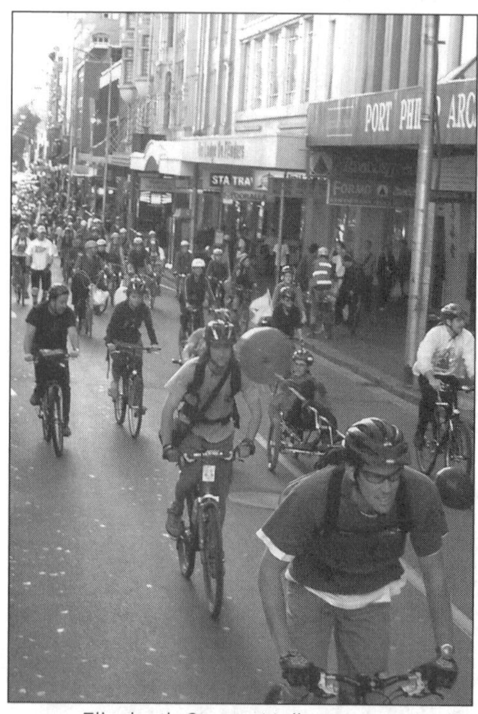

Elizabeth Street, Melbourne Australia

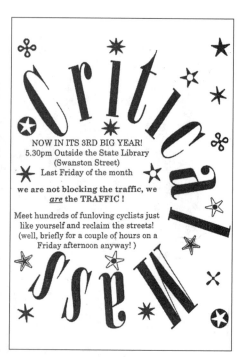

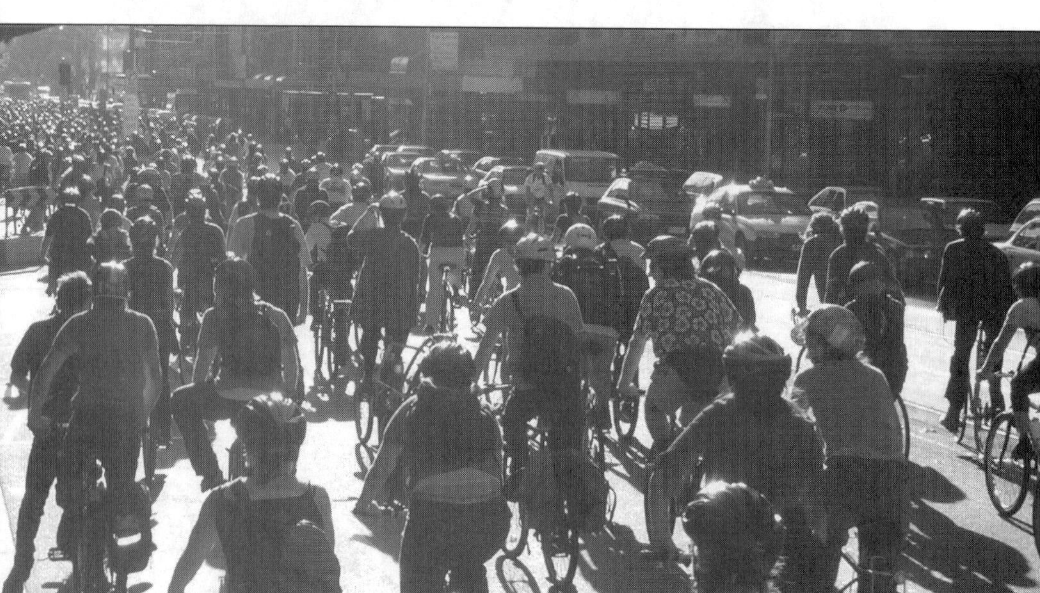

NOW IN ITS 3RD BIG YEAR!

we are not blocking the traffic, we *are* the TRAFFIC !
Meet hundreds of funloving cyclists just like yourself and reclaim the streets!
(well, briefly for a couple of hours on a Friday afternoon anyway!)

Melbourne photos © by Steven Stevenson

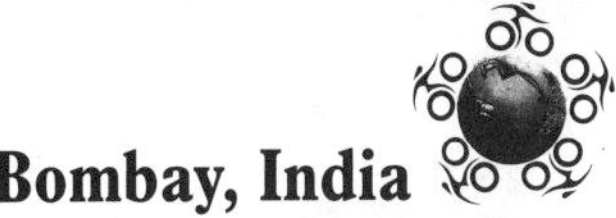

Bombay, India

MUMBIKERS TAKE TO THE STREET

ANONYMOUS, FROM THE WEB

The first Critical Mass Mumbai rally got off to an upbeat start on Friday, January 28th, 2000. Approximately 25 bicyclists, mainly students, rallied in South Mumbai's commercial district for a little over an hour, spreading the powerful message of socially just and sustainable development.

The press covered the event as an anti-pollution rally. We are grateful for this exposure, but at the same time we would like to assert that for some of us, this was not the only reason we were on the streets. Sure we were on the streets to demand our right to clean air. But we were also on the street to ask why our city is splitting apart. Why a disproportionate amount of the state's budget is spent on improving the infrastructure that will benefit a tiny fraction of the public while the rest of the population is ignored. Why development is measured by how much we spend and not how many's needs are served.

Critical Mass intends to be a catalyst for different individuals and groups to network and build relationships based on common interests. It is a public meeting where most everybody can attend. It is a regular, yet enjoyable meeting that simultaneously sends a social message even as it happens. During the ride, individuals and groups are free to distribute information and literature on who they are and any support that they would need for upcoming initiatives. It puts groups and movements in contact with energetic, interested youth who are looking for creative and positive ways to make a difference. This will enable social and environmental groups to build their constituency (and maybe volunteer) base. The cycle ride gives people and groups the opportunity to collaborate with other groups that are fighting different symptoms of the same problem.

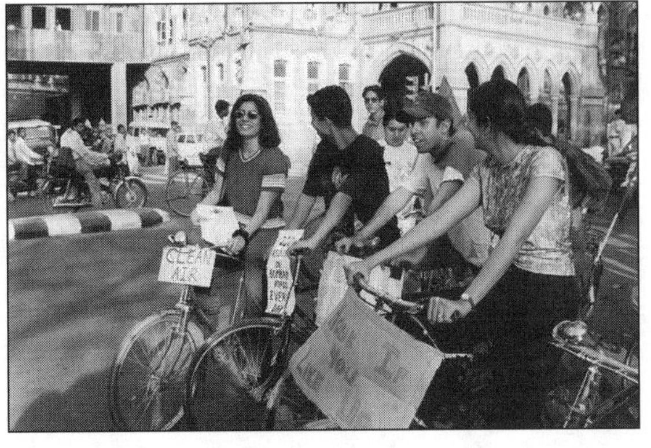

All in all, a monthly bicycle ride through the city is a decentralized yet coordinated action where no one is in charge and everyone is free to share their ideas, work and vision for a better future. Mum-baikars and MumBikers need this space to talk about alternatives to the destruction of our social and natural fabric. Let's make it happen! Since everyone does not have email access, please share this email with your friends and colleagues. If you want to know more about Critical Mass please let us know. The next Critical Mass takes place on Friday, February 25th at 5pm. We assemble outside the Nehru Planetarium.

LANCASTER CRITICAL MASS: DOES IT STILL EXIST?

BY DAVE HORTON

Lancaster Critical Mass is dead, long live Lancaster Critical Mass! Critical Mass hit the streets of rush-hour Lancaster on the last Friday of January 1995. Over the next couple of years it became a regular fixture of the local activist scene; we grew to know and love the Mass as a familiar monthly event. But as the last one took place over two years ago, surely Lancaster Critical Mass is now dead, surely it no longer exists?

The history of Critical Mass in this relatively remote corner of north west England is an intriguing one. There had been bike protest here before Critical Mass's "official" arrival—during Green Transport Week, in May 1994 for example, around eighty people took part in a city centre bike ride which could've been called "Critical Mass," but wasn't. Although Masses were by that time already regular monthly occurrences in other parts of Britain, it wasn't until the start of the following year that activists here—having heard and learnt about the rides in Birmingham and London—decided to bring the phenomenon to the streets of Lancaster. That first ride, in January 1995, saw four brave souls pedal around the city in blizzard conditions. Things could only look up; and they did.

Every month through 1995 and 1996, Lancaster Critical Mass hit the rush hour traffic of the last Friday afternoon of the month. Cyclists would meet in Dalton Square, with the statue of Queen Victoria at its centre and the Victorian Town Hall rising above, and ride out onto the city's ordinarily congested one-way system. Some months we had a police motorcycle escort, some months a surveillance helicopter flew overhead, and some months we were left almost completely alone. Lancaster is a small city, and Critical Mass here never became the kind of large scale protest event it did elsewhere. But a regular contingent—mostly drawn from the city's alternative networks—always put in an appearance, and good months would see sixty or seventy people turn out.

So what's happening now? Why, if it was an important and valued part of local activism, did Lancaster Critical Mass stop occurring on a monthly basis? Because Critical Mass came, during the middle of the 1990s, to be a regular fixture on Lancaster's activist calendar, its disappearance as a monthly event later in the decade is easily regarded as somehow a failure, a visible symptom of an erosion in activist energies and visions. Yet Critical Mass here has not in fact disappeared; rather, it has metamorphosed into an irregular but very effective tactic which now forms one part of the local alternative movement's mobilisation repertoire.

There's a whole bundle of reasons contributing to this shift in form of our local Critical Mass. During the mid-1990s, the regular monthly Mass was riding on both the wave of activist indignation over the British Government's road-building frenzy, and high excitement over the widespread and well publicised

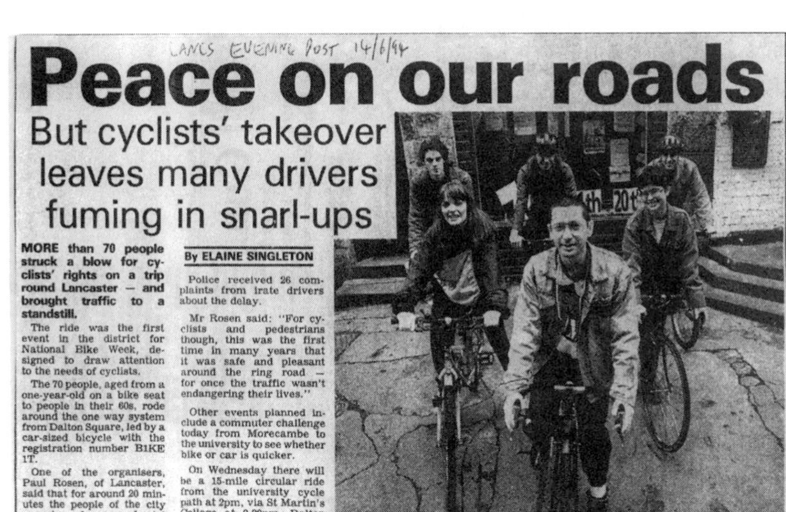

LANCS EVENING POST 14/6/94

Peace on our roads

But cyclists' takeover leaves many drivers fuming in snarl-ups

MORE than 70 people struck a blow for cyclists' rights on a trip round Lancaster — and brought traffic to a standstill.

The ride was the first event in the district for National Bike Week, designed to draw attention to the needs of cyclists.

The 70 people, aged from a one-year-old on a bike seat to people in their 60s, rode around the one way system from Dalton Square, led by a car-sized bicycle with the registration number B1KE 1T.

One of the organisers, Paul Rosen, of Lancaster, said that for around 20 minutes the people of the city experienced peace and quiet on the ring road, free from noise, pollution and danger.

Mr Rosen said on the last leg of the ride the cyclists were stopped by the police to tell them they were holding up the traffic.

By ELAINE SINGLETON

Police received 26 complaints from irate drivers about the delay.

Mr Rosen said: "For cyclists and pedestrians though, this was the first time in many years that it was safe and pleasant around the ring road — for once the traffic wasn't endangering their lives."

Other events planned include a commuter challenge today from Morecambe to the university to see whether bike or car is quicker.

On Wednesday there will be a 15-mile circular ride from the university cycle path at 2pm, via St Martin's College at 2.20pm, Dalton Square at 2.45pm, Glasson Dock, Galgate and back to the university.

And on Sunday there will be a 16-mile ride setting off from Green Ayre, near Sainsbury's, at 11am.

Paul Rosen with some of the bicycle squad

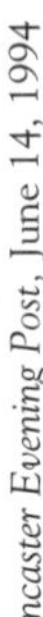

Lancaster Evening Post, June 14, 1994

opposition to it. The mainstream media fell in love with images of treehouse-dwelling and tunnel-digging roads protesters, and quite suddenly it was even a little bit sexy to be an environmental activist! Every road building project was being met with fierce and sustained resistance, and Reclaim the Streets events were breaking out up and down the length of the country. Many Lancaster-based activists had engaged in roads protests elsewhere, and now wanted to express their opposition to car culture more locally. And we had—actually still have—our own local road scheme to get stuck in to. The City and County Councils, together with our local Members of Parliament and the Chamber of Commerce, spent most of the 1990s throwing vast amounts of time and money at outlandish proposals for a Lancaster Bypass; the insane social and environmental consequences of this scheme have done more than anything else to animate a whole range of local groups and campaigns, and to turn the car—here as elsewhere—into an intensely politicised object. For many of us, it is regarded as the principle saboteur of and obstacle to convivial day-to-day life; a powerful symbol of the desecration and desolation of our communities.

That was the mid-1990s, and it felt like it would last forever, that monthly dose of communal warmth, the adrenalin rush of taking our rightful space and slowing down the pace of the city. But times have changed and key activists have moved on since then. These days, Lancaster—with a bunch of dynamic, young and eager Green Party City Councillors, and a Green County Councillor—is earning a reputation as a "green city." And just possibly, the institutionalisation of this highly energised group of green activists has increased the cultural gap and reduced the amount of communication between the more 'radical' and more 'reformist' activists within the local area. We've also just got a Millennium present, a little late but better than never; there's a brand spanking and actually quite brilliant new crossing of the River Lune, the Millennium Bridge, devoted to cyclists and pedestrians. More widely, the local network of cycle paths is—albeit very gradually—improving and expanding. There's some sense, then, that—at least in our roles as cyclists—we've won some important gains. Although plans for a Lancaster Bypass remain an important focus of activist opposition, and will continue to be met with the contempt they deserve, in general roads and cars can feel a bit like "yesterday's issue;" other concerns—such as oppositon to genetic contamination of our food—have come along, and many activists are increasingly turning their attentions to globalised protest as part of the "anti-globalisation" movement.

But, in spite of everything, Lancaster Critical Mass is not yet dead. Instead, it has shifted in form and so retains its relevance to a changing wider context. As part of the Global Day of Action Against Corporate Capital on June 18th 1999, for example, a Critical Mass formed an integral part of Lancaster activists mischievous festivities. Amidst a range of other local actions, and while another contingent of Lancastrians took to creating some timely mayhem in the financial district of London, seventy of us took to our bikes and reminded the people of Lancaster, one more time, that the future really can look different.

In this new guise as an occasional action, Critical Mass is highly effective partly because it has already—in its previous incarnation—entered local folklore. We are that anarchic bunch of militant cyclists who disrupt the totally legitimate journeys of decent, law-abiding citizens and bring complete chaos to the city centre. All by ourselves, clever things, we created what has become known locally as "Black Friday," one beautiful afternoon in 1996 when motorised traffic within the city ground to a complete and utter halt, finally—though not, unfortunately, permanently—paralysed by the sheer weight of its own collective stupidity. So today, merely the mention of those two fine words—Critical Mass—is enough to generate hysteria among certain sections of the local press, always on the lookout for the most unlikely and overblown reasons to explain Lancaster's traffic problems.

But Lancaster Critical Mass is not, and never has been, solely an attempt to influence transport policy. On the surface, rides are comprised of cyclists, concerned with and publicising the ascendancy and domination of car culture, and the consequent marginalisation—almost to the point of extermination—of the bicycle on city centre streets. But in Lancaster it is, in general, a ragtag assortment of social and environmental activists—some of whom have to borrow bicycles—who take part, and the rides have never attracted more than one or two club racing or touring cyclists. And the local cycle campaign group, Dynamo, have always had an ambivalent and uncomfortable relationship to the Mass. Some Dynamo activists have been keen and central participants, but others express outright hostility to the "unreasonable" and confrontational approach implicit within the claiming and taking of space without a formal invitation from the authorities. From their perspectives, Critical Mass risks alienating those local decision-makers with whom we should be building good, productive working relationships; the Mass is an incomprehensible and confusing collection of strange and unspecifiable "anarchist types," whose understanding of and sensitivity towards local bicycle politics is naïve or non-existent.

So whilst Critical Mass certainly represents an important intervention into debates surrounding urban transport and the future of our cities, I think its primary importance, at least in Lancaster, lies elsewhere. Here as everywhere people live and work with roughly compatible but distinctly oppositional political and value positions. Most of the time, they exist independently of one another, perhaps getting angry at the same news stories, showing support for the same issues and campaigns, whilst unknowingly crossing paths in the local wholefood co-op or sitting at adjoining tables in our green-friendly vegetarian café. Such individuals share an alternative culture, but—for as long as they remain anonymous to each other—are unable to develop joint projects from their shared ways of life, values and goals. Critical Mass made—and continues from time to time to make—visible and tangible the connections between them, transforming anonymous inhabitation of an imagined community into meaningful and possibility-laden participation in a realtime face-to-face community.

Critical Mass here has always been an occasion for the coming-together of the city's ordinarily dispersed constituency for social change, a coming-together which creates a highly visible demonstration of an alternative culture and produces those pleasures associated with immersion in good company. This alternative culture is of course always there, but it ordinarily remains out-of-sight, hidden from public view. The vast majority of the time, we go from day to day doing what we can to make the world a more socially just, greener place and experimenting with, and trying to forge, new and more appropriate ways of living. And then, just occasionally, we throw a party, come together and cause a scene.

During the mid-1990s the ordinarily invisible networks of Lancaster's alternative culture mobilised in a demonstration of unity once a month. These monthly gatherings publicly announced a locally existing alternative; we demonstrated to ourselves, to each other and to the district more widely that we were a community carrying a different agenda. Critical Mass gave us the opportunity to parade, indeed flaunt, our (internally actually quite diverse) politics. It provided an affirmation of ourselves as a political community with demonstrable values and tangible goals. And today, ten years on from Critical Mass's inception in San Francisco and due to the occasional instigation of a handful of enthusiastic individuals utilising the Internet and activist word-of-mouth and attaching fliers to bikes parked around the city, Critical Mass rides still put in irregular appearances and demonstrate to all the continued existence of a local culture of resistance.

As a regular event, Critical Mass was very powerful in helping to sustain, as well as to extend, a local subterranean movement network reflecting a distinctive if diverse kind of cultural politics. Critical Mass pulled in lots of different individuals, with quite a range of orientations to the world, and allowed them to participate in a joint project. Critical Mass provided us with an opportunity to set aside those minor differences which often keep us separate, and to unite instead along our similarities. And acting together, protesting and having fun, brought us closer together—making us more likely to stop to say 'hello' in the street, go over for a chat when we spotted a now familiar face in the green café. And, ironically, being lumped together as Critical Mass—one homogeneous crowd of people—by the local press helped to cement this sense of ourselves as a "we" which outlasted the duration of the Mass.

A BICYCLE CARNIVAL
TO SHOW

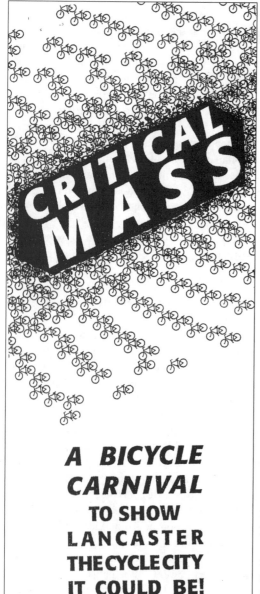

THE CYCLE CITY
IT COULD BE!
Meet Dalton Square, 4.30pm
Last Friday of Every Month
All Cyclists Welcome

Lancaster Critical Mass xerocracy

This still remains the case, albeit in slightly diluted form, today. The real beauty of Critical Mass, at least as it ordinarily tends to play itself out here in Lancaster, is its continuing ability to bring together a broad bunch of people. It acts as a real umbrella event, with progressive social and environmental activists of many persuasions joining together for a gentle pedal. Partly, of course, this is because Critical Mass is a relatively low-cost action—it demands no discernible commitment beyond turning up with your bike, intent on having a good time. And herein lies the undoubted importance of Critical Mass; it is a tool not only for enhancing the activist identities of individuals, but also for building a wider sense of political community. By bringing together people who might not otherwise and ordinarily meet, it helps to generate a stronger sense of solidarity within local social movement networks. Of course it's easy to romanticise the past, but back in the days when the Mass was always either just about to happen or had just happened, it felt like I knew more people. I could tell you which people were involved in what kinds of visionary action, and it seemed as though activists in general knew one another better. It was, put simply, a fantastic community-building mechanism.

Once the boldest move—the greater act of deviancy—of taking back space from cars is accomplished, all manner of smaller acts become thinkable. Reclaimed space becomes the setting for a festival in which the ordinary rules of interaction are subverted—the blowing of whistles at passers-by replaces the impatient growl of engines; suddenly the separation and safety constructed by the "windscreen" is gone—face-to-face interaction becomes not only possible, it's unavoidable. During Critical Mass we pedal out the kinds of lifestyle and society we want, in the present.

These days, I no longer automatically know what I'll be doing on the last Friday afternoon of the month. Critical Mass feels a bit like a barometer for the more general health and vitality of the local protest scene. Those of us with the fondest memories of Critical Mass during its regular phase are no doubt much more prone to bouts of nostalgia, when we start ruminating on the need for another Mass to perk things up a bit—stimulate everyone's spirits and energies, contacts, maybe some fresh projects. Often, and of course this is also a cop-out, we are also the ones now trying to turn our activist experiences into a means of paying the bills, or struggling hard to be good counter-cultural parents; and we are generally beginning to lose touch with "the spirit of the times."

The more inward-looking and subcultural orientation implicit in the community-building function of the Mass is not to say, though, that it doesn't also and always retain a strongly outward-looking orientation. Rides never fail to engage with and creatively prod the imaginations of appreciative onlookers. All kinds of fliers have, over the years, been produced and handed out to waiting (most often very patiently—motorists in Lancaster are habituated to, and so remain largely passive in the face of, hold-ups) motorists and passing pedestrians. And on the whole I think we have always been greeted with an appreciation borne of the recognition that something needs to be done about the congestion and pollution which daily strangles the life from Lancaster city centre.

And the Mass never fails to construct a space, carved out of the ordinarily car-dominated city streets, which has a powerful impact upon all those who experience it. Despite the whoopees and whistles of the Mass, the street turns amazingly quiet; the sound of the voice is slight compared to the incessant and oppressive grind of motorised traffic. Quite suddenly, and in a way which has never failed to surprise me, the street becomes a participatory space. Time is slowed right down, almost like it's standing still, and an alternative set of urban rhythms becomes discernible. To hear in broad daylight on an ordinarily traffic-choked street the sound of another person laughing, without knowing why, is to experience the desirability of a transformation in urban space. Critical Mass signals to the rest of Lancaster the presence and possibility of an alternative. The answer—both to city centre gridlock and to existing unsatisfactory forms of community interaction—can be put into practice, here and now.

Undoubtedly, Critical Mass within Britain forms an important part of a much broader anti-roads movement, which—whilst it continues today—was at its most intensely vibrant during the mid-1990s. As such, it has contributed to shifting understandings of the place of the car in our cities. Today, for example, almost no-one in Britain would dispute both that the car is a problem, and that the personal freedom to drive where you want, when you want must inevitably come to an end. But Critical Mass, or something very much like it, still clearly has an important place within the protest cultures of Britain's cities. In Lancaster, as an occasional rather than regular action, Critical Mass is no longer these days always referred to as Critical Mass. The various fliers circulating in advance of the ride of June 18th 1999, for example, mentioned an 'Urban Promenade' and 'The Call-it-what-you-want' ride. Importantly, though, the idea that lots of people riding around our city centre is an incredibly effective way of taking action is now firmly embedded within the repertoire of a generation of activists.

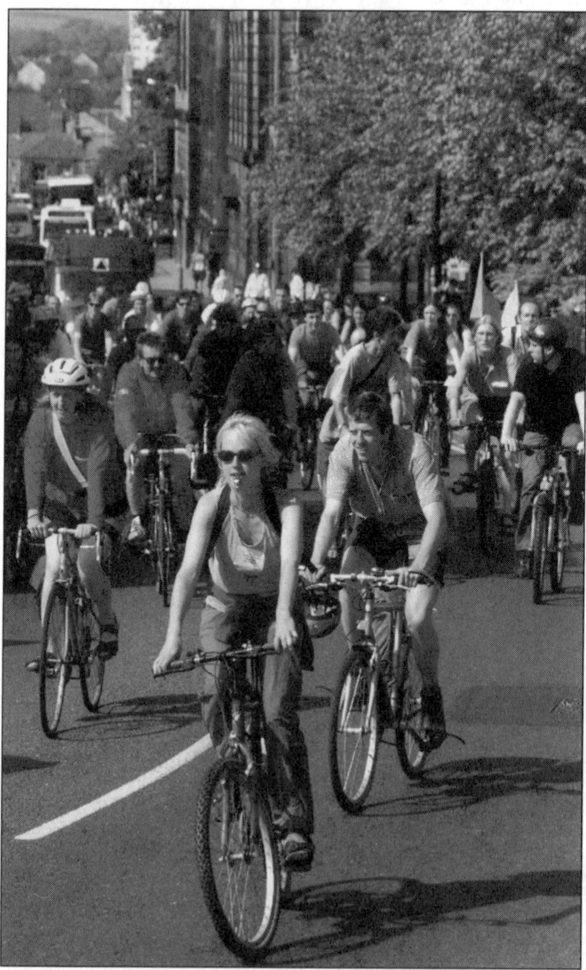

Lancaster England, c. 1996

Wherever it takes place, the Mass announces actually existing alternatives to "business-as-usual." The priorities and values of subterranean networks, committed to the cultivation of liberatory struggles for social and ecological justice, are paraded and—as in all good parades—succeed in stopping the traffic. And most importantly, Critical Mass helps to build and nourish those moral and political communities which engage in very many different protests, plans

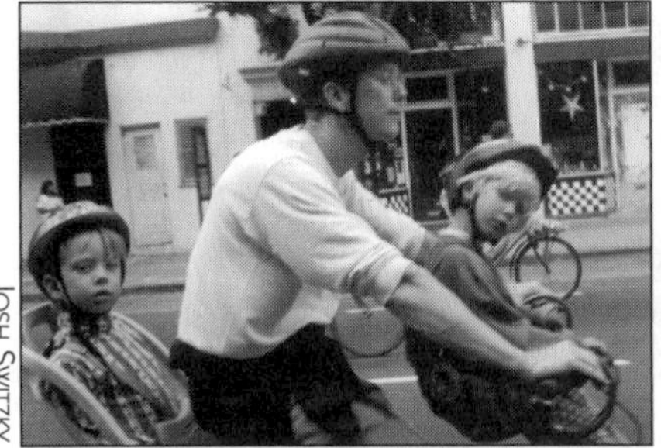
Josh Switzky

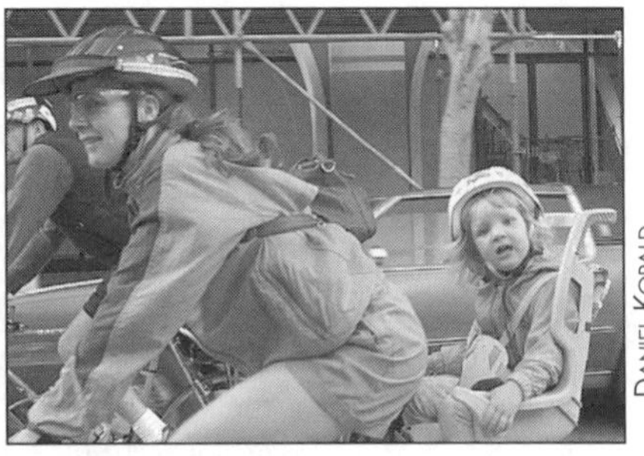
Daniel Kopald

Kids in San Francisco Critical Mass, 1999

and projects for grassroots social change.

So what are the possible future paths for Lancaster Critical Mass? I think its capacity to make protest participatory will almost certainly see its continuation as an important strategy in future days of action. But there are also clear ways in which it could be made, should there be a bicycle entrepreneur so inclined, more populist and large scale. It's always felt ironic to me that, given Critical Mass is consistent with all kinds of government policy—to do with Local Agenda 21, reducing car dependency, building participation in sustainability and reinvigorating city centres—it has sometimes met with such hostility from the authorities (actually, in Lancaster it feels like we provide the local constabulary with a rare opportunity to test their procedures for dealing with civil disturbances).

With its developing car-free transport infrastructure, the local district is becoming more popular with leisure cyclists. Such people form a potentially mobilisable base for mass participation bike rides which might inculcate the idea that cycling is a viable means of transport in the next generation, who are currently growing up with the idea that cyclists are an extinct or at least endangered species of road user. More intense local promotion of "Car Free Day" and similar events might also see something not unlike an officially sanctioned Critical Mass bringing more people by bike into and around the city centre. But, in the more immediate future, I have a feeling that Critical Mass will dust itself down and wheel itself out for another dose of bicycle carnival sometime fairly soon.

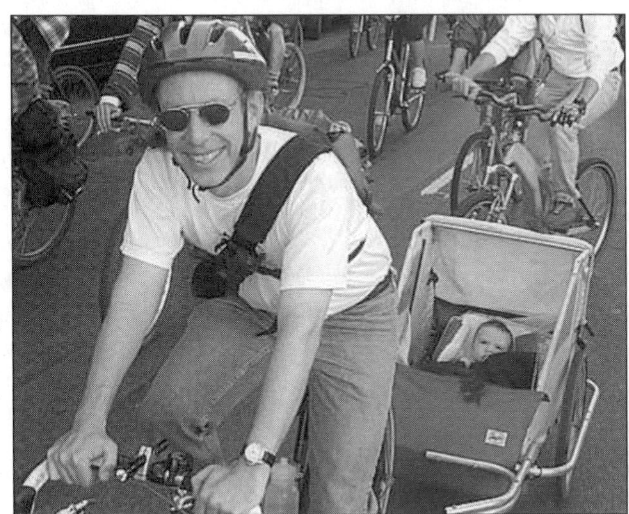
Daniel Kopald

Kids in San Francisco Critical Mass, 1999

London, England

CRITICAL MASS, LONDON STYLE

SEPTEMBER 14, 1995, AUTHOR UNKNOWN

Sit back, close your eyes and imagine a thousand people bicycling down the wrong side of the road! It's no daydream, its Critical Mass in Jolly Ol' England. Started about two years ago, the Critical Mass in London has reached epic proportions, approaching the magnitude of San Francisco's. By my estimation, there were about a thousand riders in the August [1995] Mass, almost doubling the previous month's ride. London's streets tend to be much more narrow than those found in American cities such as San Francisco, so the overall impact on the rush-hour traffic was enormous. The Mass seemed to stretch through London's streets for miles, and took close to 20 minutes to pass.

Kudos for the non-organizers of the ride, for it seemed incredibly well structured. Typical of British etiquette, we were never allowed to split up, for the front would usually stop in the middle of a busy intersection or circus (busy traffic circle) and patiently wait for the back to catch up. Also, cyclists frequently exalted the presence of pedestrians and made a mini-ceremony of allowing them to cross the streets undeterred by bikes.

Confrontations from both sides were non-existent; motorists in Britain are much more hesitant to either yell or beep their horns, almost all patiently waited for the Mass to wind its way past as if they "understood." In consequence, the mood of the ride remained jovial, but nonetheless effective, as thousands of Londoners and tourists stood in delight as traffic Hell zones like Trafalgar Square and Piccadilly Circus were completely free of cars, noise, and pollution for a handful of precious minutes. It was amazing to peacefully ride through some of the same areas of town that had been so chaotic and polluted as I had previously walked through them on foot. Although I have heard of problems with the police on past rides, in August the cops, on motorcycle, seemed unobtrusive and simply did their jobs by stopping traffic on busy roads in the front, or by bringing up the rear.

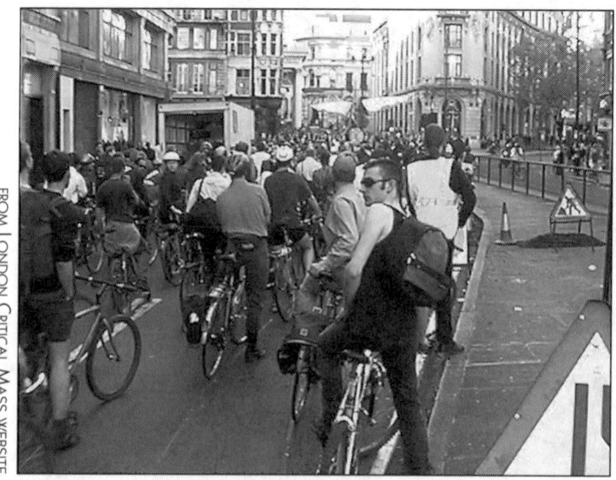

FROM LONDON CRITICAL MASS WEBSITE

London Critical Mass, April 1994

Pro-bicycle/anti-car activists in England's capital have shown both their

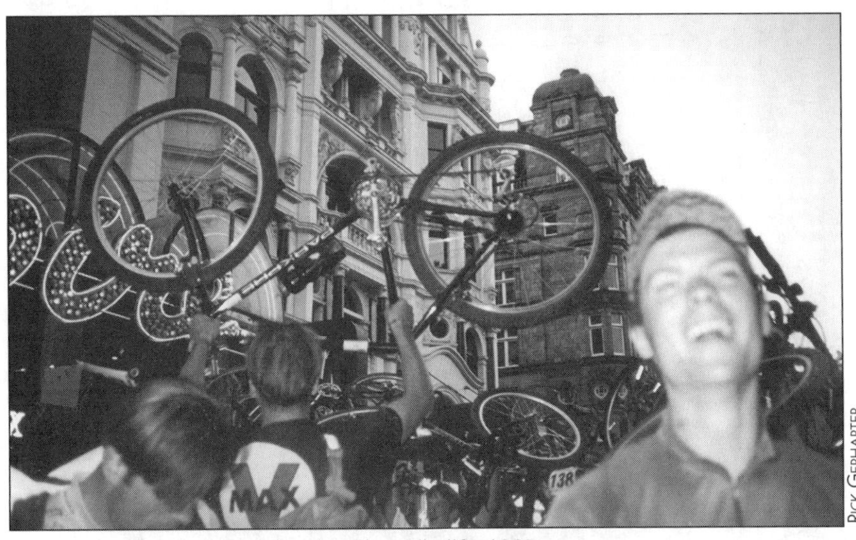

RICK GERHARTER

London Bikelift, 1995

sense of humor and commitment to other forms of activism while doing Critical Mass rides. August's ride was simultaneously a protest against France's desire to resume nuclear weapons testing in the South Pacific. You better believe there were a couple of pretty freaked out security officers at the French Embassy when a thousand people on bikes showed up to give them hell. Additionally, on a previous ride, Critical Massers celebrated the 40th anniversary of McDonald's by bringing the Mass through the restaurant's drive-through over and over again, frustrating motorists wishing to feed their fat faces.

Although its air is probably Britain's most polluted and its Street the most chaotic, London is not the only site for Critical Mass rides. The burgeoning pro-bicycle movement has found the strength to host Critical Mass rides in 16 other cities, including Oxford, Bath, Cambridge, Liverpool, and Edinburgh and Glasgow in Scotland. Also, cyclists have joined with the long standing anti-roads movement In Britain to create a powerful force as they demand that the government build less roads, fund more public transit projects, promulgate bicycle transportation, and create more livable communities.

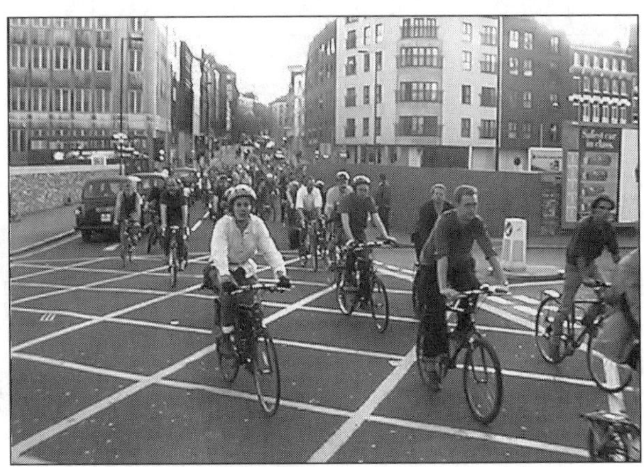

London Critical Mass, April 1994

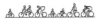

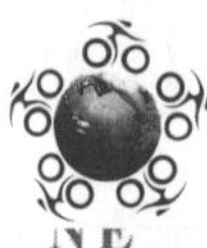

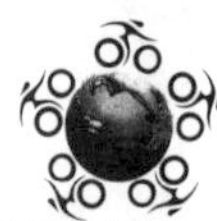

Global Gallery

SATURDAY, JULY 29, 2000 3

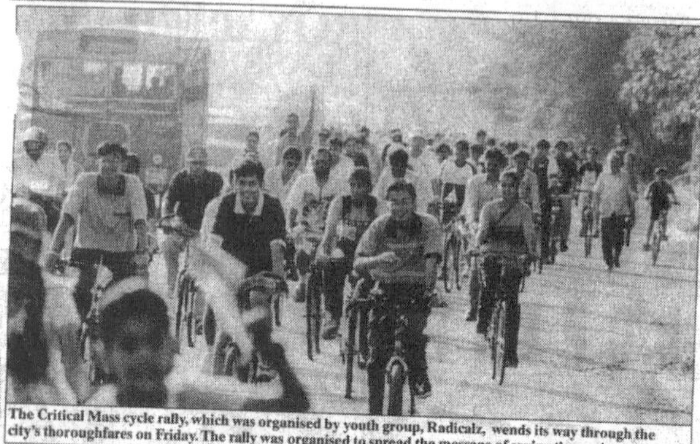

The Critical Mass cycle rally, which was organised by youth group, Radicalz, wends its way through the city's thoroughfares on Friday. The rally was organised to spread the message of saving the environment.

Cycle rally bearing green message gets good response

By A Staff Reporter

PUNE: The 'Critical Mass cycle rally' organised by city youth group, Radicalz, evoked an encouraging response here on Friday evening, showing that citizens still cared about the environment in Pune.

About 250 cyclists, aged between 10 and 60, pedalled over 15 km in the rally, which began from the University of Pune at 5.15 pm, went past the Shimla office, district court, Zilla Parishad, Ambedkar road, M G road and East street, before ending at the B J Medical college grounds at 7.00 pm.

Critical Mass is an international phenomenon, where people in large numbers cycle on the last Friday of every month across 200 cities of the world, spreading awareness about the need to save the environment.

The Radicalz group, comprising young city collegians, decided to

from Pune, India, Saturday, July 28, 2000

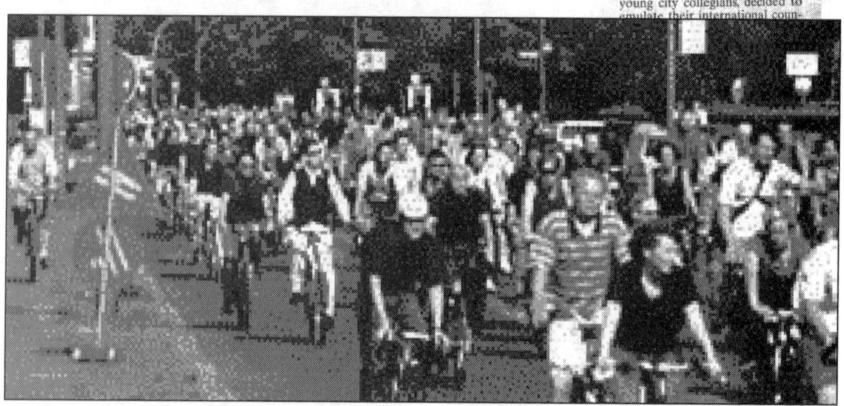

Berlin, Germany 1997

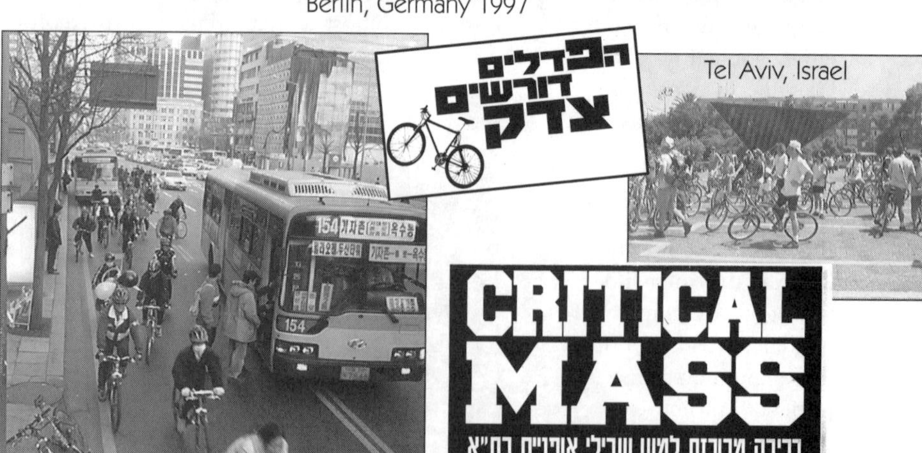

Seoul, South Korea

Tel Aviv, Israel

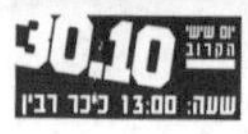
יום שישי
הקרוב
30.10
שעה: 13:00 כיכר רבין

כל יום שישי אחרון של כל חודש מתאספים רוכבי
האופניים לנסיעת מחאה למען שבילי אופניים בת"א
התארגנות מכיכר רבין בשעה 13:00

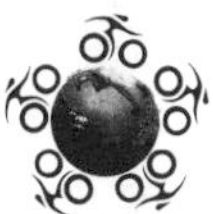

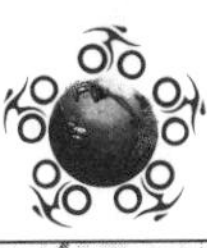

Global Gallery

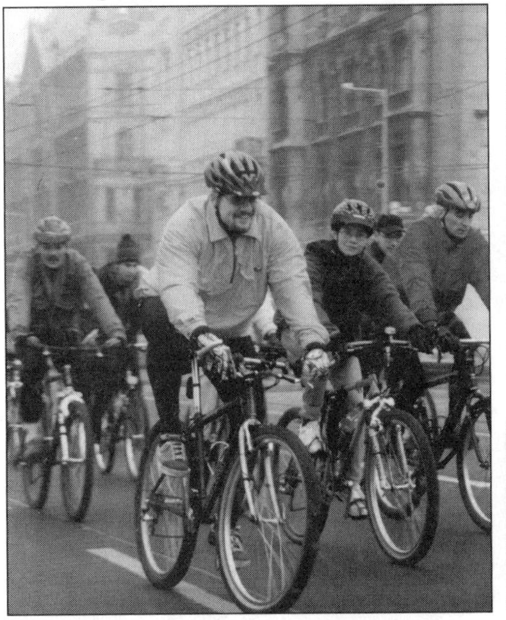

Budapest, Hungary

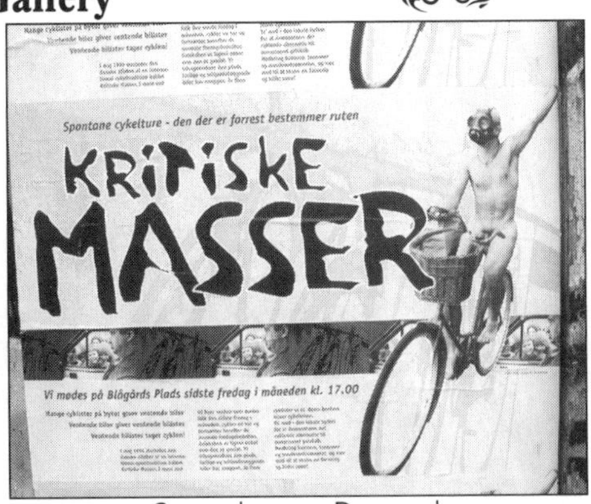

Spontane cykelture - den der er forrest bestemmer ruten
KRITISKE
MASSER
Vi mødes på Blågårds Plads sidste fredag i måneden kl. 17.00

Copenhagen, Denmark

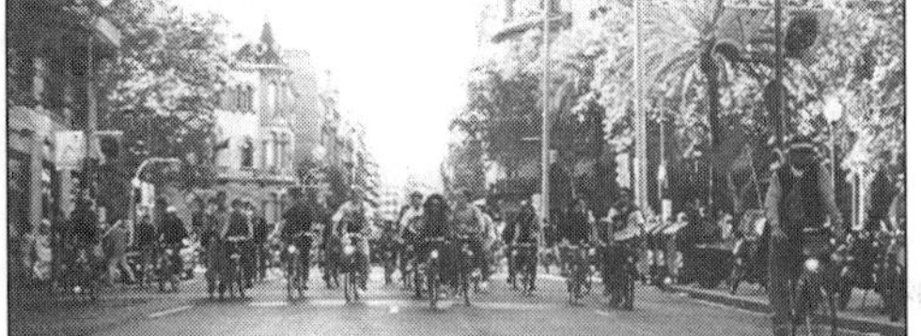

Barcelona, Spain

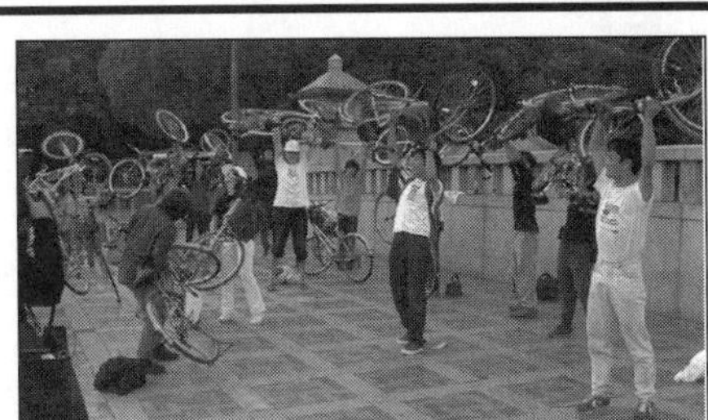

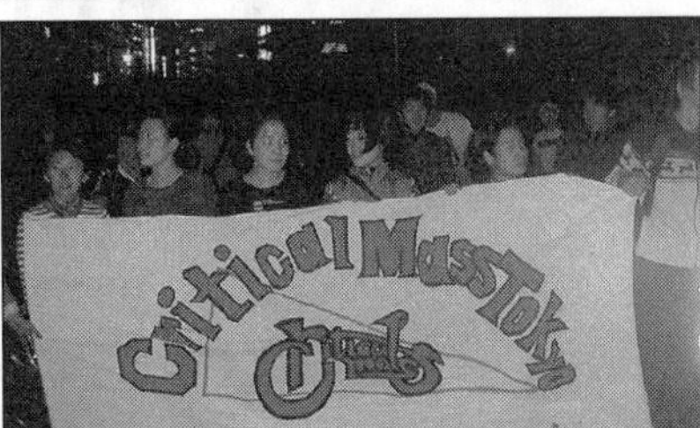

Critical Mass Tokyo

Tokyo, Japan
The inaugural Tokyo Critical Mass ride was well attended by 35 or so cheering, bell-ringing cyclists. Setting out from Harajuku at 4.30pm "The Mass" wound its way through Shibuya and on to Hibiya Park, finishing around 6pm.
—November, 1998—

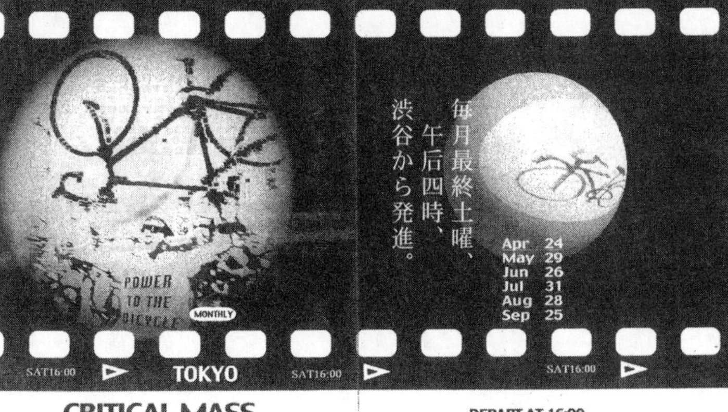

CRITICAL MASS

DEPART AT 16:00
FROM
THE FRONT OF NHK-HALL

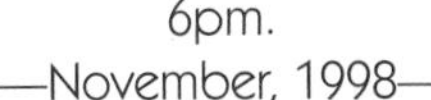

DEFINING ANARCHY

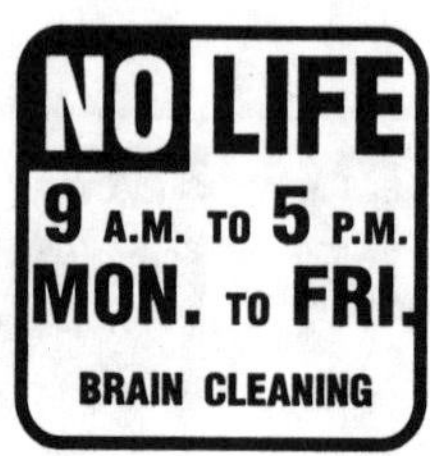

CRIT MASS

BY BERNIE BLAUG

I love Crit Mass for its anarchic nature. No one leads it, no one controls it, no one plans its routes and no one is its spokesperson. Whenever anyone has attempted to take control of any part of it they've always been unsuccessful—and I, for one, am glad of that.

Depending on who you ask, you'll always get a different description of what Crit Mass actually is. To some, it's a pro-bike, anti-car monthly action. To others it's a friendly, social, casual cruise. And, to yet more it's an opportunity to ride *en masse* through downtown and the neighborhoods—and for a change outnumber the cars. To me, it's all that and more.

Its anarchic nature has also made it difficult for the cops and mainstream media to pin it down. Doubtless the cops would love it if there were "leaders" they could hold accountable, meet with before, during and after the monthly rides—and threaten if they weren't getting things to their liking. Whenever anyone has tried to step forward and speak for all Crit Mass riders, frustration and confusion have nearly always quickly followed. I think its very nature of no leaders, bosses or appointed spokespeople is the main reason the Ride has lasted a full decade.

The media would also like spokespeople, or at least an office, they could go to for quotes and insights, but alas, for them, that's also proved elusive. Instead, if they want to write about it they actually have to go out and engage cyclists on the ride itself and really pursue the story, rather than compiling it all from their offices.

The police, and to a lesser extent, the media seem to have come to their senses in the past year or so and realized that it's easier to let the Ride go ahead, rather than trying to outlaw, restrict or re-route it. After all, it's only a couple of thousand people going on a bike ride. . .

Anarchy: The very word (especially after 9/11) invokes many images for all of us, nearly every one of them now negative. I feel Anarchy is not about chaos, murder, mayhem, etc. (as it's invariably portrayed in the mainstream media). To me, Anarchy is all about self-responsibility, self-empowerment and not needing

SAN FRANCISCO
SFPD
PEACE DEPARTMENT

NOTICE OF PARKING VIOLATION PD

MAKE | DATE | TIME CHECKED | TIME ISSUED

LICENSE NUMBER 1 2 3 4 5 6 7 U V P

BODY | LOCATION (APPROX.) OF VIOLATION

STATE | TAB MO | YR

COLOR

NOTE: FAILURE TO CHANGE OUR TRANSPORTATION HABITS MAY SUBJECT US ALL TO A GRIM FUTURE

V.I.N | VNVTW

I CERTIFY UNDER PENALTY OF PERJURY THAT I'M NOT JUST BEING MEAN. I REALLY JUST WANT TO HELP THE POOR SOUL WHO IS OWNED BY THIS VEHICLE. STAR

HUMAN ·

	√	VIOLATION	PENALTY
1		PARKING IN BICYCLE LANE 22500H VC	200
2		TALKING ON A CELLPHONE WHILE DRIVING 23103E VC	411
3		PARKING ON THE SIDEWALK 22500F VC	175
4		BRAINWASHED BY TELEVISION 010101A VC	9.95
5		DRIVING AN SUV 38505 VC	350
6		TRYING TO MAKE UP FOR YOUR LOW SELF ESTEEM BY DRIVING AN EXPENSIVE CAR	999

	√	VIOLATION	PENALTY
7		ROAD RAGE 23103A VC	357
8		STUCK IN GRIDLOCK ON A BEAUTIFUL DAY 23333A VC	500
9		POLLUTING THE AIR & WATER 38390A VC	275
10		WHINING ABOUT HIGH GAS PRICES 12345A VC	15.14
11		MAKING THE EARTH A WORSE PLACE FOR YOUR CHILDREN 2034BC VC	850
12		COMPENSATING FOR YOUR ANATOMICAL **SHORT**COMINGS 52153A VC	4.5"

OTHER	CODE	SECTION	PENALTY
			$
			$

DESCRIPTION: (DETAILS OF VIOLATION)

DO NOT WORSHIP CASH SEEK ENLIGHTENMENT

STAR NO. ☐ 5200 ☐ 5202 ☐ 5204

HUMAN'S SIGNATURE CVC

REMOVE THIS STUB BEFORE MAILING

BEN SEIBEL AND BETH VERDEKAL

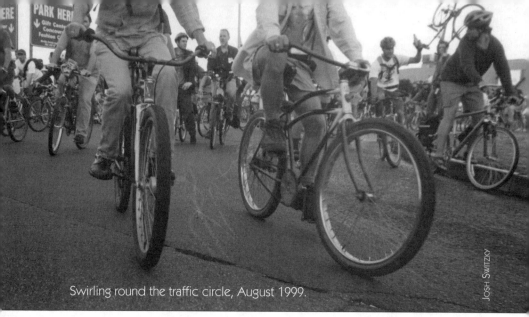

Swirling round the traffic circle, August 1999.

JOSH SWITZKY

(or wanting) authority figures to constantly tell us how to act, feel and think. I've been a regular mass rider since the 2nd SF Crit Mass (in 10/92) and have been on over 50 of 'em altogether. Obviously, not everyone on every ride has acted like an angel, but for the most part, Crit Mass riders know the difference between right and wrong and act accordingly—with or without police presence.

Critical Mas is an organic, spontaneous, inspiring, anarchic thing of beauty. VIVA LA MASS!

HOW CRITICAL MASS CHANGED THE (AMERICAN) WORLD

BY ANNA SOJOURNER

Critical Mass is not a protest but a demonstration, in the simplest sense of the word. It is a demonstration of social space, the rarest bird in America. It works, because people automatically feel it's right, though many of us have never before experienced free public space. Critical Mass cuts through the noise and inertia of the American transportation system and teaches us to carve a wedge of our city for ourselves. It feeds us a reality we use to create a vision.

With no knowledge of history or sense of possibility, we assume that the way things are is the way things ought to be. Just because our home is friendlier to autos than humans doesn't mean it ought to be that way. Critical Mass gives us knowledge and a sense of possibility bigger than any rhetoric, any architectural model, any developer's ad campaign, or any promise. We humans want social space, we need it, take to it like ducks to water. After 10 years of massing, we found out that the society we want isn't so unobtainable after all. That's liberation. Thanks, Mass.

CYCLING UNDER THE RADAR—ASSERTIVE DESERTION

BY CHRIS CARLSSON

> *"An unusually loose netwar design—one that is eminently leaderless yet manages to organize a large crowd for a rather chaotic, linear kind of swarming—is found in the pro-bicycle, anti-car protest movement known as Critical Mass (CM) in the San Francisco Bay Area."*[1]
>
> —David Ronfeldt and John Arquilla
> *Networks and Netwars: The Future of Terror, Crime, and Militancy*
> Rand Institute

> *"Anarchist spontaneity, anonymity, leaderlessness, and ubiquity are a mischievous mirror of the fluidity and omnipresence of capital in its most advanced post-industrial form. . . a counterpower whose morphing, mobile affinities speak back against a financial command that is vaporous, nomadic, and strikes across all points on the social horizon."*[2]
>
> — Nick Dyer-Witherford
> "Global Body, Global Brain/Global Factory, Global War: Revolt of the Value-Subjects" www.thecommoner.org

Bicycling is a particularly solitary activity. Not everyone rides a bike; in fact, it's a rather small minority. And of people who do choose to bicycle, an even smaller minority choose to participate in Critical Mass. At first glance bicycling seems an unlikely place to find a political movement of people animated by a passion to change how we live. But the fiercely individualistic folks who choose to bicycle AND ride in the monthly Critical Mass are among those at the forefront of today's social revolts.

Even though bicycling in modern cities is extremely isolated and dangerous, every day thousands of people choose to embrace the bicycle as their means of personal transportation. Why? What does it mean that so many people are willing to choose something so discouraged by the structure of society—both its physical layout and its psychological assumptions? What is the meaning of this limited and largely invisible form of social opposition, this growing desertion from the hyper-exploitation of the car/oil nexus? And how does Critical Mass take this expression and deepen its meaning and power?

Famously, the motivations of Critical Massers are as numerous as the number of riders. Ask anyone why they are on a Critical Mass and you'll get a response from a long list of possible answers. But what people think they're doing is less interesting than what it *means* that a specific fraction of the population has found a form of political and social expression in the Critical Mass phenomenon.

In Critical Mass we discover partial and beginning answers to questions most of us haven't even begun to ask. Some have called our times the "end of history," others a "New World Order," still others the emergence of something beyond any nation-state called "Empire," or "globalization." Whatever one might call it, the assumptions and dynamics of society are undergoing dramatic change, a change that the popular press has done little to explore or explain beyond clichés and platitudes derived from looking in the rearview mirror. Critical Mass has grown alongside the emergence of a new global system as one manifestation of its flipside, a new form of social opposition.

Nobody asks for your ID, your money, your soul or your brain at Critical Mass. It is a living, collective affirmation of the human drive for authentic, unmediated community. People arrive, excited to join a temporary, mobile occupying army of noisy rolling revelers, relishing the sounds of people laughing and talking, hooting and whistling, tinkling bells and spinning gears. You are invited to talk to strangers and they usually answer with sincere enthusiasm. The Critical Mass experience is contrary to "normal" life thanks to the absence of buying and selling, and the equally important lack of a hierarchical structure.

People who seek personal autonomy find each other on bicycle at Critical Mass. It is a breeding ground for people who are ready to start living in a world shaped to facilitate cooperation, generalized prosperity, and ecological sanity as opposed to cutthroat competition, war and the barbarism of worldwide famine and environmental devastation. Critical Mass is a place to taste the imaginary (but suddenly and briefly real) power of collective spirit, to feel you are alive and aware as you help create a true and uncorrupted sliver of autonomous, self-directed public space. You taste a radically public and directly democratic potential in the euphoric sharing of a freely created convivial space predicated on individual engagement.

The New Shape of Class Conflict

Critical Mass participants are largely members of what has been termed the "Cognitariat," the human "know-how"—technical, cultural, linguistic, and ethical—that supports the operation of the high-tech economy[3]. This includes programmers and secretaries, office managers and account executives, but also waiters, bike messengers, students, gardeners and musicians. Most San Francisco riders work in the cubicular world of corporate America, shuffling information and maintaining software and hardware for the globe-spanning corporations that most benefit from the new shape of the world, or the ubiquitous nonprofit corporations that have sprung up to address the yawning chasms left behind by capitalist development.

Our era is characterized by a rapid enclosure of human life within the boundaries of buying and selling, i.e. the world of commodification. Commodification has expanded into new realms and more and more of life: from childcare and psychotherapy to personal trainers and dogwalkers, the markets never close anymore with supermarkets open 24/7 and financial markets trading at all hours across the planet. The side of this that we are usually aware of, at least in part, is shopping, where we get the goods we need to live by exchanging money for them. But shopping is also an arena in which our choices can define our identity and sense of self, where we make our individual mark on the world. We seem oblivious to the side of commodification in which we are the commodity, wherein our ability to work is the only real product we have for sale and where our creative contribution to making the world is sold to purposes beyond our choice or control.

What this omnipresent Economy also represents is a radical expansion of the terrain of exploitation. Classical revolutionary analysis focused on work, especially factory work, as the site of maximum exploitation—hence the point at which revolutionary opposition (by workers) was most likely to erupt and where it would find the most power to counter the power of capital and its owners. While it is still true that profits are derived from the coercive relations of wage-labor in workplaces across the planet—and it is still a crucial area of social and political conflict—our era is better understood as one in which a general level of profitability is maintained through a system of "social labor"—a real enclosure of all living activity into the logic of buying and selling. As I write this in mid-March 2002, the U.S. press trumpets the end of the economic downturn that followed the dotcom bust and Sept. 11 attacks. Enron, Global Crossing, Arthur Andersen—individual businesses teeter and collapse, but the incessant participation of U.S. consumers, endlessly expanding their debt load, blindly trusting the fundamental reliability of the modern Economy, keeps the system from falling into an historically familiar abyss.

> *"This is a new proletariat and not a new industrial working class. . . 'proletariat' is the general concept that defines all those whose labor is exploited by capital, the entire cooperating multitude . . . In the . . . context of Empire, however, the production of capital converges ever more with the production and reproduction of social life itself; it thus becomes ever more difficult to maintain distinctions among productive, reproductive, and unproductive labor. Labor—material or immaterial, intellectual or corporeal—produces and reproduces social life, and in the process is exploited by capital. . . Th[is] progressive indistinction between production and reproduction . . . also highlights once again the immeasurability of time and value. As labor moves outside the factory walls, it is increasingly difficult to maintain the fiction of any measure of the working day and thus separate the time of production from the time of reproduction, or work time from leisure time. . . the proletariat produces in all its generality everywhere all day long."*[4]
>
> —*Empire* by Michael Hardt and Antonio Negri

People working in corporate America often change jobs. These days, dissatisfaction or oppression does not lead people to get organized and fight back. Instead, people quit and look for a new job. The dramatic transience in workplaces and neighborhoods has eroded a sense of community, and undercut the belief that we all share similar predicaments and experiences. Efforts by companies to ameliorate a modern life drained of genuine sociability with the fake life of the "corporate family" don't fill the void. Flight from the inequities of work life leave Americans more isolated, confused and ignorant of class dynamics than ever.

Incongruously, as the totality of life has become increasingly absorbed in socialized economic activity, our personal experience (at least in the modern metropolis) is one of increased isolation. We are far less likely to know our neighbors or have lasting connections with co-workers than was common in previous eras. We feel alone in an ever more integrated system of making our world together. We are driven by the accelerated pace of daily life to a state in which we have no time—no time to socialize, no time for our kids or our lovers, no time to stop and think. Between working and shopping, and expanding periods of transit between every economic activity, we hardly have time for anything beyond sleeping.

Our atomization as individuals leaves us helpless in the face of a system that incessantly proclaims itself as the best of all possible worlds. If we are not satisfied, something must be wrong with us, because everyone else agrees, or so the absence of visible dissent seems to indicate. But this hollow consensus is extremely shallow. It is undercut by real life experiences every day. As long as those experiences are understood as personal failures rather than systemic necessities, we continue to participate "willingly"—lacking any alternative, trapped by bills, debts and fear of falling.

The contagious pleasure of a movement like Critical Mass threatens the precariousness of today's world, which depends on cooperative participation by the majority of people as workers and consumers. Critical Mass is an unparalleled practical experiment in public, collective self-expression, reclaiming our diminishing connectedness, interdependency and mutual responsibility. CM provides encouragement and reinforcement for desertion from the rat wheel of car ownership and its attendant investments. But even more subversively, it does it by gaining active participation in an event of unmediated human creation, outside of economic logic, and offering an exhilarating taste of a life practically forgotten—free, convivial, cooperative, connected, collective.

In the social factory, resistance can erupt in arenas outside the traditional sphere of the workplace. When old-style leftists despair over falling rates of unionization and strikes, they are failing to appreciate the wider terrain of class conflict taking shape in this new period of history. Critical Mass underscores the primacy of transit as an arena of contestation. Bicyclists have withdrawn from the exploitative relations of car ownership and the degrading second-class citizenship (and waste of time) imposed by public transit. But this revolt is personal and invisible—until the creative eruption of Critical Mass proclaims these myriad isolated acts to the world as a shared act. It is a public declaration that suddenly reveals individual choices as social, political and collective responses to the insanity that passes as inevitable and normal. In creating a moving event, celebrating and being a real alternative, Critical Mass simultaneously opens up the field of transit to new political contestation, and pushes it to another level by pioneering swarming mobility as a new tactic.

When someone becomes a daily bicyclist s/he makes an emphatic break with one of the basic assumptions and "truths" of the dominant society: that you must have a car to get around. The actual experience of urban cycling refreshes the cyclist mentally and physically. That experience in turn inoculates the bicyclist against the disdain heaped on cyclists by "normal" people, often while they're driving. In addition, it begins to undermine all sorts of received truths, packaged and delivered by entertainment conglomerates with a vested interest in maintaining our dependence on steadily consuming their products in pursuit of an elusive happiness, or at least a satisfaction that we can't seem to get.

Bicyclists remove themselves, at least while riding, from the overwhelming saturation of the media. Instead of being told about traffic and weather, celebrity traumas, spectacular crimes, government proclamations, the latest scores and the whole seamless web of marketing and entertainment that calls itself 'news', the cyclist sees the dark clouds gathering, speaks to the neighborhood grocer, chats with the local kids on the corner. The bicyclist is experiencing life directly, avoiding the calculated mediation foisted on citizens by the ever-present babble of TV and radio. Short-circuiting the self-referential presentation of an edited and finally false "reality," the cyclist's critical attitude, already strong enough to get her on a bicycle, begins to reinforce itself.

Bicyclists reject "simulatory conditioning. Revulsion against the power of a commercially driven media to saturate consciousness, structure social interactivity and standardize creativity has become a major theme of the new dissidence, for which culture jamming, ad-busting, and subvertisements are familiar forms."[5]

The Empire Strikes Back

> *"Whether such movements will remain only a spectral, haunting, deconstructive discomfort to capital, or develop the substantial capacity to make 'an exit to the future' is uncertain. The more vital they become, the more reality their projects assume, the more hollow and wraith-like will the market values they oppose appear, and the more lethal the force it will bring against them."*[6]
>
> —Nick Dyer-Witherford

It's not surprising that in cities and towns across the world, but especially in the U.S., whenever a group of ten to fifty bicyclists (or more!) have appeared on the streets, riding in a leisurely social atmosphere, the police have responded with a predictable and disproportionate fury. The mighty forces kneading our lump of earth into a shape that assures their wealth and power cannot ignore Critical Mass. Wherever it erupts, with few exceptions among the 250-odd cities and towns across every continent where groups have ridden as "Critical Mass," local and state police have responded quickly and punitively. Many individual cops are personally offended by cheerful bicyclists thumbing their noses at the automotive debt ball-and-chain they themselves have embraced so ardently. But the visceral hatred of a few zealous police is just the local manifestation of a much larger systemic fear of rebellion.

We can perhaps understand the individual motorist who quickly turns his everyday road rage against these visible rebels on bicycles, trapped as he is in a vehicle that symbolizes his freedom while actually imprisoning him—in debt and anxiety, but at that moment, in a metal box in a traffic jam. He has traded a great deal of his life to "own" this car—and now a contingent of revelers, by their simple pres-

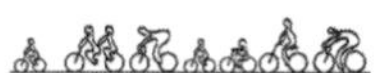

ence, shatters the untenable illusion of his freedom. It is an illusion that he is already struggling to maintain against all evidence even before the bicyclists started shouting about the emperor's obvious nakedness. Needless to say, the motorist is outraged.

In a contrasting scenario, the motorist sympathizes with the passing bicyclists but as she waits through one, two, maybe three traffic light cycles, her time is slipping away. Her tension soars as impending appointments with family or job are delayed. Trapped in gridlock, exasperated by free-spirited bicyclists who don't seem to care about her situation, her mood darkens. She, too, resents the visible cause of her delay, and joins the more belligerent motorist in wanting to at least reprimand the cyclists—who they see as childlike, unrealistic, irresponsible—that There Is No Alternative!

So the local police dispatcher gets a barrage of complaints by cellphone from angry motorists—people who have come upon a disruption, an unauthorized procession of people who are filling the always congested thoroughfares with bicycles—what's more, they're having fun! The offended motorists are in a hurry—as always—but for once there is an identifiable culprit behind their daily humiliation. As if the pressure of work, bills and family weren't enough, now they're stopped in traffic by a boisterous bicycling traffic jam.

The police, facing another routine Friday of fender benders and flat tires, spring into action. Highways hold more cars than they were meant to, the daily traffic jams being a public version of the thickening arteries and slowing blood flow of the obese commuter/consumer who keeps the body politic wheezing along, dependent on cars and malls, wars and work. But the police, like the citizens trapped in their cars in another routine traffic jam, know that something more dangerous is happening than just a few dozen bicyclists riding home together.

The police recognize their duty to raise the personal cost of participating in such an affront to social consensus. Tickets, arrests, harassment, even police violence, have all been applied to Critical Mass participants from Austin, Texas to Portland, Oregon to Minneapolis, San Francisco, Los Angeles and New York. In city after city, authorities do their utmost to contain and quarantine the contagion. This includes a range of responses from police repression to attempts to create CM leadership structures through negotiation, even up to official permission and sponsorship. But so far, Critical Mass has eluded these familiar techniques, still rolling free in dozens of locales.

In many places, including San Francisco, police have gone through periods of ignoring Critical Mass, assuming it will either peter out on its own without the antagonistic energy provided by police repression, or just become so routine that boredom drives away the personalities who originally cracked open the social space for Critical Mass to flourish. Periods of benign tolerance have left the event room to grow and expand, but have also absorbed the event into the "normal" fabric of life, a once-a-month predictable ritual that changes nothing. If the participants fail to make the experience a dynamic, rejuvenating, visionary happening, slowly and inexorably the power of Critical Mass diminishes. But in many places, San Francisco especially, when Critical Mass is left alone it con-

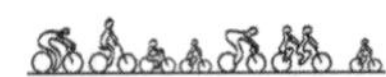

tinues to inspire new and old participants, providing an incomparable lesson in practical anarchy. It is a leaderless, amorphous reinhabitation of the urban landscape in a temporary community outside of economic logic.

Critical Mass: An Exit to the Future?

> *"...the classic formulation that sees action on the streets as more real than its symbolic forms is wrong: in this case, it is the street action that is symbolic. But to recognize this is not to say such movements are insignificant: on the contrary, they are the constituent moments of new identities and agents, the big bubbling cauldrons out of whose mists emerging subjects defect from capital's value schemes in scores of directions, transformed by their confrontation with capital's security forces, by their combination with other[s]."*[7]
>
> — Nick Dyer-Witherford

> *"Autonomous movement is what defines the place proper to the multitude. . . Through circulation the multitude reappropriates space and constitutes itself as an active subject. ."*[8]
>
> —Michael Hardt and Antonio Negri

Critical Mass since its beginning has identified itself as a celebration more than a protest, and is for many of its participants a prefigurative experience, both calling attention to and actually creating a taste of a different way of life. The vibrant grassroots culture is the best proof of this. Costumes, flyers, posters, art shows, concerts and parties all have promoted and extended Critical Mass into areas of life beyond mere bicycling, and have given creative voice to hundreds of riders. The wildly popular Halloween ride has brought out a profusion of clever costumes every year in many cities. Critical Mass participants often bring art to the streets outside of the social ritual of Halloween. Dinosaurs have popped up in a number of cities, especially along the west coast of North America (from Vancouver to LA), making the obsolescent car/oil system the butt of a sharp visual pun.

Critical Mass is also a practical lesson in direct action for all its participants, focused on the moment and the immediate experience rather than towards representatives, government, politicians or demands. Critical Mass has often provided participants a breathtaking experience of

> *"inherent risk. [The] excitement and danger of the action creates a magically focused moment, a peak experience, where real time suddenly stands still and a certain shift in consciousness can occur. Many of us have felt incredibly empowered and have had our lives fundamentally radicalized and transformed by these feelings. Direct action is praxis, catharsis and image rolled into one."*[9]
>
> —John Jordon

Critical Mass is an experience that goes beyond symbolic action, in spite of its enormous symbolic importance. It is a public demonstration of a better way of moving through cities. But during the time it is underway, it is more than a demonstra-

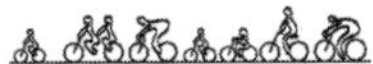

tion. It is a moment of a real alternative, already alive, animated by the bodies and minds of thousands of participants, who are not waiting for the world to be changed... They are changing it. The world CM'ers live in is already different because we participate in Critical Mass. We have harnessed a mysterious but simple and direct social power to invent our own reality. At this moment, our choice to bicycle leaves the realm of mere refusal and becomes a creative act, a mobilization of what we might call "collective invention power." Tellingly, collective invention escapes the rules and limits of the market entirely.

Bicyclists refuse the nonsensical "necessity" of driving as a first step in a series of personal choices that taken as a whole, represent a new type of political contestation, not only oppositional, but visionary. It is an act of desertion from an entire web of exploitative and demeaning activities, behaviors that impoverish the human experience and degrade planetary ecology itself. Bicycling is simultaneously a withdrawal from an important sector of economic activity. Time spent making money to pay for a car is now freed up for other parts of life. Though miniscule, each individual's active disengagement with the expectations of economic self-enslavement is a material and psychological blow for human freedom.

Apart from the individual psychological explanations, clearly as a new form of leaderless, mobile temporary occupation, Critical Mass strikes deep fear into the system. It represents a desertion from one piece of a coercive order that keeps us working for them AND trapped in an individualistic worldview. It also manifests a positive reinhabiting of an ever-more degraded urban landscape. And most threatening to the system, CM is tangibly fun, nourishing a human capacity for sharing pleasure unmediated by buying and selling, and as such it is a dangerously exciting precedent.

Footnotes

1. Ronfeldt, David and Arquilla, John. "What Next for Networks and Netwars?" pp. 336-337 in *Networks and Netwars: The Future of Terror, Crime, and Militancy*. Rand Institute: 2001
2. Dyer-Witherford, Nick. "Global Body, Global Brain/Global Factory, Global War: Revolt of the Value-Subjects," p. 14. www.thecommoner.org: January 2002.
3. Dyer-Witherford, *op.cit.*, p. 17. See also Dyer-Witherford's footnotes to Virno and Hardt, and Franco Berardi, "Bifo/Berardi, interview on "The Factory of Unhappiness," http://www.nettime.org. Posted 11 June 2001. Also, Jean-Marie Vincent, "Les automatisms sociaux et le 'general intellect.' *Futur Antérieur* 16 (1993): 121.
4. Hardt, Michael and Negri, Antonio. *Empire*, p. 402-403. Harvard University Press: 2000
5. Dyer-Witherford, *op.cit.*, p. 18.
6. Dyer-Witherford, *op.cit.*, p. 30.
7. Dyer-Witherford, *op.cit.*, p. 29.
8. Hardt and Negri, *op.cit.*, p. 397.
9. Jordon, John. "The art of necessity: The subversive imagination of anti-road protest and Reclaim the Streets" in *DiY Culture: Party & Protest in Nineties* Britain, ed. George McKay, Verso: 1998, p. 133

A QUIET STATEMENT AGAINST OIL WARS

BY CHRIS CARLSSON, FROM A FLYER DISTRIBUTED AT SAN FRANCISCO CM, OCT. 2001

Critical Mass has not seen a lot of xerocracy (opinionated flyering) lately. And yet, just by its persistence, it continues to define and keep open an important social and political space. Now that we are once again faced with open war, hot and murderous, our mass bike-in automatically takes on a greater political meaning.

Over the past nine years, Critical Mass has been a steady, important rejoinder to the madness of the car/war society that depends on oil and other fossil fuels. Uprisings in Mexico, Nigeria, Venezuela, and the ongoing conflicts in the Middle East all underscore the permanence of war in our era. Critical Mass is our way of gathering publicly to repudiate the insanity of the Orwellian world we live in, where War is Peace.

We all feel some kind of pressure to "do something" either along with the patriotic campaign, or against it. But part of bicycling together is the calming and contemplative experience it inherently provides. As fear and panic have been exacerbated by the crescendo of militaristic posturing, what better response can we make than to calmly ride our bicycles through town, discussing world events and our part in them? We must stand our ground, clear our minds of the fear that is being intensively marketed to us, and resist the social control the authorities try to maintain with it.

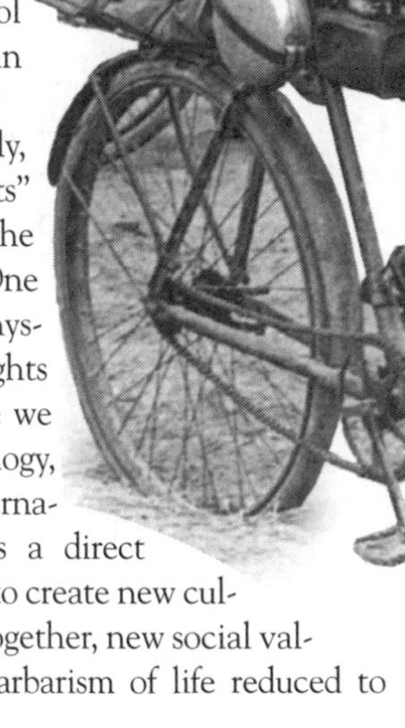

We have to think creatively, not just about the distorted "facts" we're being fed, but also about the uses governments make of war. One of the crucial functions of a war hysteria is to drive all other thoughts out of our minds. No longer are we to concern ourselves with ecology, alternative transportation, alternative sources of energy. War is a direct assault on the painstaking effort to create new cultural norms, new ways of being together, new social values that transcend the banal barbarism of life reduced to commodities for sale.

Now more than ever we need to talk to each other, to share what we know, what we believe, and what we can imagine. Riding in Critical Mass we are already taking a small, simple step towards a better world, a place of abundance, security and camaraderie. In the months ahead—of ongoing war against mysterious "internal enemies"—we may find that bicycling will become an even more important tool in preserving and extending our abilities to resist a blindly repressive state. During the last open war, the Persian Gulf War of 1991, local bicyclists played an important role as highly mobile scouts for the huge anti-war demonstrations that crisscrossed the city for several months.

While we can still ride openly together, let's renew our friendships and our trust, knowing that our social bonds are under assault and will need the strength to bend so they won't break. Wars destroy humans and the physical infrastructure of human societies. They also disrupt and destroy human communities, not just elsewhere, but here. In those disruptions are also openings and opportunities. Amidst the hysteria of the past six weeks have also been extraordinary openings to revisit assumptions, explanations, and our sense of how life came to be this way.

Many people are understandably concerned about our safety in the wake of the developments since mid-September. Much to the horror of anyone not predisposed to a simplistic, patriarchal authoritarianism, the U.S. government has taken the bait and is following precisely the worst course of action it could have possibly chosen in the wake of the attacks.

We have to step back from the frenzied hysteria that has been cultivated to gain popular support to "do something" with our expensive and brutal military machine. When we take a deeper look at the context of current events, we can see that the government's strategy is only rhetorically interested in combatting terrorism. The effort to subdue Afghanistan (a mission fraught with disastrous historical precedents) has more to do with central Asian oil and narcotics than terrorism, which is only a convenient excuse for a military campaign that the Bushies came into office determined to pursue.

If it was terrorism that the Bush gang wanted to uproot, a much different policy would be on the agenda, one that included a transformation of our material relationship to oil and our political relationship with Middle Eastern countries. Counting on the political and historical ignorance of Americans, the men propping up Dubya arrogantly assume they can militarily defeat any opposition to U.S. efforts to control world oil and narcotics supplies. They even dare to use the pretext of a national emergency to force through restrictions on civil liberties, to railroad new trade legislation, and open Alaska's National Wildlife Refuge to oil drilling. (The sad fact that there is a de facto one-party state in the U.S. is another topic altogether.)

Grassroots opposition can expect to be visited by government surveillance and repression. Meanwhile, intelligent political discussion is only available on alternative radio programs and internet sites far from the one-note mass media that most people rely on for "news."

In the face of one of the worst propaganda onslaughts in U.S. history, we must demand the truth. Let us ask ourselves, who decides? Who benefits? Who loses? Why this and not that?

Of Oil Wars and Leaked Memos

BY CHRIS CARLSSON, FROM A FLYER DISTRIBUTED AT SAN FRANCISCO CM, SPRING 1997

In 1991, over 100,000 San Franciscans participated in anti-Gulf War demonstrations, often on bicycle. Well, as we ride along in our typical Critical Mass, we are still connected to wars elsewhere. The connections between our symbolic and active protest against the consumer end of the auto/oil industry and the hot wars in Mexico and Nigeria are considerably less immediately visible than the Gulf War, but in many ways, the concealed struggles are more interesting. The Zapatistas are fighting for a new model of social power, based on bottom-up democratic communities and extensive discussion and consultation before decisions are taken. Their struggle, centered in the Mexican state of Chiapas among Mayans uprooted by centuries of colonization and marketization, is adjacent to Mexico's large oil reserves, a fact well known to all who live and work in that part of the country. Meanwhile, in neighboring Tabasco state, over 20 oil facilities were besieged for weeks by angry peasants and oil workers in mid-December 1994, protesting fraudulent elections, a corrupt government, and widespread pollution. Not surprisingly, Chase Manhattan Bank sponsored a report to a group of large investors in mid-January, in which it was openly suggested that the Mexican government had to eliminate the Zapatistas to regain the confidence of investors, and that the ruling party, decades-long dictators in a one-party state, should seriously consider the ramifications of allowing real elections to erode their power. Treasury Secretary Robert Rubin's former firm, Goldman Sachs, has also chimed in with conservative advice for the Mexican government. The walls of San Francisco's Financial District surely obscure banal everyday acts just as horrific as these calls for mass murder emanating from Wall Street.

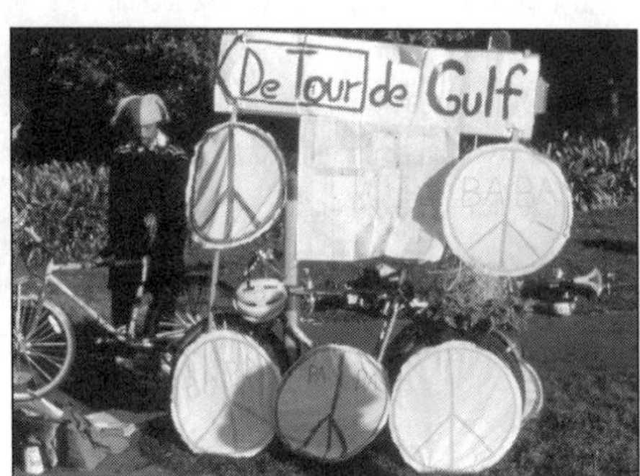

1991 Bay Area Bike Action ride against the Gulf War

A Greenpeace letter quoting from a restricted memo authored by the Chairman of Internal Security, Rivers State Nigeria: "Shell (Oil Co.) operations are still impossible unless ruthless military operations are undertaken for smooth economic activities to commence."

Shell has been drilling for oil in the Niger Delta for 36 years. The Ogoni people have been protesting to protect the Earth and their lives.Their non-violent protests have resulted in 1,800 deaths, Greenpeace reports—because money is at stake. Over 80% of Nigeria's revenue comes from oil, and Shell is the big money generator.

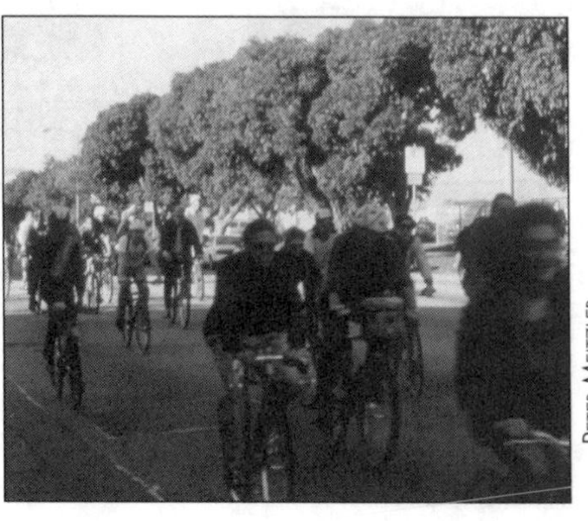

PETER MEITZLER

Ken Saro-Wiwa Murdered by Nigerian Military Dictatorship

The Nigerian military dictatorship murdered Ken Saro-Wiwa and eight other Ogoni activists in early November 1996. Fake murder charges have failed to disguise their real "crime": organizing the Ogoni people to demand a cleanup of the ecologically devastated Niger River delta (football field-sized pools of waste oil litter the landscape with the consequential cancer and health epidemic in their wake), and to demand that Shell Oil compensate the Ogoni people for the $30 billion of oil pumped from their lands since 1958.

In spring 1994, oil workers, gov't. workers, college students and most of Nigeria went on strike and fought running battles with the military. When European oil companies cut production by 40% in sympathy, San Francisco-based CHEVRON and New York-based MOBIL flew in additional foreign workers to keep the oil flowing from their wells and increased production to 120%. This saved the life of General Abacha's dictatorship.

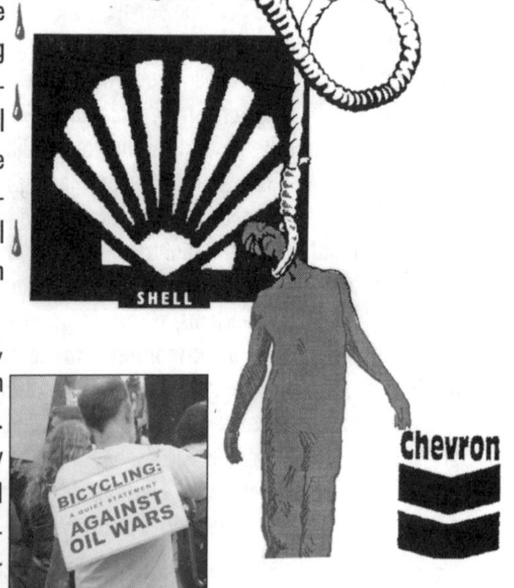

San Francisco, California

Worried about terrorism?
Want to know what you can do?
Help fight back, ride a bike!

Where do terrorists get their money?

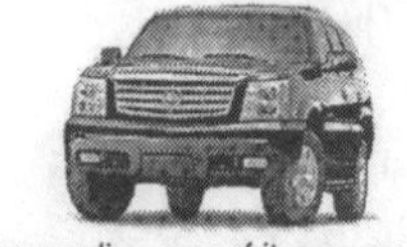

If you buy gasoline, some of it may come from you!

CRITICAL MASS
LAST FRIDAY OF EVERY MONTH
5:30 AT WEST WASHGINTON & THE SQUARE

Madison, Wisconsin

Chapel Hill, North Carolina

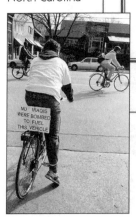

Boston, Massachusetts

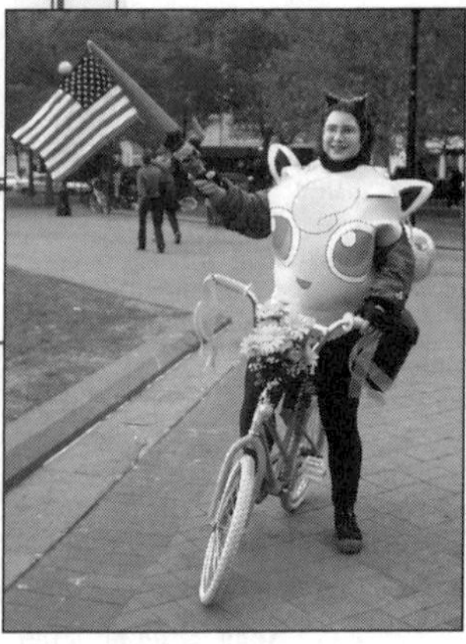

FROM THE GROUND UP

By Bill Stender

"Hey, I dont WANT to drink and drive, but how else am i gonna get my F-ING CAR HOME?" said the late comedian Sam Kinison. It was very funny to me, at least the way i heard it...I think the joke was that he doesn't consider the notion of not drinking. But maybe it was supposed to be about the even more outrageous notion of not driving. Why is drinking and driving so righteously condemned when the number of lives taken by the mistakes of impaired drivers represents only a tiny fraction of the total taken by the car overall?

The devastating impact of the automobile upon our planet, our nation and our communities has been well documented, and ignored. The end of oil and the harsh economic effects that will follow have also been well presented and yet the US Senate, ironically amidst a Middle East war, recently rejected the call for increased fuel efficiency standards. Conservation or alternative energy is given mere lip service or dismissed out of hand. Denial and double-speak are the answers we get to questions of global warming, dependency on foreign oil and spiraling traffic congestion. If Sam Kinison were a politician, he might say; "Hey I don't WANT to lead the world down a dead end, but how else am I gonna get my F-ING CAMPAIGN FINANCED?" The corruption and co-optation of our democracy by big money is common knowledge, fodder for comedy routines.

Popular indifference allows this to continue and has been made possible by the relative comfort of the Average American. Gas brings us a lot. But this indifference will crumble if it were to run out. And what then? Will society turn into a scene from Mad Max, with rampaging desperados racing down the road pillaging each other's precious drops of gasoline? Oil is synonymous with economic

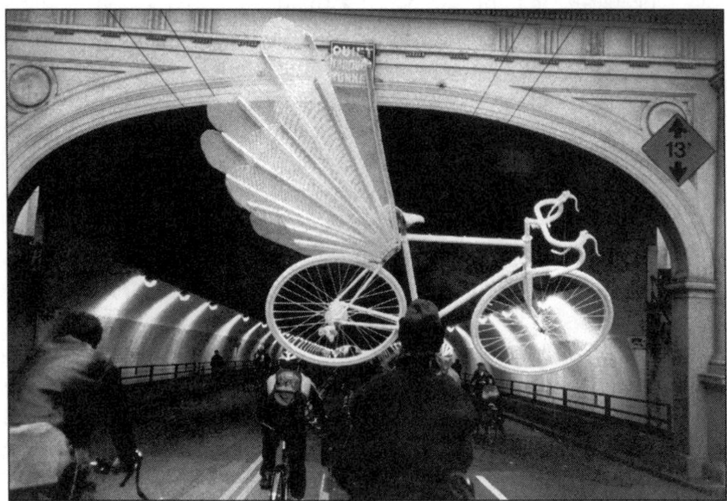

The Bike Angel enters Stockton Tunnel as part of Critical Mass in summer 2001.

progress, expansion, performance and power and is even equated with Freedom itself by advertising. Are there no alternatives? Will prosperity and happiness disappear along with the oil?

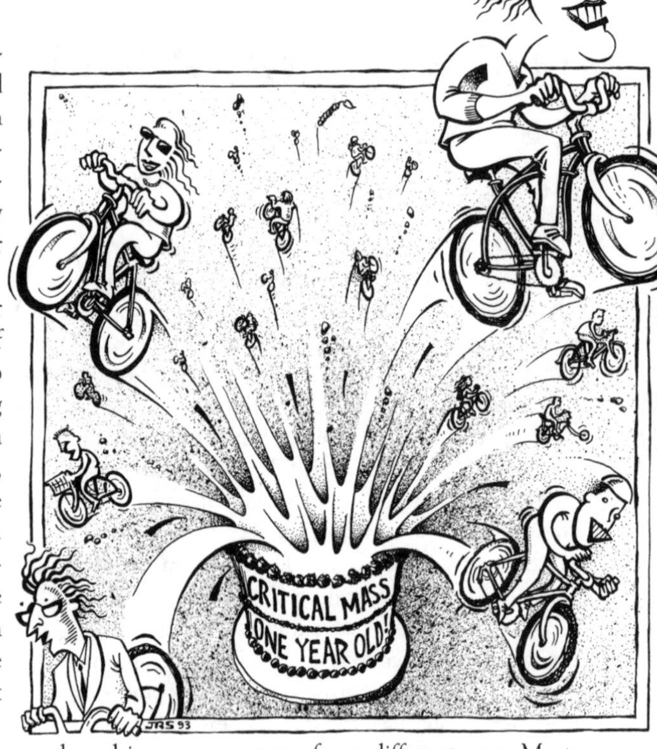

JAMES R SWANSON

There will be no clear demarcation of the "end of oil," so there will be no cataclysmic restructuring of society. As the price of a particular lifestyle goes up, more and more people choose different ones. Fortunately the development of different and more fulfilling lifestyles has been ongoing alongside the dominant lifestyle brought to us by our sponsors.

Critical Mass is, among other things, a prototype for a different one. Most notably, Critical Mass is an experiment in a true democracy—an experiment with what a society could be like—and it is exciting! It appears to the motorist, stuck in their congenital traffic-jam, as simply an affront to their right to proceed. While it does challenge this perceived right, CM is really challenging impediments to something much deeper—the right to proceed with an alternative vision for life in general, the right to choose a life worth living—a vision jammed by a recalcitrant central government promoting policies and enforcing ethics created in the interest of a small group of very rich benefactors.

Critical Mass does not directly articulate any challenge to the status quo, it simply exists alongside the state of things. CM recognizes no authority within its ranks, has no central goal, bylaws or dues. There are no requirements to join Critical Mass beyond enjoying yourself and behaving as a good citizen (of Critical Mass) and even that enjoys wide latitude. The biggest crime against the gathering is an insistence on some central program; a route, rules of the road or insisting on allegiance to a singular political cause.

One might expect this lack of leadership and organization to be a short-lived experiment but instead it seems to be the secret to its success. With the subtle pugnacity of a sapling, the movement has grown and enjoys firm roots in the traditions of democracy and social libertarianism. It may be difficult to perceive, stuck in the traffic jam that we have inherited, that eliminating centralized command and control is a potential solution to the most vexing problems facing the nation and world. Yet the organization of CM demonstrates the potential of self-organization in place of central authority.

The best solutions to all kinds of problems across the nation have long come from the ground up. Communities take their problems in hand and find a solution. Grassroots organization, as in tackling the problem of drinking and driving, eventually forced the laws to change at the top, one state at a time. As we watch the erosion of middle class prosperity, once insulated by cheap oil from the harsh realities of relentless expansion, we'll see people looking more closely at viable alternatives, new ways to make things work. And it is almost guaranteed that the answers will again be found by groups in one's own community rather than on Capitol Hill.

Critical Mass resonates with so many because it exemplifies this very act of taking matters into one's own hands. It does not protest for change, it simply changes. Critical Mass doesn't try to force anyone to join or do anything, it simply does its thing. The police have often responded with arrests and harassment of the participants, but this has only encouraged CM to grow. There is an instinct to protect the right to freely assemble. Perhaps it *is* an *inalienable* right. CM takes that right at face value and exercises it. Critical Mass challenges Authority by ignoring it.

Or perhaps it doesn't so much 'ignore' Authority as render it irrelevant. No pledge of allegiance nor singular goal is necessary. In the recognition of our commonality, in voluntary and enjoyable participation, everyone gets back what they put into it—there is pride of ownership. Organization from the ground up allows maximum individual expression as well as a cohesive group. Expectation for leaders to make things better is removed (and reduces the disappointment when they fail).

"Governments are instituted among Men, deriving their just powers from the consent of the governed..." so says the Declaration of Independence, but the next step is the common recognition that there are no 'just powers' of government, there's only the consent of the governed. While governmental bodies may serve specific logistical purposes, they needn't be confused with a need for Overseers.

Critical Mass can claim success. It has grown and spread worldwide. It has served the end of bicycle activism, environmental activism, of generating social awareness and building community. It has done so without any leaders or agenda or mission statement or membership. Yet it enjoys the strongest of allegiances and wisest of leadership. It is therefore a model and a harbinger of a new way for the brave new oil-less world. Critical Mass says; don't fight the power—BE the power! It's funny, basking in that power, Kinison's joke appears quaint.

ASSHOLE

Name: ______
Address: ______
City: ______ State: ______ Zip: ______

PAYMENT ENCLOSED: YES NO
COURT DATE REQUESTED YES NO

YOU WERE OBSERVED:
- Speeding
- Driving With No Common Sense
- Driving With No Regard For the Lives of Others
- Not Using Your Turn Signal
- California Stop
- Road Raging

YOU ARE:
- Parked Illegally
- Blocking Pedestrians
- Obstructing A Fire Hydrant
- Impeding The Flow Of Traffic

DEPARTMENT OF MANNERS
Your NOT Special!

WOULD YOU RATHER:
- Drive Friendly?
- Get A Real Ticket?
- Be Charged with Vehicular Homicide?
- Ride YOUR Bike?

//////328953-FU2 850295\\\\\\

A UNIQUELY DEMOCRATIC EXPERIMENT

BY MICHAEL KLETT

Critical Mass is democracy at its best. As the participants change, so does the nature of the beast. It changes from month to month and season to season just within the same city. Each ride is different from city to city, depending on the size of the ride and the attitudes of the riders and the authorities. The ride constantly synthesizes the amalgam of desires and allows for collective and individual responses to motorists, pedestrians, bus riders, authorities, and the various neighborhoods through which it passes. Within Critical Mass itself there are no leaders; organizers yes, we are all organizers—but we're not in charge. That has been the key to its success.

Slackers, geeks, and a good dose of the old and new left fill the ranks of Critical Mass riders. In a society where riding a bicycle to work is seen as almost subversive, once a month the subversives create a structure which works well. The seductive freedom of a Critical Mass ride is a powerful attraction to many people, but it is definitely not for everyone.

In San Francisco, the riders have refused to let the media, police or mayor define us. People have consciously tried to channel the energy and focus of the mass in various directions through xerocracy. Over the past ten years various events, memorials and protests have been included in the themes and routes for the Mass. Political issues have been proposed sometimes but were rejected or ignored by the majority of the riders. Some rides in San Francisco split into two groups, one with a political mission and one without. It can be quite stunning to see the literal flow of a true democratic process.

During rides there has been some coordination among a few to lead to a suggested destination. Discussion and cajoling percolate through the Massing crowd. Often a small group of 'leaders' will have to turn around and rejoin the 'mass' that has decided to turn a different way.

Critical Mass is a unique laboratory for experimenting with group dynamics. The tendency of a group to act like a herd can lead to a dull ride. Luckily, the wide variety of people usually creates enough of a carnival atmosphere to get people interacting on a level rarely seen downtown. Someone dressed as a well-sponsored professional racer has a good laugh with someone who finally got around to pumping up the tires of the bike that sat in the back of the garage for ten years. Self-appointed bicycle diplomats banter with the people waiting for a bus.

Routes were intentionally designed to cover different parts of the city for the first several years, visiting the tunnels occasionally. San Francisco's Broadway and Stockton tunnels are both typically filled with cars and exhaust. When Critical Mass takes over one of these tunnels for a few minutes, it underscores the stark contrast between the destructive atmosphere of cars and the playful sprawl of bicycles. The downhill directions are especially fast and fun in the tunnels.

The initial thrills of reclaiming tunnels from cars soon wore out when riders led

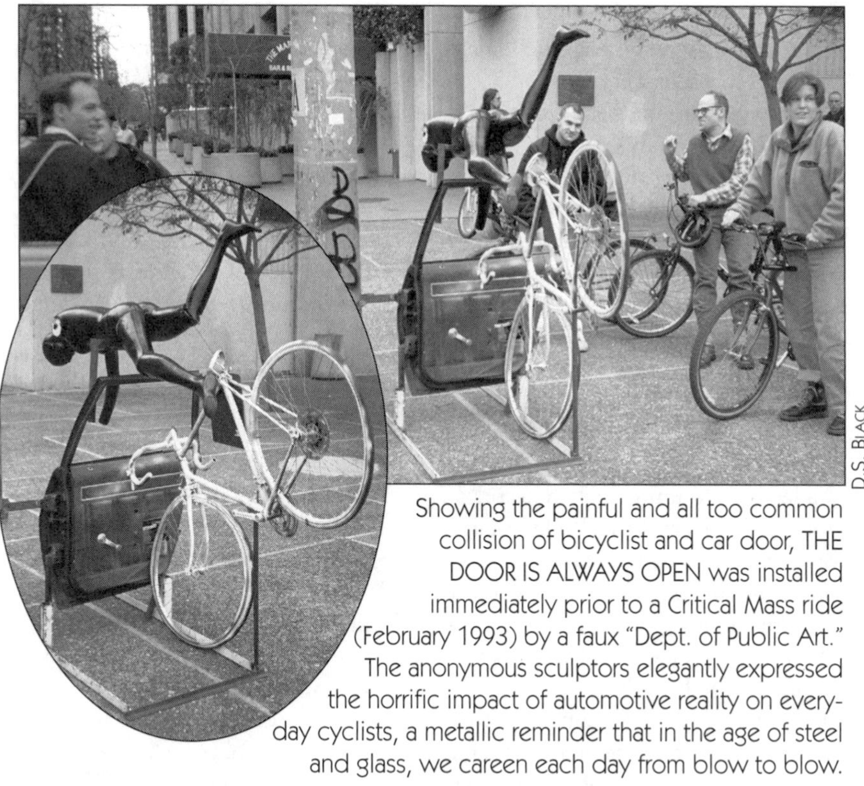

D.S. BLACK

Showing the painful and all too common collision of bicyclist and car door, THE DOOR IS ALWAYS OPEN was installed immediately prior to a Critical Mass ride (February 1993) by a faux "Dept. of Public Art." The anonymous sculptors elegantly expressed the horrific impact of automotive reality on everyday cyclists, a metallic reminder that in the age of steel and glass, we careen each day from blow to blow.

Critical Mass back the same way month after month until it became aggravating and boring. This same pattern was repeated with Pacific Bell Park. During baseball season, ride after ride would be steered to the park despite the disruption of the Mass through all the ballpark traffic. As route planning and xerocratic map publishing subsided in the past few years, the cyclists who found themselves at the front often didn't have any idea of where to take the ride for maximum fun and political impact. Experienced city cyclists have had to rush to the front to assertively direct the ride from time to time to avoid the problems of repetition and boredom.

Unfortunately, the conduct of the police can often set the mood for each Mass. It takes a lot of discipline among the participants to think ahead of the police tactics. The most effective methods have been to keep everyone upbeat and polite. Kash once said, "Inside every car, there's a person trying to get out." Critical Mass works best when it is *for* bicycling rather than *against* cars, when the group as a whole feels cohesive and creates its own mood and agenda.

It became apparent early on that it was pointless to directly confront authorities blocking our paths. We tried a route that would split between a mellow route and a more challenging hilly route and then rejoin at a later point. This was to prevent the ride from being too boring for the hammerheads, too difficult for less experienced riders and to limit the fragmentation of the ride. The police overreacted and set up a huge phalanx blocking one intended route at the split. After raucously protesting, the mass continued in one group but the lesson was learned—the cops were fixed and we were mobile. The ability to go somewhere else, and quickly, has been exhilarating and expedient.

Belligerent and aggressive individuals (nicknamed in the early months the "Testosterone Brigade") involved in the rides have been confronted about their behavior, especially when mob psychology starts to take over. Threats and mistreatment from motorists and police have been met with solidarity and patient good humor whenever possible. The non-intrusive use of cameras and video recorders is very effective in diffusing heated situations. Angry or bewildered drivers have often done stupid and dangerous things which have incurred the wrath of a group of riders.

Each participant is urged to be responsible for herself or himself. As the monthly rides got bigger and bigger, Critical Mass in SF got to be the hot thing to do. Many people would come down to the start of the ride and look for a map or a leader to tell them where to ride. They were uncomfortable with the idea of group decisions and the fluidity of everything. After being asked where the ride was going time after time by new people, I began to respond with 'Where do you want it to go?' and 'Didn't you make a route?'

Critical Mass has successfully avoided external cooptation for ten years. Attempts by people to sell things, except for a few home-made t-shirts, have been thwarted more by indifference than outright hostility. This has helped allow us to avoid the trap of being branded as this year's model. Of course people come to be seen at a hip event. One of many examples is Roberta Achtenberg, a 'liberal' politician who came to court votes—now vice president of the San Francisco Chamber of Commerce!

For a while we had the corporate scouts like *Wired* magazine come by looking for a way to package the next hip thing and help sell ad pages. For the most part we were too amorphous and unpalatable for them to co-opt. The major corporate media tried their best to portray CM as a dangerous group of anarchists. Funny thing was, that seemed to attract more and more riders. Every time Willie Brown, the mayor, tried to smear the event, he made himself look ridiculous.

A significant detraction to the image of Critical Mass (and the pleasure of participating for many riders) is the insufferable self-righteousness of some of the participants. Nothing turns people away faster than the attitude of many "principled" people. There isn't much point in screaming "CARS SUCK" at someone sitting in a traffic jam on a Friday night. They don't *want* to be there.

They won't stop and consider taking mass transit or bicycling if they feel that someone is depriving them of their rights. If, however, they are delayed by a cohesive, fun-loving group of revelers, they might decide that on the last Friday of the month (if not other times), it would be better to take the bus or train. Decades of car-oriented city planning won't be reversed overnight. Critical Mass powerfully demonstrates an alternative to current reality. In-your-face taunting and posturing only hardens people's positions and increases defensiveness and reflexive hostility.

Someone could do a long study of the psychology of bicyclists, who see themselves as a wronged and threatened group, suddenly finding themselves in the majority while on a Mass. But let's put things in perspective—a bike is usually just a tool. It can be a means of self-identity, but hopefully a rider's identity extends to more than being a cyclist. We want to completely change the world and people's fundamental ways of interacting with each other. To let the discourse degenerate to an us-versus-them situation, bicycles versus cars, allows the media and others to reduce Critical Mass to constituent or lobbying politics. In their world, society is divided into groups fighting to grab a piece of meat, where one group only wins by denying something to another group.

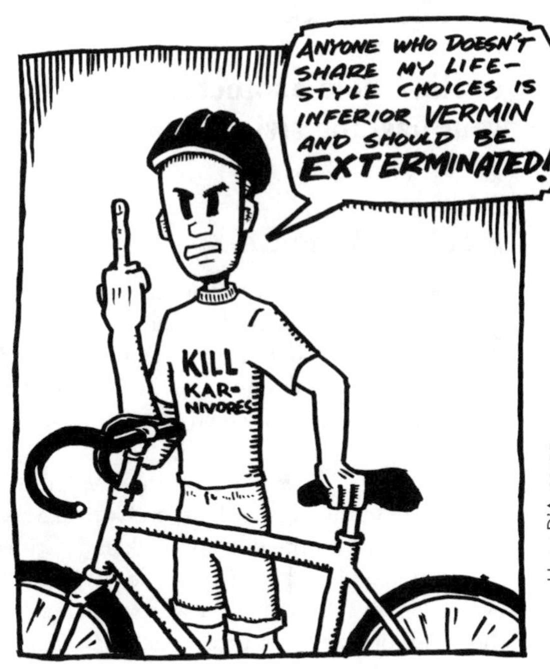
ANYONE WHO DOESN'T SHARE MY LIFE-STYLE CHOICES IS INFERIOR VERMIN AND SHOULD BE EXTERMINATED!
KILL KAR-NIVORES
HUGH D'ANDRADE

Bicycles are liberating by nature but it is not all sweetness and light. The commodification that this society injects into any form of enjoyment pervades cycling as thoroughly as anything else. Mountain bikes have probably sold more SUVs than anything else. The image of bicycle riding is everywhere in advertising, promising the freedom that comes from one more purchase. The titanium industry arose from war. Shimano is the leader of disposable parts and planned obsolescence. *Bicycling* magazine runs more pages of car and trucks ads than content.

It is difficult to remain cynical when riding a bike, if only for the duration of a ride. The alienation of the daily grind, the lack of any real choice or control most people have in their lives, gets put aside for an hour or two. At other times, of course, we are too wise and hip to permit ourselves the luxury of relaxing our masks of indifference.

There has been a decade-long process of Critical Mass in San Francisco defining itself. It is many things to many people, as varied as its participants. It provides a rare experience of democratic self-organization within a constantly changing mass of people. Any particular ride is never predictable even when it turns out to be less than exciting. That is the inevitable byproduct of a leaderless, open event defined anew every month by hundreds and thousands of people coming together freely without a formal agenda or structure.

San Francisco (or your town) is well worth a Mass.

UNLEASHING PUBLIC IMAGINATION

or How 'bout another shot of existential whup-ass for your flagging civic libido?

BY JOSH WILSON

Free Your Mind ...

Critical Mass had to happen. It makes sense. It already was there on the streets. It just needed a name, and a few core ideals around which to concentrate: Spontaneity, community, participation, respect, quality of life.

These core ideals unite Critical Mass with a number of parallel cultural phenomena, the origins of which seem to be a genuine urge for a humane, democratic, creatively engaged society.

Critical Mass is turning off the TV. Critical Mass is punk rock in a garage somewhere in the Mission District. Critical Mass is an underground rave at 3 am in a warehouse by the docks in Oakland. Critical Mass is a D.I.Y. art gallery in an office abandoned by a failed dot-com. Critical Mass is the Internet when everyone still talked about it as an idealized public commons. Critical Mass is thousands of extravagant freaks gallavanting around the Nevada high desert at Burning Man each year.

More specifically, Critical Mass and all these cultural phenomena are distinct faces of the same urge towards the democratization of imagination —that is, the nurturing of creative expression, in all its forms, from the community level up, rather than from the commerce/industry level down.

Of course it's imperfect. It's easy to put down a happening garage band as a tempest in a teapot that'll never crack the mass market. It's tempting to dismiss ravers as being stuck in a trite, "lite" world of dippy-trippy pop diversions. Burning Man practically begs to be denigrated as an expensive desert retreat for a moneyed alternacultural elite.

But all that cynicism belies an essential, unifying truth about underground music and participatory art: In each instance, the mundane "daily grind" is transformed into a perpetually unfolding moment of creative realization. The same is true of Critical Mass—it is, of course, nothing less than the sudden, breathtaking transformation of public space by a collective act of will and imagination.

Breaking through to this moment—of positive imagination made manifest, of transformative creative expression—is to catch a glimpse of paradise on earth. That freedom, and the personal and collective power that comes with it, is our birthright as humans.

All over the world, humanity's dreams have been turned into commodities. We dream in Kodachrome of Pepsi, the WB and Lexus. Our romantic and sexual desires are sublimated into acts of consumption, and focused on commercial surrogates. Our dreams have been co-opted by consumerism and advertising, beaten down by cycles of debt and "wage slavery," benumbed by news broadcasts of human suffering so unspeakable, yet so mundane.

As a result we are party to an ongoing cycle of environmental degradation and terrible human suffering, most notably of late, as a result of "First World" corporate collaboration with corrupt, unstable "Third World" governments in the name of what some people, in all seriousness, call the "Free Market."

But the seeds of change are sprouting anywhere the public imagination is restless enough to strive for a new, beautiful way of being. Regional culture and personal transportation, while seemingly separate, are all part of the same quality-of-life equation. Thus, independent music, community art and bicycles are crucial expressions of a burgeoning movement towards genuine democracy—uncommodified, uncompromised, inclusive, responsive to individuals, families, communities and regional cultures.

It isn't easy. Much of it will die on the vine, under-watered and malnourished. But why not try? As often as this is a "top down" situation—with vastly powerful government and corporate entities imposing their version of reality as a series of tidy, shrink-wrapped purchasing options—we are equally gifted with grassroots-up choices that are simple, efficient, clean, safer and more, ahem, "empowering" ...

Critical Mass is—for me, anyway—a near-perfect example of direct democracy and grassroots culture in action. Like the independent media, art and music

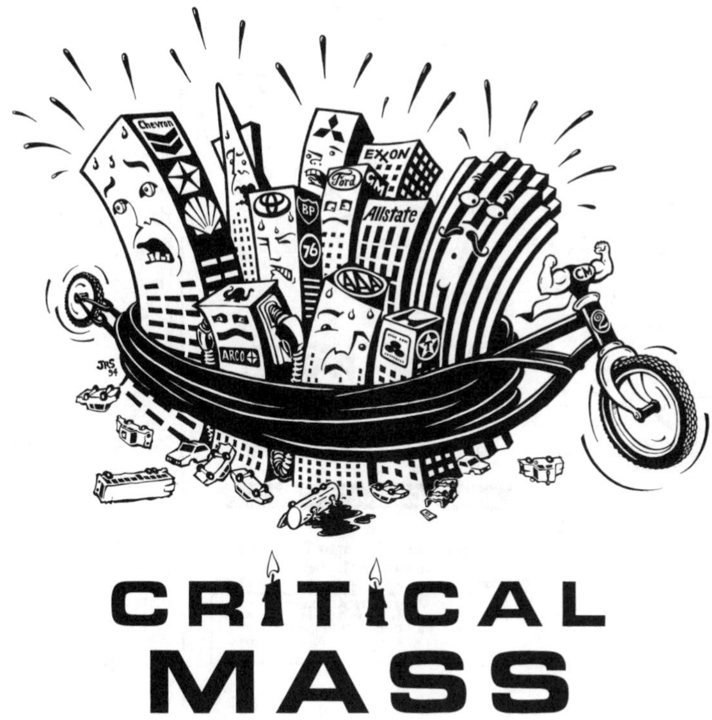

James R Swanson

movements, the Mass has its sloppy and ugly moments. But the culture seems to be highly adaptable and conscious, seems to have learned how NOT to be a mob, but rather an evolving, responsive and responsible social phenomenon.

I know this. I have seen it happen. I have participated in this process, and have served as a link in the neural network that makes up the mind of our culture.

Guess what? You have too. You're part of the great collective unconscious of humanity, with its perpetual stirrings into waking life. Moments of wakefulness erupt when we perceive the world of human culture and human choice for what it is—the product of imagination and will, the manifestation of our dreams and nightmares.

In San Francisco, where Critical Mass first "happened," personal and public transportation is a horrible mess, with alluring fantasies of a climate-controlled, surround-sound, luxury-sedan commute obscuring a nightmare reality of gridlock, road rage, depersonalization and a staggeringly destructive petrochemical industry.

San Francisco is beautiful and wild, yet cramped and in many ways hideously deformed. Contradictions abound. Everything that is good and bad about humanity is here, resplendent and grotesque. The idealism is heartfelt and searching, the hypocrisy so facile. Not long after moving here the depth of the contradictions was made clear, and my choices became apparent.

On the one hand, San Francisco has produced music, literature and social movements that have changed the world. On the other hand, the commercial media establishment here has entirely marginalized the thriving independent music and

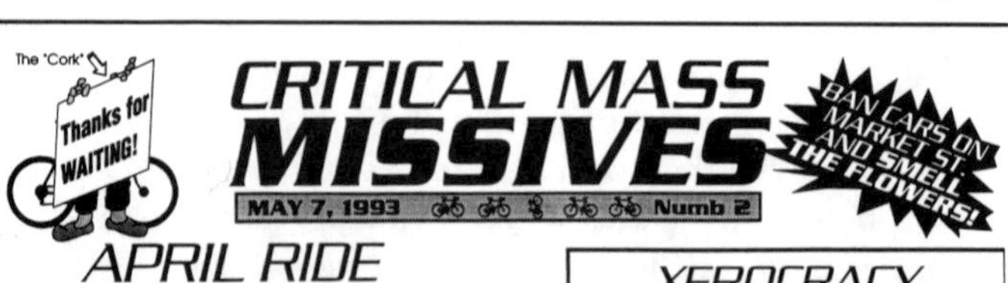
The "Cork"
Thanks for WAITING!
BAN CARS ON MARKET ST. AND SMELL THE FLOWERS!

CRITICAL MASS MISSIVES

MAY 7, 1993 Numb 2

APRIL RIDE AFTERMATH

More than 350 euphoric bicyclists gathered at Dolores Park after the April 30 Critical Mass ride. The relaxed socializing was abruptly interrupted by the news that a bicyclist had been hit by a car back at Guerrero & Market. Then the news arrived that bicyclists were being arrested at the scene.

A woman's bicycle was crushed under the wheels of a BMW. The BMW had some windows smashed, the mirrors ripped off and many dents. There are wildly contradictory accounts of what actually happened, but as this goes to the copier, it seems that the woman whose bike was crushed has been charged with malicious mischief, her boyfriend is charged with battery, and the motorist has been designated the victim! Eyewitnesses disagree over whether the driver provoked the bicyclists by ramming them in an attempted vehicular homicide or if he was provoked by angry, taunting bicyclists. In any case, the police refused to take statements at the scene from eyewitness bicyclists on the grounds that they were "biased," whereas motorists were not!

Regardless of the truth of the events, this one incident does not define the Critical Mass ride. Four hundred bicyclists passed thousands of cars during an hour and a half without incident. Nevertheless, lessons can be taken from this experience: The Critical Mass ride depends on being a mass. When people fall behind unintentionally, or hang back deliberately to taunt motorists and guilt-trip people for not sharing the same lifestyle choices, tensions quickly rise and motorists feel they can "punch through" the now dispersed Mass. "Corks" (people with signs saying "Thanks for Waiting!") will be on hand in the future to make intersection blocking fast, easy, and COURTEOUS!

The Critical Mass ride is self-defeating when it is self-righteous. SELF-RIGHTEOUSNESS IS REPULSIVE! We are not riding to impose our choices on others but to demonstrate our choice, our right to this choice, and the miserable conditions we now face, as well as a show of our pleasure and camaraderie at being together. Critical Mass riders individually must establish and maintain behavioral norms that we would like to prevail in society IN GENERAL!

Why get on our bikes and reject automobiles? Partly because cars impose a social isolation, with many people alone in cars, often insecure and lonely. Our ride is a public antidote to this bored isolation, but few people would abandon the false security of their cars to join a bunch of bicyclists who are berating them for being in the car in the first place! We have to be smart about human motivations, and turn our rage and frustration about the absurd organization of this society (and our particular anger at autos) into an irresistable impulse toward human society and social pleasure. (Those few who have been aggressive blockers and taunters have a special responsibility to help those who lose their bicycle and/or freedom as a result: legal defense and bike replacement are already tasks at hand, unfortunately.)

The ride is well received by the public when we maintain our cohesion, our sense of fun and play, and we do not needlessly antagonize people or arbitrarily interfere with their ability to get where they're going.

HEY! We got on bikes in the first place, at least in part, because it's better and faster than cars and buses. Aren't we about ending gridlock? Well?...

PROTESTING CARS is one thing.
Berating *PEOPLE IN CARS* is
stupid, wrong-headed, and
COUNTER-PRODUCTIVE!

COMBAT--*DON'T REINFORCE*--
ISOLATION & ALIENATION!

XEROCRACY RULES OK?

Critical Mass is a monthly organized coincidence wherein hundreds of bicyclists happen to find each other and ride home together! There is no organizing committee, nor is anyone in charge, per se. Ideas are shared through a Xerocracy, that is, anyone can make copies of their ideas and opinions and spread them around. If you do so, you become one of many Xerocrats! Be prepared to discuss your missives and defend your arguments!

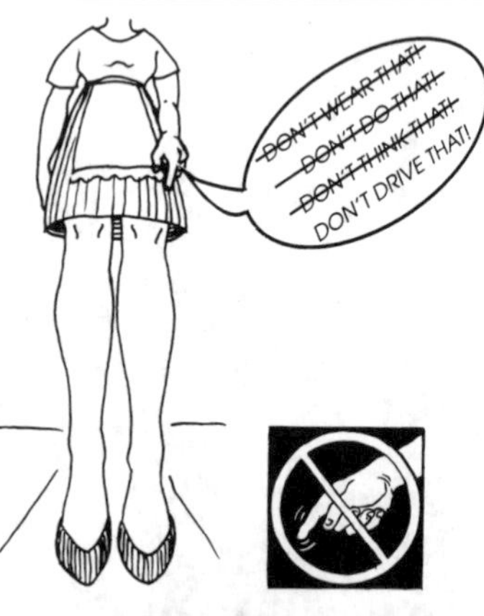
DON'T WEAR THAT!
DON'T DO THAT!
DON'T THINK THAT!
DON'T DRIVE THAT!

DON'T YOU HATE NAGGING?

May Critical Mass Theme:
Summer Gear
(shorts, Hawaiian shirts, scuba gear, BBQ, etc.)

MAY 28 CRITICAL MASS
Head to Dolores Park after the ride (7 p.m.) for the 1st Annual
***BAR-NONE BICYCLIST* PICNIC!**
It's a potluck, a picnic, music, a BBQ(?), a social scene!
If you can bring an Hibachi, a Weber, food/drink to share, please do!

arts communities, and turned this town's legacy of social innovation into the kitschy cliché of beatniks in berets and tie-dyed hippies.

The Bay Area is renowned for its natural beauty and quality of life. But you can take a short ride up Twin Peaks and see a brown layer of smog over the city and the Bay. You can experience the personal hell of "Car Wars" and the road-rage generation, whether you like it or not, down on Market St., on Mission St., riding along the coast, through the Presidio, or just around the neighborhoods. Speeding SUVs, cabbies on a mission, BMW drivers with status and vengeance on their minds, clueless dingbats yabbing in cell phones and slamming into the next car's fender ... or worse.

The first Critical Mass riders "dared to dream different," and while this new dream has never been perfect, it is so very much better.

... And Your Ass Will Follow!

My personal story of bicycle salvation is simple enough, starting with memories of zooming along quiet streets as an adolescent in suburban New Jersey's summer twilight, and continuing through two dismal years in Washington, D.C., where a post-collegiate career in nonprofit environmental activism became less enjoyable than the actual bicycle ride to work each day.

Before too long it became obvious that I needed to switch jobs and become a bicycle messenger, an epochal decision that has influenced my life choices to this day. After leaving D.C. and winding up in San Francisco in September, 1992, my car, while parked on a hill in the Sunset District, was totalled by a big sedan piloted by an uninsured driver. It was a fortuitous accident, saving me heaps of cash in tickets, gas and repairs. It also compelled me to develop a relationship with the fair city by the Bay, intimate like only a sweaty, exhilirating bicycle ride can be.

About the same time my car was totaled, thus neatly resolving my transportation issues, I became enamored of the indie and underground music scene—weird local bands, jazz and hip-hop interactions, local bars with stages stuck in the back, and, of course, college/community radio. I fell in with a local station, KUSF over on the University of San Francisco campus, and before long was playing my own weird records at 3:00 am for all the wacked-out night owls of the Bay Area.

Bicycling fit in well with the lifestyle—riding to clubs and concerts was the best way to avoid interminable waits for the MUNI bus after hours in some sketchy armpit of town. It was fun and rock 'n' roll and good exercise, and the Bay Area itself is so damn beautiful that rides across town or across the Golden Gate Bridge are equally thrilling. Falling in with Critical Mass was inevitable.

It was just plain fun. I never really perceived it as confrontational, although it became obvious later that the political statement resonated to all levels of society. Individual reactions to the experience of riding *en masse* vary widely. Many cyclists became ecstatic simply from the community experience, reliving carefree childhood moments, while others wanted to be involved with the ride more intimately—wearing costumes and bringing along mobile sound systems, or drawing route maps and trying to guide the experience more directly.

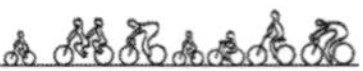

Pedestrians and drivers were generally supportive. Kids would lean out apartment windows and bang on pots as we rode past; old men outside barbershops waved; dull faces behind semi-translucent windshields would unexpectedly break into grins.

Others were not delighted. Some pedestrians and drivers got impatient, even downright crazy. The heaviest and worst interactions brought the San Francisco Police Department into the mix. There were chaotic moments, including a notable police riot [July 1997] that occurred in the wake of Mayor Willie Brown's limousine convoy experiencing a Critical Mass-induced traffic delay. That took several months to shake out, and made the national headlines.

Throughout it all, email debates raged about the methods and reasons for Critical Mass. Should the Mass cork (block) intersections completeley till it passes? What if there's an ambulance in the oncoming lane, or a working delivery driver about to miss a deadline? Is the Mass a political act? If so, what's the message? And who's it targeting? The entire car culture? The Mayor? Individual drivers wasting resources by commuting alone? But wait, aren't other commuters our allies, rather than our enemies? They're stuck in the same mess as we are, right?

And what about the confrontational bicyclist assholes who start fights with testy car drivers, who cut off pedestrians and run lights with shouted curses in their wake? There are plenty of morons on bikes, and I've been one myself. Trying to "make the light" is a dangerous habit. Not waiting for pedestrians is stupid and harmful. (Then again, there are a lot of dumbass pedestrians out there as well.)

What about the police, ideally there to serve and protect, but often acting to harass and detain? I remember once, in the wake of the Willie Riot, waiting at a traffic light with several hundred other cyclists, preparing to ride the Broadway Tunnel. Suddenly there was a police officer in the way, assaulting one of the vanguard riders and halting our progress. I looked up the hill to my right and was shocked to see a phalanx of cops running down the hill at us, flipping down their riot masks in case the bicyclists waiting patiently at the stoplight were to suddenly pull out mace and molotov cocktails. They stopped at the bottom of the hill and kind of milled around, looking at us. I saw one of them clutching what appeared to be a handful of plastic garbage-bag ties, but which were, I realized, actually disposable handcuffs

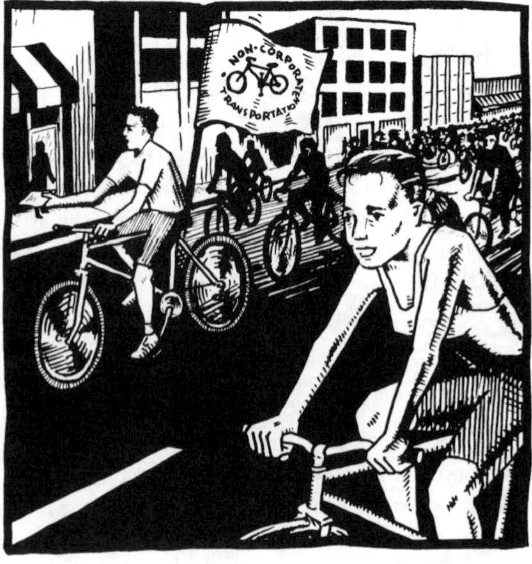

HUGH D'ANDRADE

used for mass arrests. The crowd eventually dispersed with little more than a few scuffles, all entirely the fault of the SFPD. I was absolutely furious that someone would try to criminalize me like that, and filed a complaint with the citizen's police review board. It was rejected as invalid after several months.

In the end, Critical Mass adapted slowly and awkwardly in great collective acts of innovation. Critical Mass riders learned new forms of road etiquette and sustained a casual sense of fluid community. Most of us have come to appreciate that the agenda of the ride is wide open to whatever one brings to it, so long as one is respectful, artful, imaginative, and adaptable.

This is also all true of the indie music and art scenes, and of Burning Man, all of which, like Critical Mass, flourished in San Francisco through the '90s. All these movements were and are committed to the creation of authentic culture and community in direct response to the inadequacy of existing commercialized choices.

And each of these disparate but overlapping movements have experienced shake-ups and transformations, from the notorious dot-com evictions that destroyed so many art and music venues (not to mention low-income neighborhoods in general) to Burning Man's ongoing clashes between the "temporary autonomous zone" philosophy and the urge to regulate things and make a profit.

In every instance, the communities have adapted and evolved, for better or for worse, and often both. That adaptation is an ongoing process—none of this is resolved or "over." And through it all, the choices remain clear and compelling.

Why line up for tickets to fucking Limp Fucking Bizkit when you can get all the viscera with immeasurably more inspiration, meaning, spontaneity and talent at a local punk rock show on a Friday night? Why go to Disneyland for some artificially flavored fruit juice and a few animatronic pirates, when you can walk through labyrinths of art, color, sound and fire under the jeweled night sky of the Black Rock Desert? Why sit in a traffic jam eating stress and generating toxic fumes when you can have a brisk bike ride home with a bunch of pals?

Put aside doubt. Sure, some of those garage bands are going to be lousy. Yes, it's a pain in the ass to camp out in the Black Rock Desert. Your bike ride to and from work will certainly have its off moments—be it a rainy day or an assault by a swerving, horn-blowing late model Olds.

But isn't difficulty just par for the course? We're sold dubious solutions in six-packs, payable in monthly installments and guaranteed hygenic, except for the non-biodegradable plastic trash and the oil wars burning worldwide. So many of the remedies promised by industrial consumer-culture make the situation worse, like shooting heroin to cure the pain. It does for a while, but also reinforces the problem.

Perhaps, through a combined act of imagination and will, we can develop genuine, well-rounded, environmentally sustainable, locally responsive and economically fair solutions to societal needs, rather than our current reality of morning headline horror.

Can you imagine riding a bike to work tomorrow?

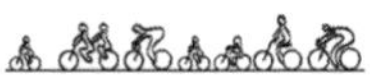

POLITICS CAN BE FUN

BY STEVEN BODZIN

On a bright, hot day at the end of September, 1992, I arrived at Justin Hermann Plaza for the first Commute Clot, ready for a routine failure. I had left over 200 flyers on bicycles around the city over the previous week. (In 1992, that meant I hit every bike I saw.) I had given out a couple dozen more in person. It was a flyer I designed, and I was happy with it, but that was par for the course.

Experience had taught me to have low expectations. I had organized important demonstrations before, like the province-wide takeover of government offices to protest the logging of an old-growth forest in Ontario. Massive flyering and press outreach did what? In the case of the group I was in, it got eight people to show up to a single-room office on the outskirts of the city, where we spent five hours being pains in the neck until the police finally agreed to arrest two people. Sure, it made the national news, and it even helped stop the logging. But after the demo, we protesters each shrunk back to our isolated selves, craving a better world but unable to convince others to take part in creating it.

I was jaded, but this Commute Clot idea seemed worth trying. It was clever, and it sounded like it could even be fun. I first heard the notion two months earlier, in the same downtown plaza. The U.S. Department of Transportation was there, promoting alternatives to single-occupant vehicles. Folding tables were scattered about the plaza, each covered with stickers and buttons bearing guilt-trippy—or even nonsensical—slogans like "Bicycle for clean air" and "DON'T BE AN SOV!" The place bored me even as I entered it. I saw it as the kind of geeky, wonky event that was designed to flop. It offered no compelling reason for anyone to stop using a car. It was just lip-service to alternatives, even as the rest of the government teamed up with industry to support the ever-growing automobile juggernaut.

I visited the table set up by the San Francisco Bicycle Coalition, a group with which I had recently gotten involved. At my first meeting, there was a go-around in which participants told what bike advocacy they were up to. I explained that I had just gotten back from a bike trip across the US and then to the Earth Summit in Brazil, and that I could see bike advocacy was one of the keys to the whole sustainability movement. But the Bicycle Coalition was still tiny. A world of activist possibilities was present and necessary for the dozen people at that table. Bikes on transit, on bridges, on freeways. Bikes for the aged, the homeless, the working poor, the rich and famous. Bike parking, bike lanes, bike safety, bike races, bike education. Proper law enforcement, bike theft prevention, you name it. It was all in our dreams, and so little out in the world. It was at once exciting and overwhelming.

At the SFBC table, I met a tall guy named Chris Carlsson. He told me his idea: A regular bike ride in the Financial District. I told him about my experience in the summer of 1990 in Boston. The locally based foreign aid group Bikes Not Bombs and an Edmonton-based activist named Tooker Gomberg got a group of people together to ride bikes and guilt-trip motorists. For the occasion, Bikes Not Bombs activist Carl Kurz and I wrote and designed a parking ticket that looked just like those on Boston windshields, but instead of "parking in crosswalk," the listed infractions were more like "oil spills" and "species extinction." After the fun and thrill of the first ride in Boston, the participants started riding every Tuesday morning. We generally had six to ten riders. We gave out our "Earth Violations" to any motorist who would take one, and we gave out "Certificates of Merit" to people on bikes, the bus, and the subway. It was a lot of fun, and we probably raised some consciousness around transportation choices. If nothing else, it was worth it for the smile on the face of the woman getting off a bus, who gushed, "My goodness, nobody's ever given me a certificate of anything before!"

Chris' style of activism was a shade different. Almost everything I said sparked him to argue with it on philosophical and pragmatic grounds. Guilt-tripping was a useless strategy, he said. Mornings are no time for demonstrations, when everyone has to get to work and nobody can stick around to hang out. Weekly rides are too frequent to draw real crowds. Raising consciousness among observers and the media doesn't matter, he said. What matters is having fun and changing reality for those within the rides. And then he started talking about "work reduction." As my eyes glazed over, I suggested he go to the next SFBC meeting.

His ideas were eye-opening. I had never encountered this particularly California type of activism. I had always seen demonstrations as means to an end, not ends in themselves. I had always placed utopia in the future, following the struggle. Chris seemed to be hinting that the struggle itself can be the utopia. I started to understand the idea of "revolution of everyday life." "The revolution will not be televised." "Be the revolution." "There is no way to peace, peace is

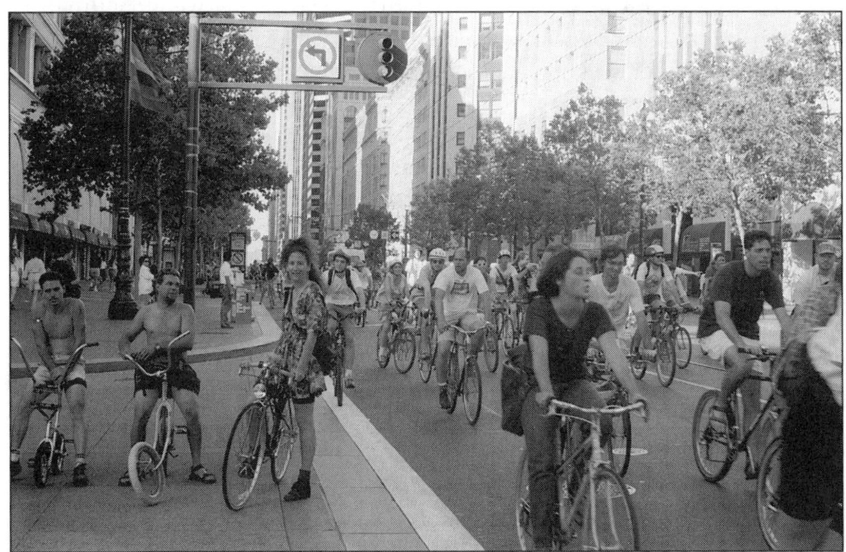

PAMELA PALMA

Market Street at Geary in San Francisco, 1994.

the way." These slogans moistened to life within me as I imagined hundreds of cyclists riding together, reclaiming the pavement for life. What could anyone do about it? Maybe it *was* possible to create the alternative world now, without waiting for some imaginary revolution. "How will you know when the revolution has happened?" my girlfriend at the time liked to ask.

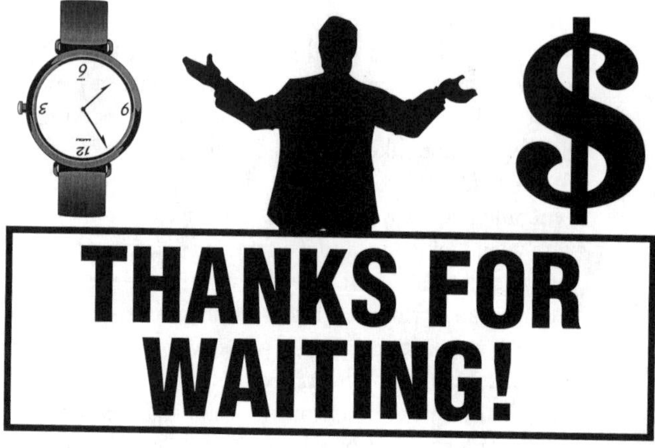

Corking sign used originally in San Francisco, 1993

Chris showed up at the SFBC's headquarters, the back room of the Pot and Pan. The place was a greasy-spoon Chinese restaurant on 9th Avenue with harsh fluorescent lights and terrible acoustics. He and his grade-school daughter stayed only long enough to ask if the SFBC wanted to take charge of this ride. He suggested, "The last Friday of every month" as an off-hand possibility for when it would take place. The discussion went quickly against sponsoring the ride, based, at least on the surface, on concerns about liability. So Chris left, and I don't think I saw him again until September 29.

Meanwhile, I was excited by the idea, and it didn't seem like anyone was doing anything to make it real. So I made up a flyer, copied it, and gave it out. It wasn't until two days before the ride that someone told me, "I saw the other flyer for that." I was surprised, as I didn't know another flyer existed. In fact, I didn't see Chris' flyer until over a month later.

So when I showed up at the "foot of Market," I expected a dozen riders to be there, and that we would meet and have fun and the whole idea might go on for a couple months before petering out. Instead, four dozen people were there, and we had a great old time, riding in the golden evening light, ringing bells, hootin and hollerin, confusing the world with our happiness.

Sure enough, politics *could* be fun. Happy social environments would win what logical persuasion couldn't. Afterwards, at Zeitgeist bar, many of us agreed we should do it again the next month.

This revelatory joy persisted and increased as the months passed. I was awed to see people drinking and smoking pot and riding in a great mass together, and to see cops ignore the ride, and later escort the ride in an accommodating way. I got a goofy smile every time I heard someone talk about "this amazing bike ride I saw the other night." Residents, riders, even many motorists seemed entertained and happy that this ride had been born. The lack of attention from cops and press made the whole thing feel like an underground growing in plain view, an alternative reality inviting everyone while living by new rules.

Naturally, these hopes soon turned in part to annoyance. As the ride grew, I felt increasingly surrounded by hypocrites, by thoughtless people portraying themselves as thoughtful saviors. Even Chris, who had conceived of many of the good ideas for the rides, was far from immune to my annoyance.

Among the xerocrats, there was a hierarchy that was only partly voluntary. The dozens of people who put their own hours and love and worry and care into rides—even into early rides, when the shape of the event was still gelling—are mostly forgotten. Today, thanks to his exceptional devotion and his willingness to speak and argue, it is all "Chris Carlsson." He is a mostly unwilling celebrity but a celebrity nonetheless. For all his disclaimers about not being "the leader," he is still given credit for the ride.

But Chris gets only a small bit of my annoyance. My greatest annoyance is with the mental patterns of the riders. Despite having this open place where a new reality could be born, most people kept living by their normal rules of life. This was particularly true around leadership. Mass started looking to me like Orwell's Animal Farm. At Mass, everyone is a leader, but some people are more leaders than others. Those of us who understood and took part in xerocracy led the gullible hordes. From the first ride on, most riders paid no attention to the overall route, expecting trained professionals to take charge of such details. I found it discouraging to learn that most people would rather attend a party than throw one, would rather sleep through life than take charge of it.

This same failure of imagination led to the growth of the "testosterone brigade." This is the name given to those macho folks who race to the front of the ride and lead it wherever they feel ready to go. From what I hear, many Masses around the world are led entirely by this pack of spiteful dogs. In San Francisco, conscious effort has tamed them somewhat, but riders have nevertheless handed power to them far too often. Power is given, not taken. The riders who followed these jerks did so voluntarily. When they were leading the ride up the 18 percent grade of Powell Street and a few of us tried to divert riders onto an easier street, the mob just powered past our little call for a detour. I ended up attacking the hill with the slow riders at the back, parents with children, a rider with a stereo system, and a pedicab driver all cussing as they pushed up the hill. I rode off in a different direction, disgusted with the lemming mentality.

I believe that as the rides grew and there grew a clearer division between followers and leaders, followers took less and less responsibility for their actions. We figured out on the very first ride that it was safer and more fun to stick together and proceed through red lights. But it was also clear that we each needed to take responsibility for ourselves and for the ride. This meant using caution. Today, many riders blithely enter intersections without looking at the lights or the cross traffic, expecting others to protect them.

Similarly, some riders release pent-up anger at cars from the safety of the crowd. These people were rightly scolded by one rider, Kash, at the beginning of a ride. He yelled to the crowd, "Some people seem to think that Mass is a good place to take revenge on cars. It's not. When I'm on my own, and someone attacks me, I take revenge. I do whatever it takes to ensure my safety and the ongoing safety of my friends. But when I'm here with my friends, this is a time to celebrate." He told the riders to kill them with kindness. And he was right. The power dynamics of Mass are not those of everyday life. Having 1,000 friends around gives cyclists uncharacteristic power, and some have no idea what to do with it. Those who use the crowd for protection as they violate the humanity of motorists or pedestrians are not taking responsibility for themselves. It is yet another disappointment.

These various annoyances led to a hilarious irony. As we flowed out of Justin Hermann on a spring ride in 1993, I was crowded in and I felt like a sheep. I felt surrounded by people who were taking part in revolution without any revolutionary sensibility. Rather than following their boss or their fashion magazine, they were following a route map that I had handed out. And it just came out—I started chanting, in my best sheep's bleat, "Four wheels ba-a-a-ad, two wheels go-o-o-od." I was making fun of people. Yet the chant was taken up, sheeplike, by those around me. It was painful to take in so many simultaneous layers of irony.

Finally, the "social space" that was one of Mass' goals is only as good as the riders. Yes, we show that public space can be more than a traffic sewer. We live it as a social space, a political space, a place for the *polis*. In doing so, we could help revive democracy and civic life. I have met people after Critical Mass, including real friends. But in my usual after-work Friday evening haze, I am often in no state to energetically reach out and meet new people. When I have been, it's been rewarding. But like so many other things, you only get out of Mass what you put into it. When I'm feeling grumpy or tired, I often find the ride alienating. I see many people casting about fecklessly for connection, like high schoolers in the cafeteria, nervously seeking a place to sit. Critical Mass is a civic space, but the ride itself is a poor place for intimate connection.

Finally, there is the relationship to the wider world. When I meet people who have seen the ride, they are often excited to learn that I do it. Spectators tend to have good feelings toward it, just as they do toward murals or a free clinic. But that's about it. One non-participant recently summed it up well: "It's one of those things I'm happy to see, but I don't have time for. It's part of the San Francisco I want to live in, but that doesn't really exist anymore. I'm just glad that some people are doing it." For many people, it is a comforting bit of counterculture spectacle, a salve that reminds them that they live somewhere really hip and cool and cutting edge, even if they spend their days at work and their nights surfing the Web. This is a condescending, compartmentalizing attitude that keeps any radical act from really breaking through.

For participants—the people who matter—Mass has helped inspire a decade of remarkably evolutionary activism, from Reclaim The Streets (now honored as an FBI-listed international terrorist group) to Seattle's anti-WTO swarms. But for me, the ride has hit a point of diminishing returns. It is time to get beyond Critical Mass, to take the next step. We need to keep our imaginations open to what that can be.

WHY THEY'RE WRONG ABOUT CRITICAL MASS!

The Fallacy of Bicycle Advocates' Critique

BY ADAM KESSEL

"I have no problem with waving and smiling. I have no problem if the entire flow of traffic is going the speed of the Mass. I take offense at the times you run red lights, the times there are open spaces in front of the Mass and you still take up four lanes. I take offense at the claim you are celebrating biking, when you're really trying to take revenge on what you perceive to be wrongs visited upon bikers by motorists."

—Mr. Hat, Frequent Pseudonymous Poster to the Boston Critical Mass E-mail List

"The reason I didn't like it is because many cyclists did not follow respectful share the road rules. They were out to harrass cars. If I were in a car, I'd be really pissed. ... They went against all the Effective Cycling rules."

—Rebecca Kushner, 4/11/00
(Public Posting to CM E-mail List)

"Their act is violence perpetrated upon the community. If their intent is to [resist by non-violent means], I invite them to join an advocacy group such as the Bicycle Federation of Wisconsin which is working daily to eliminate the barriers and reduce the frustration felt by all cyclists and lots of motorists."

—Charles Gandy, Executive Director of the Texas Bicycle Coalition.

"The Critical Mass rides [...] are misdirected, childish efforts at bicyclist advocacy."

—Kenneth O'Brien, Maine Area Effective Cyclist Advocate

"But which unjust laws are CM riders fighting against?"

—Paul Schimek, Effective Cycling Instructor #422

A robust Critical Mass movement inevitably bumps up against fairly vocal folks who would prefer we stay off the streets at rush hour and not ruin the meager gains that have been won for bicyclists over the past few years. Disapproval is particularly acute when Critical Mass is just getting started in a city, where the staunchest Critical Mass critics are often the most dedicated bicycle advocates. After a while, some of the grumbling dies down and these advocates begin to accept CM's presence, if not actively encourage it.

These criticisms present a useful gateway into how and why Critical Mass works. They bring to the forefront contrasting models of social change and particularly highlight the difference between so-called "liberal" or "reformist" modes of change and "radical" or "revolutionary" modes. Critical Mass actually brings out distinctions between these modes while at the same time encompassing them.

First, I'd like to make the usual apology that this is just my take on things. Anyone who claims to know the one true nature of Critical Mass is probably missing the point.

There is, in my view, a widespread misunderstanding, reflected in some of the quotes above, that a Critical Mass ride is trying to "demonstrate" something to someone or convince people to change their minds about things, as if it were a novel form of reasoned argument. If we were to accept this view of the "purpose" of Critical Mass, we would indeed be fair targets for a lot of criticism. If we're trying to change people's minds, why do we get in their way? Shouldn't we be doing everything possible to make everybody *like* bicyclists? Sure, we hand out flowers and hold up funny signs during the ride, but wouldn't it just be *nicer* if we would keep to one lane and refrain from impeding the "regular flow" of rush hour traffic? We could still "make our point" but at the same time broadcast "a more positive message."

From the point of view of an urban bicycling advocate, the ride itself has an overall neutral effect on the state of infrastructure, education, and enforcement favorable to bicyclists. There are numerous positive effects. People see a lot of bicyclists having fun, they hand out informative flyers that do influence people's opinions, and so forth. Maybe a few pro-bicycle politicians jump on the bandwagon and take advantage of the opportunity for publicity about a sustainable transportation initiative. There are also, of course, some negative effects in terms of traditional bicycling advocacy, which are described in great detail elsewhere. In my view, these positive and negative effects balance each other out.

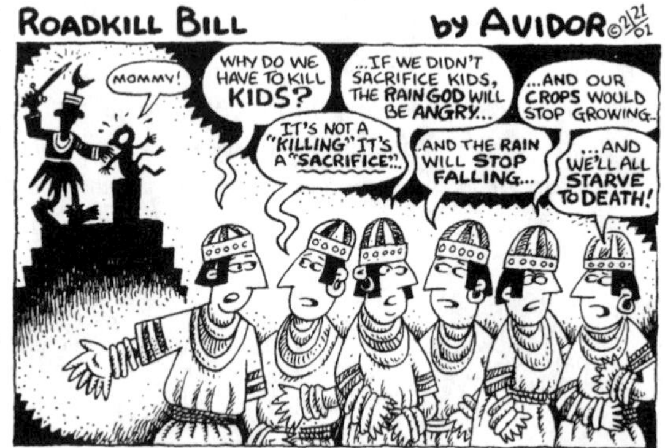
ROADKILL BILL
by AVIDOR ©2/21/01
MOMMY!
WHY DO WE HAVE TO KILL KIDS?
IT'S NOT A "KILLING" IT'S A "SACRIFICE"!
...IF WE DIDN'T SACRIFICE KIDS, THE RAIN GOD WILL BE ANGRY...
...AND THE RAIN WILL STOP FALLING...
...AND OUR CROPS WOULD STOP GROWING..
...AND WE'LL ALL STARVE TO DEATH!

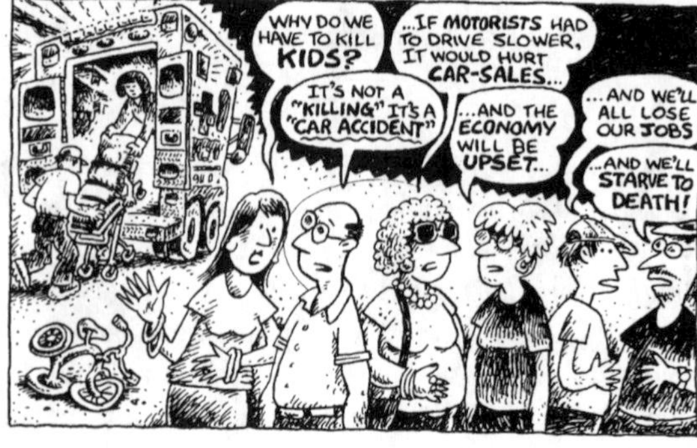
WHY DO WE HAVE TO KILL KIDS?
IT'S NOT A "KILLING" IT'S A "CAR ACCIDENT"
...IF MOTORISTS HAD TO DRIVE SLOWER, IT WOULD HURT CAR-SALES...
...AND THE ECONOMY WILL BE UPSET...
...AND WE'LL ALL LOSE OUR JOBS
...AND WE'LL STARVE TO DEATH!

If your main concern is bicycle advocacy, the main difference CM makes emerges in the time between rides, when otherwise depoliticized cyclists

Come join the pedal-powered party. Bring your momentum. No RSVP required.

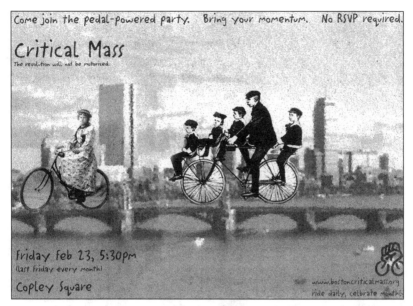

The revolution will not be motorized.
Friday Feb 23, 5:30pm
(last Friday every month)
Copley Square
www.bostoncriticalmass.org
ride daily, celbrate monthly

are inspired to take action; to write letters to their representatives and city councillors; to argue with their neighbors, families, and friends; to become increasingly aware of the primary role that auto-centric transportation and land-use policy plays in setting foreign and domestic priorities, in separating out rich from poor and black from white, in causing more deaths, injuries, and illnesses than all of our other major epidemics combined. If the point is to advocate for better policies via widely accepted democratic channels, Critical Mass contributes to this mode of change by building an army of better advocates.

I've spent a great deal of time at meetings of regulatory agencies, planning and zoning boards, and other decision-making bodies that determine what our environment is going to look like, which in turn has enormous impacts on our daily lives and social interactions. It is absolutely clear to me that these organizations do not make their decisions based on reasonable arguments, on trying to do the right thing "for the citizens of the city," whether environmentally, socially, or economically. Zoning, development, traffic planning—all are politically driven. This means they reflect the underlying distribution of power in society. And I can assure you that bicycles as a mode of transportation are totally off the radar (at the very best, a token afterthought). Until bicyclists are organized—and I believe Critical Mass is a powerful tool for organizing and politicizing otherwise disenfranchised bicyclists—there will be no sea change. We will celebrate excruciatingly small victories. But we can do much better.

Advocacy alone, however, is not how social change—or collective determination of uses of public resources—occurs. Few historical examples come to mind of an oppressed class of people winning over the general public on the basis of their likeability. Nor does progressive change occur as a result of convincing, well-reasoned arguments and good-natured debate. The labor movement was not built by a concerted effort to convince capitalists that the workers were friendly people who deserved better pay. *De jure* racial discrimination did not end because of an effective public relations campaign highlighting the merits of African-Americans. struggles for democracy and human rights under dictatorial regimes have never been won because the underdog rationally convinced the dictator to abdicate power.

NO EXIT
© Andy Singer
DRIVE TO WORK / WORK TO DRIVE
I HATE DRIVING... BUT I NEED A CAR TO GET TO WORK
HONK!
I HATE MY JOB, BUT I GOTTA MAKE CAR PAYMENTS
QUIET DOWN!
PETE SINGER

Why should the situation be any different for the Critical Mass community? Although our interests are varied—bicycling seems to be only one small but essential part of what unites our movement—our situation is clearly that of an interest group that traditionally has been poorly represented in the American political system. Our success is linked to our numbers, our strength, our power, and ultimately our unity, but it is not particularly dependent on good public relations and a non-threatening demeanor.

Even some in the mainstream acknowledge the critical, more radical, role the Mass plays in effecting change. A highly respected professor of urban planning at UC Berkeley recently published an article in which he said that the prospects of achieving bicycling advancements in the US are specifically tied to the ability of grassroots political pressure brought on by such groups/movements as Critical Mass (Martin Wachs, *Transportation Quarterly*, "Discussion of 'Bicycling Boom in Germany: A Revival Engineered by Public Policy' by John Pucher," Fall 1997).

Social progress—whether in civil rights, environmental protection, economic justice—never occurs without a group that pushes harder, that reframes the questions and recenters the debate, that occasionally acts "as if" what they wanted to be true *were* true. This is the more radical role Critical Mass plays in social change. I do not ride with Critical Mass (necessarily) to make a good impression on people, to convince drivers

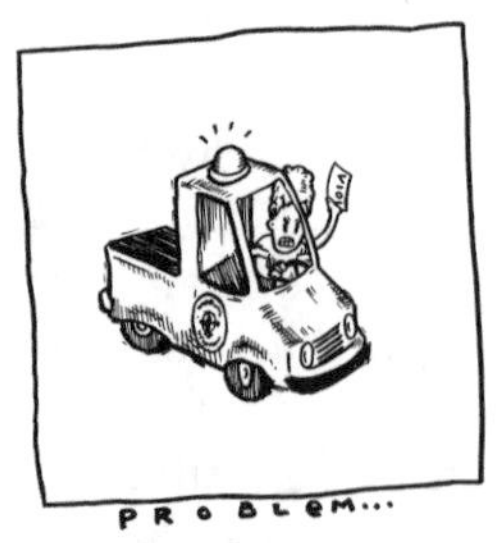
PROBLEM...

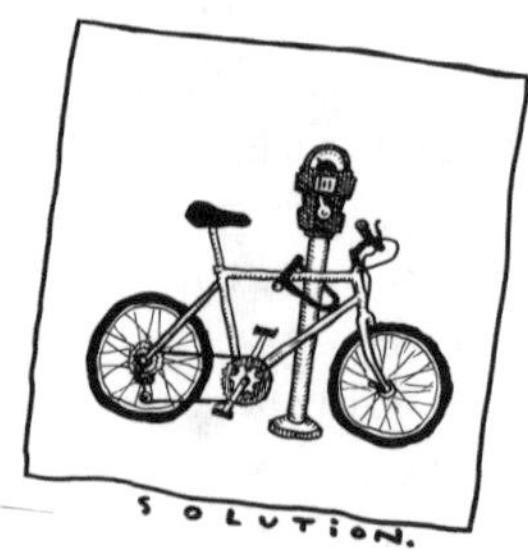
SOLUTION.

HUGH D'ANDRADE

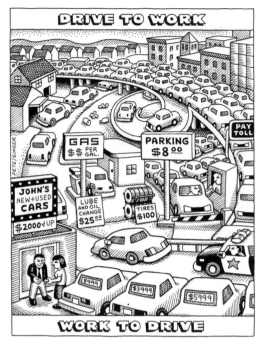

of anything in particular, to "advocate." I ride because I find the mass creates a temporary autonomous zone (to borrow a slogan from Hakim Bey); a place where bicycles do have the right of way—and not just on paper; a non-imaginary safe, quiet, clean, and fun use of the public good, the streets which we all pay for and the air which we all breathe; a place where the streets are designed for bicycles, not cars. Critical Mass does not ask the question of whether bicyclists should have "equal rights" to the streets, where "equal rights" means "just like cars." Instead it presumes that the public space should be for us, the people, and then gives the cars a chance to figure out how to fit in.

The transformation that occurs on the streets during Critical Mass rides is not the result of more bike lanes or bike racks, traffic-calmed streets or better signage, nor does it come from better laws on the books or better enforcement of existing laws, nor does it even come from increased respect for bicycles from those operating motorized vehicles. Instead it emerges from the fact that we are present in large numbers, and we have made a collective decision that this is how we want things to be.

Activists often refer to "direct action" as a means of accomplishing political goals. In fact, this can mean two different things: in one sense, direct action is "taking to the streets," demonstrating and protesting. In its more powerful sense, however, it is the action of taking control over the conditions that we live in. Inasmuch as the mainstream media has provided positive coverage of the recent wave of antiglobalism actions initiated in Seattle in 1999, it has focused exclusively on the first sense: large numbers of people demonstrating their beliefs and protesting against the powers that be. Participants in these demonstrations, however, often return with a much more profound sense of empowerment from the decentralized, consensus-based decision-making processes that have evolved around these events. They realize that the world we envision may be possible on a large scale; not only that, but that this world *exists* on large scale, in various pockets at various times. Critical Mass is powerful as these protests are powerful, not simply because it demonstrates some idea, but because it *enacts* that idea.

Critical Mass's radical nature lies in its *process*. It is a means of moving, not a particular destination. It claims, first and foremost, that we do things ourselves, and that this way of doing things is fundamental to liberty. Effecting change ourselves, rather than urging the duly-elected representatives to do something about it, is a very dangerous way to do things, and has certainly met with a good deal of resistance from the police. Some would argue that it is less democratic: isn't this the few imposing their will on the many? Others predict that legitimization of this mode of social change will inevitably lead to anarchy, where everyone who wants to accomplish anything will take to the streets, break windows, and set fires.

It's important to remember, however, that democracy is not necessarily premised on majoritarian rule. Sometimes extraordinary counter-majoritarian actions are essential to protect the very mechanisms upon which democracy depends. It is quite clear that the Supreme Court, in ordering the desegregation of Southern public schools in *Brown v. Board of Education*, was not enacting the will of the majority. Even though the body politic would not have voted to eliminate segregation, the action was essential to the furthering of democracy, something that even the most conservative have finally come to admit. Similarly, living in a society that is predominantly based on auto-centric and environmentally unsustainable patterns of development, where we might even vote for the policies we get, doesn't mean it's not more democratic for a small, determined group of people to act against the will of the majority.

CM's critics often focus—nearly pathologically—on the degree to which Critical Mass does or does not follow "the law." They claim they would support and even participate in CM, if only we stopped at all red lights, kept in one lane, and followed the rules set out for us. Of course, it's not the occasional misdemeanor or traffic violation that causes all the tumult: it's the fact that there are hundreds of bicyclists riding together in what is traditionally car territory, having fun. Although we might be able to get some sanctimonious reward out of

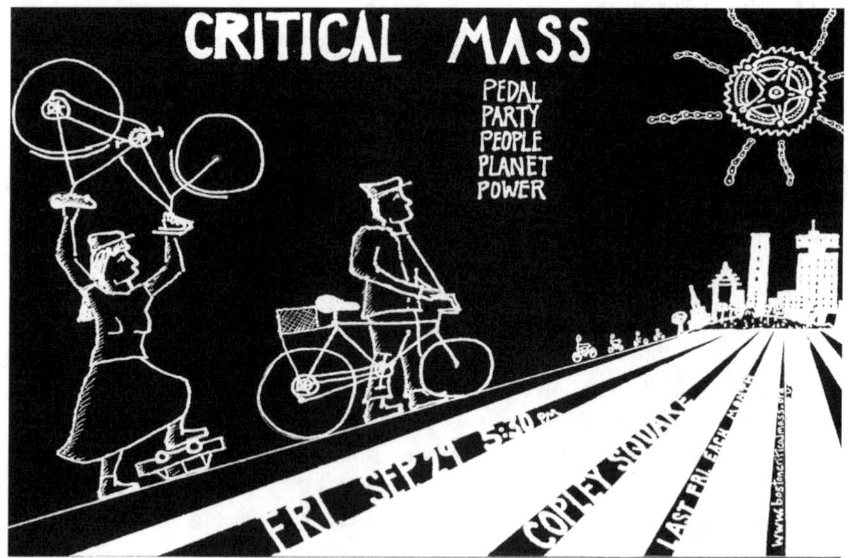

CRITICAL MASS
PEDAL
PARTY
PEOPLE
PLANET
POWER
FRI SEP 29
COPLEY SQUARE
LAST FRI EACH
www.bostoncriticalmass.org

reminding the drivers that we are just following the rules of the road, I doubt it would make any difference in making the ride less controversial, nor even in reducing the incidence of conflict with the police.

There is a deeper issue at stake here, though. Laws are only as powerful as we allow them to be. The decisions as to what rules we are to live by are not passed down, engraved in stone, from the gilded halls of the legislature. They are fluid; we make them every day by deciding which rules to respect and which to ignore. For example, a local religious group recently attempted to press charges against a movie theater screening an allegedly blasphemous film. The court clerk asked the group several times if they really wanted to pay the filing fee. Because they believed the law to be what was contained in the officially published state statutes, they paid the fee and eagerly approached the Judge with their argument. They were sent promptly out the doors, minus their filing fee. Why wouldn't the Court enforce the Law? Because the people had stopped believing in it a century ago.

When Critical Mass is attacked as leading to anarchy, we might have to agree. CM does not delegate decision making power to duly-elected officials; it is not always entirely law-abiding; and the unplanned, spontaneous nature of the rides might accurately be described as "anarchistic." But anarchy is much more of a method than an ideology, a way of experiencing the world rather than a political system. Most importantly, it realizes that the force which stops us from breaking windows and setting fires is not the threat of violent police retaliation but rather mutual respect and voluntary adhesion to practical norms of behavior. In my experience, Critical Mass has only become "anarchistic" in the negative sense when faced with extraordinary violence from the police, which is much more the exception than the rule. If we learn anything about the potential of large scale anarchistic movements from Critical Mass, it is that they are predominantly non-violent, and do a much better job at self-policing than any group depending on outside forces to keep them in line.

Environmentalists are often accused of being motivated by a "social agenda." They will deny the accusation, claiming that their arguments are based in scientific fact, are in fact grounded in demonstrable "truths." But I think we would do better to admit the accusation. It is precisely our "social agenda" that makes the movement appealing and powerful. What good is saving the world, if you don't first create a world worth saving? Critical Mass grasps this reality and engages in it, by putting the social agenda in the forefront. Sure, we want cleaner air and more efficient transportation, but we only want it if we can radically restructure our relationships and our work in the process.

Of course, the critics are welcome to disagree with anything I've said here. If they want to shift the direction of Critical Mass in a more "positive" sense, they can bring more of the type of people they'd like to see riding, the last Friday of every month wherever their local mass convenes. Fundamentally, CM organically adopts the character of those who contribute most to it. It is powerful not because of the message it sends or the image it conveys, but because it engages and empowers its participants, welcoming anyone who wants to chip in.

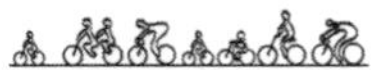

GOOD FOR THE BICYCLING CAUSE

BY DAVE SNYDER

Critical Mass is one of the best things to happen to the Bicycle Coalition specifically, and the bicycle movement generally. I say this as the executive director of the San Francisco Bicycle Coalition (SFBC), the city's mainstream bicycle advocacy group, even while I recognize that Critical Mass has angered thousands, maybe tens of thousands, of Bay Area residents, especially motorists. I say this even though, to this day, most people who know about bicycle advocacy from television can't tell the difference between Critical Mass and the SFBC, forcing me to clarify countless times in discussions, "No, we don't organize that Friday night ride. We're the mainstream citizens' advocates for safer streets." We've recently begun an expensive public relations campaign to promote "peaceful coexistence" between motorists and cyclists, in part to associate our organization with that message in the public eye instead of with Critical Mass.

Taking into account the negatives, Critical Mass, at its most raucous heights, is still great for the bicycling movement. Look at the media coverage we got!

The bicyclists' demand for safer streets for riding got more positive coverage in the media around the July 1997 meltdown than any other time in the past 100 years. Sure, it came with more negative coverage, too, but if you look at the coverage carefully, you'll note that the negative coverage was about the ride. "Crack down on the unruly bicyclists!" When the media got to covering our agenda, it was overwhelmingly positive. All the opinion columnists felt they had to take sides, and even the most rabid car advocates had to admit, "sure, the bicyclists deserve more space on the roadway." When your enemies cede you that point, you know you have won! When's the last time the League of American Bicyclists got quoted in *USA Today*? After Critical Mass.

STOCKTON

ASS APPEAL An eclectic group of anarchists and policy wonks, Critical Mass is forcing S.F. to create a bicycle-friendl

Local: *A bicycle movement gets City Hall's attention*

Two-wheel revolt spins populist message

San Francisco Weekly, December 7, 1994

The SFBC had a minor role in the development of Critical Mass, but a major role in the interpretation of the event in the media. We used the attention

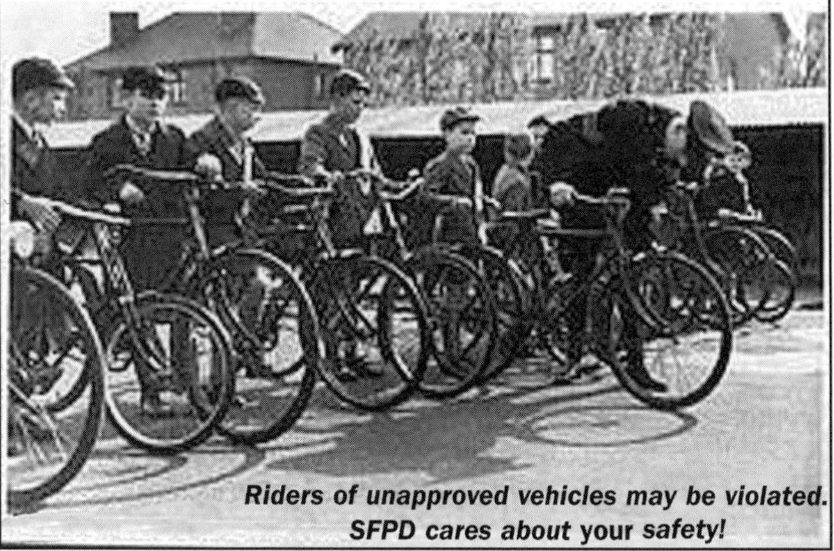
RIDE ONLY POLICE-APPROVED VEHICLES
Riders of unapproved vehicles may be violated.
SFPD cares about your safety!

MATT HOOVER

focused on the event to direct interest to our agenda, which we promoted as central to the future livability of San Francisco. We demanded a network of safe streets for bicycling, with the thousands of Critical Mass riders implicitly showing broad and enthusiastic support for that agenda.

It took us a while to start working the media like this. Initially, we were happy the SFBC was left out of the negative coverage of Critical Mass. We weren't Critical Mass; we had nothing to do with it; we shouldn't have been in those stories and we weren't. Then we got an unsolicited call from a progressive public relations firm called SPIN offering us help with the media: "You guys are getting crushed, just crushed! Let us help you."

They helped us realize that a story about bicycles is a story about the Bicycle Coalition, that the public will connect our organization with the ride whether we're mentioned by name or not. Since promoting bicycles is our mission, if we're not putting our spin on bicycle-related events we're not doing our job. They helped us develop a media strategy that paid dividends for years. Their advice was simple: "develop your message, and stick to it like glue."

Our message was core to our mission: "Bicyclists need the city to develop its proposed bicycle network." If a reporter asked, "what do you think of Critical Mass?" we would answer, "bicyclists are really upset because the city has a plan to create a safe bicycle network and they're not implementing it." After sitting on the sidelines for much of the summer of 1997, we got into the thick of the public debate (at least the public debate as reported by the media) and helped frame the issue. In October 1997, a survey of 600 registered San Francisco voters revealed that our message was working: 76% of respondents answered "yes" to the question, "do you think the city should build more bicycle lanes."

This huge support, immediately after the Critical Mass meltdown, proves the point. If anyone ever tells you that "responsible bicycle advocates" should discourage uncontrolled gatherings of thousands of bicyclists taking over the streets in massive civil disobedience of traffic laws, they're wrong. It is in fact irresponsible not to *encourage* such a display of bicyclists' might.

Our tardiness in spinning the media message to our story reflected ambiguity about our role in Critical Mass that started in the summer of 1992 before the very first ride. The committee that called themselves the San Francisco Bicycle Coalition debated our role and decided to keep the Bicycle Coalition out of it. We never endorsed the ride, though our promotion of it is considered by some to be tacit endorsement. We've never condemned the ride, though we've published criticism and worked hard on occasions to encourage non-violence and respect on the ride itself. We did buy the cake for the ride's first birthday party in September 1993, a decision that stands as the most debated pastry purchase in the history of the Bicycle Coalition. And while the worst fears of the original naysayers were actually borne out, and bicyclists got more negative media coverage than we could have imagined, the full truth revealed how wonderful Critical Mass has been for our agenda.

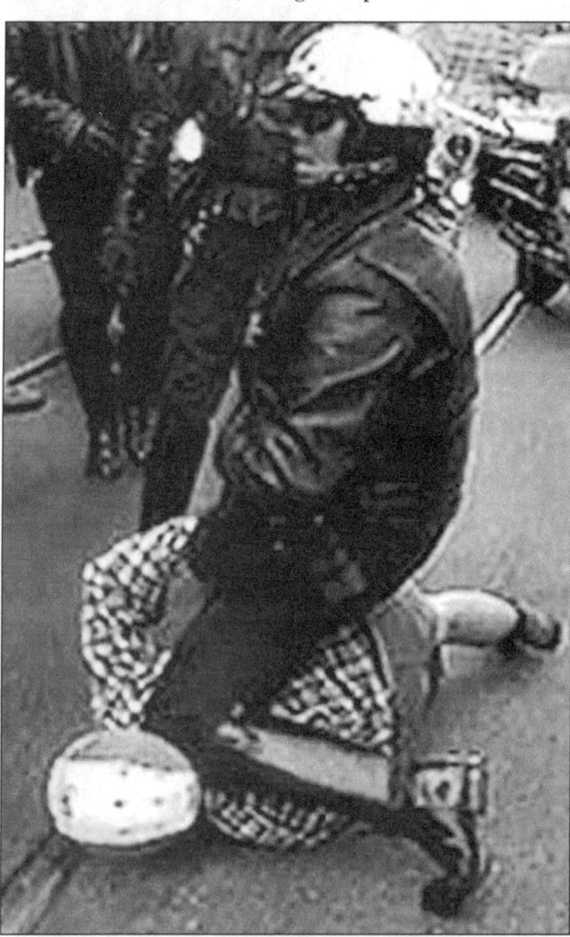

At Mayor Willie Brown's instigation, police attacked Critical Mass in July, 1997. Here is one SF's "finest" on a woman barely over 5 feet tall, who offered no resistance to the unprovoked attack on Market Street.

We are closer than ever to our goal of making San Francisco one of the safest and easiest cities to ride a bicycle in, west of Amsterdam. With a little over 1 million people in the daytime packed into no more than 49 square miles, San Francisco is one of a handful of U.S. cities that has the density to support a profound shift to bicycling as a major transportation option.

It was thanks to Critical Mass that we got to put such a bold demand on the official agenda. Critical Mass forced the politicians to ask us "what is it you folks want?" We said, "well, those folks aren't us folks, but since you asked, here's what we want: the bicycle network. Now." We were promised hearings on eight bike lane proposals of our choosing, most of which required removing traffic lanes. A half dozen city traffic engineers dropped what they were doing to analyze the proposals. When a supervisor's aide was asked "why is the city responding so attentively to the bicyclists," her answer was to the point: "who else can turn out 5,000 people on the streets to protest bad conditions?"

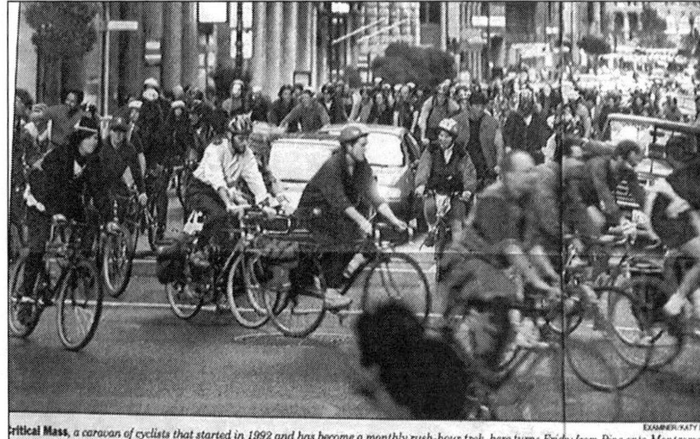

ritical Mass, a caravan of cyclists that started in 1992 and has become a monthly rush-hour trek, here turns Friday from Pine onto Montgomer

CYCLIST CYCLONE HITS CIT

By Dan Brekke
OF THE EXAMINER STAFF

OK, a confession. I put my bike in my car and drove — *drove* — to bicycle ride dedicated to the proposition that

Critical Mass winds through town, insisting that bikes are here to stay

that, and the fact the ride ti traffic for a few minutes one ing a month (if you look at an intersection), have drawn th attention of official San Franci

San Francisco Chronicle, October 22, 1994

I should also thank Mayor Willie Brown, whose promised police crackdown and colorful insults against Critical Mass helped fuel much of the publicity. We launched the "Stop the Backlash" campaign, and SFBC membership grew from 1,100 to 1,500 in three weeks! (It's 3,300 today.) I even got to thank the Mayor for that, as we shared an elevator later that year. He asked me, "how's that campaign for the bike network going? Making any progress?"

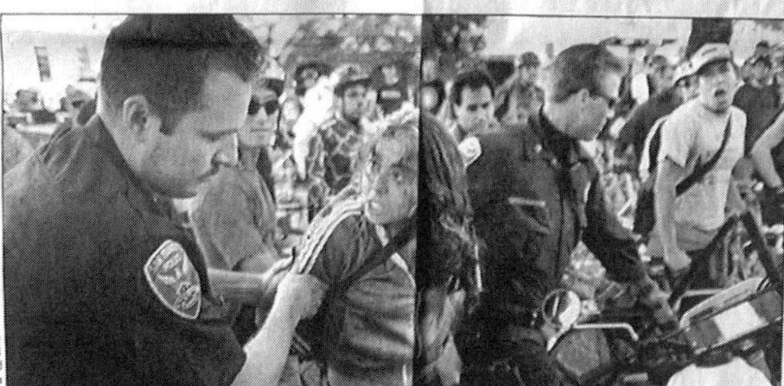

Wild ride for Critical Mass

those complaints.

Hall was arrested for allege using his $4,000 camera to assa Officer Alec Cardenas. Hall has i sisted that police apparently f threatened that he might be phot graphing officer misconduct.

"There was a crime committe there — the assailant was a poli officer who tried to abridge m First Amendment rights," He said afterward. "The criminals a still at large, and they wear badge and guns."

Hill had been near the Powe Street cable car turnaround whe he saw Hall's arrest. When a polic officer arrested Hall, a female by stander grabbed his camera an threw it into the crowd, shoutin for someone to take the film to th newspapers.

Hill caught the camera and, be lieving that Hall's First Amend ment rights were being threatened tried to flee. He was arrested o suspicion of felony theft. He sa

Dozens of cyclists chased off I-80 on-ramp; three arrests; one officer injured in acciden

By Marianne Costantinou
OF THE EXAMINER STAFF

It was a short ride, only a hundred yards. But it was as f they needed to go — for now.

As motorists honked in supp and fellow cyclists cheered wi and held their bicycles high o their heads, several dozen bike ers raced up the entrance ramp I-80 Friday night, asserting th longstanding demand to have cess to the Bay Bridge — and a where else cars can go.

Motorcycle cops turned b

San Francisco Examiner, August 1, 1998

UCCM: UNIVERSITY OF CALIFORNIA CRITICAL MASS

BY BETH VERDEKAL

I first found out about Critical Mass from a San Francisco Bicycle Coalition (SFBC) newsletter in February 1993 when I was 24. I was blown away by the article and rode that month. Loved it! I called Dave Snyder (SFBC Director) and asked how to get involved. I had a Gulf War flyer I wanted to get out to the public and saw Critical Mass as the perfect venue. Dave told me to call "Jim and Chris's office." I talked to Jim [Swanson] and he said I could do my hand printing of the flyer at their office that Friday. When I walked through the door with a car tire strapped to my back via messenger bag, Chris Carlsson (CC) turned around and said, "I thought that it would be you coming by." Coincidentally, CC and I had talked on my first ride. By night's end the flyers with red tire tracks freshly applied were drying throughout the office and I was hooked in to a new phase of my life. (The image of the Gulf War soldier came from a magazine article. The caption said the soldier was crying because he had just found out his buddy, in the body bag to his left, had been killed by friendly fire.)

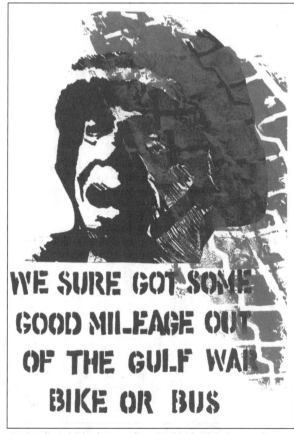

Beth's first Critical Mass flyer in 1993. The tire track was achieved with bright red paint.

Critical Mass was a free-for-all. As a bicyclist with near death experiences riding in the City, I, like other cyclists, had lots of angst to vent. CM was the perfect venue for a budding activist to blossom. Never in my life had I seen such a one-to-one ratio of my effort resulting in effect.

My get-it-done skills were used to the limit making flyers, 'zines, contributing to *Missives*, getting copies made, handing them out. The monthly deadline kept myself and others going at a heavy pace for years.

I schmoozed like never before, like at the copy store where I got deals. It was incredibly fulfilling to load a heap of anti-establishment/we've-got-a-better-idea propaganda into my bike basket. I wore dressy outfits when I passed out the flyers at the beginning of the ride not only because I liked them, but also because I knew they were eyecatching and would help me break the ice with riders. I'd gear up the crowd for our suggested route by calling out interesting tidbits on the suggested route, or words of caution regarding cops writing tickets.

For June 1994, I got the idea to take Critical Mass down Lombard Street (San Francisco's famous touristy, curving red brick street). Mass was still new to riding any serious distance. We had just gone to the beach the previous month. Some thought the ascent to Lombard would discourage all riders from participating in the route. I was so jazzed with the idea, though, that I refused to take 'no' for an answer. CC insisted I ride around to find a mellow route. After a little recon we found a way. Only one short block was steep enough where people might have to dismount. Woohooo!

That month I beamed as I passed out the route sheet, making sure riders were aware of a dangerous intersection at the bottom of a speedy downhill.

Faces lit up as people crested the hill and pointed their tire down the view we've seen a xillion times on postcards sold everywhere in SF. We had over 1000 riders that month. At the bottom shining faces turned upward to watch the rest of Mass as they poured through the winding way like soda pop through a crazy straw. Everyone was yelling, whistling and tinkling bells. Even the cops were chuckling and grinning ear to ear. I was ecstatic!

On the flip side, I laid myself out there pretty thin in grasping for connection the only way I knew how—by doing. I simply had loads of energy and I had no idea of where to go with it. So I pumped it into being An Activist. I was so obsessed with Critical Mass's success, I rarely took any of the people I worked with too personally. Even much of my bonding with my then boyfriend, JRS, was heavily involved with CM. After a ride the crew would gather and dissect the event like a bunch of food critics.

"The route was good, but the cops! What do we do about their harrassment?"

"I loved when we rode around at the Palace of Fine Arts, that's a great ending!"

"Who took us up Leavenworth? That hill sucks!"

We'd buy six packs, smoke pot and go on and on all night. I'd wake the next morning scheming for the following months. I'd fizzle by the following mid-week, but would start ramping up two weeks before the next Mass for *Missives* prep. Then it was more talk, more partying and another ride. I locked myself into a routine that was emotionally safe—me strategizing with "mine" to win over "them"—a type of Activist Purgatory. This dialogue went on for years until the activism that followed the 1997 riot wound down, along with my relationship with Jim.

I went through a heavy phase of self-loathing for all the time I'd spent with people around Critical Mass but with whom I never really connected personally. My heart ached. All the time I had sacrificed to fulfilling a self-imposed duty to change the world, when it was me inside who really craved the change. Where did I come off thinking that my FIGHTING for the earth was going to bring peace? And why did I find it so hard to drop planning/strategizing for CM in between rides?

The activism I embraced in CM fell right in line with the dichotomy mainstream society fosters—the "us/them" alienation mentality. I, like other cyclists, made a conscious choice to be on a bicycle and not to embrace the car ownership endorsed by society at large. And as I biked, I become more and more aware of my choice to put myself in danger daily. As I began to meet people and told them of my transportation choice, they reflected the WOW aspect of me just getting around by bike: The Danger, the Guts, the Commitment. I began to feel like I was someone who was a cut above the Average Shmoe. I met others who had the same personal sentiment and my pride grew stronger with their reinforcement. The Us/Them Mentality had its hold by now.

After a two year break from the weekly hang-outs I so urgently embraced, I came to see the limits of that paradigm. The box around "My Identity" and "Their's" limited personal interaction before it ever had a chance. How could I interact with my fellow US dwellers on a common level if I already have a grudge because of their chosen means of transportation? The issue is not how we get around, but the circumstances which shape those choices. The lack of transportation choices is more important than questioning how people choose to make their lives livable (the symptom being their choice).

The very fact that how we get around can cause such a social rift is a sorry indication of how easily we are estranged from our neighbors. How confined we must all feel to so strongly react to another's choice that LOOKS so different from ours on the outside, and yet is just a decision made within the same context that we all face. Who benefits when we do not empathize with each other's choices? How has this social paradigm been fostered? How do I play a part in it every day? How can I affect social change by my daily actions? By my interactions with others?

Our only hope for a true social shift is to treat each other with compassion. Compassion reflected in my dealings with others encourages people and connects to their humanity. Many of us don't agree with some very basic tenets of government and choose to live here as happily as possible. How do we reconcile our inner convictions with our inevitable compromises, see the common humanity in others who make different choices, and together make this home?

Critical Mass is a beautiful monthly petrie dish, available for experiments in human connection. Though my way of interacting has changed over the years, I still go to Critical Mass and participate in whatever feels right. This consistent forum has been crucial to my self-discovery. I am so thankful to the participants of Critical Mass for keeping this ride going. Happy 10th Birthday, Critical Mass and its riders!

Homage: *I'd like to pay homage to five CM cyclists who I miss and did not live to see the tenth anniversary of Critical Mass.* —*B.V.*

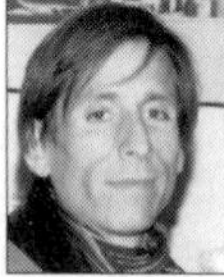

Michael Botkin was an early rider. He was a writer, an activist and a professor. He wrote articles for gay papers and *Processed World*. He had watched so many friends die of AIDS that his dead-pan humor had been honed to dark. More than once I remember a room hushed by one of his comments and then laughter bursting out. He died of AIDS in 1995.

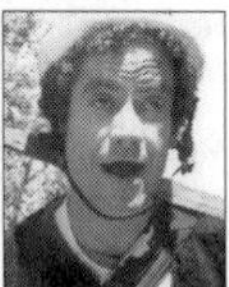

Marcus Cook (aka Fur) was on the first ride. He also wore fake fur. He wrote for a messenger 'zine *Mercury Rising* and played in a punk/funk/messenger band, L Sid (They had a cartoonist work on stage as the band played). He helped get the messengers involved in Critical Mass in the early days. He died of an overdose of heroin in January 1995.

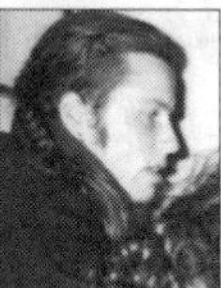

Travis Moraché, an early rider and xerocrat (he worked as manager for a copy store where he published *Broken Spoke* 'zine three times in 1993). He was a cartoonist and event coordinator. Travis was also involved in the Illegal Soapbox Society that had races on Bernal Hill, SF. His dark side led him to suicide by hanging in 1996.

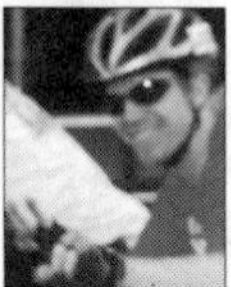

Chris Robertson. He came on the scene later, energetic and eco-minded. He rode on the AIDS ride. He was murdered intentionally by a raging truck driver in 2001 during a funeral ride for another fallen cyclist, a horrible crime that went unprosecuted.

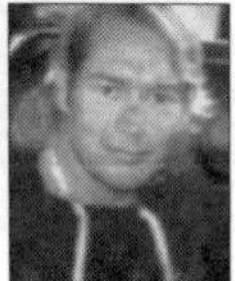

Cap Thomas, an early rider. He pretty much single handedly got bikes on Caltrain, a train that services San Francisco to the South Bay. He wore the most hideous '70s-esque tie-suit combos to countless evening meetings. His activist style was tenacious, patient and polite. No one knew he had AIDS until after his death. He died in 1994.

Thousand Bicycle Wheels *(after Rilke)*

BY MARINA LAZZARA

To the place last creating a never never or else some other kind of field that stretches out and stretches out and begins and begins over and over again until the last burns bright and burns. Today there isn't much that fits in twenty-dollar increments. Only facts, figures, the shadow of the leopard in our palms. But there's a language that is so beautiful, we don't even have to talk. We don't even have to create a never never or else some other kind.

Me? I'm priceless. I get either the place or the palace or the seclusion of plastic cards touching. Yes, I want everything. In fact, I want a lot. The dust that rises from the dirt pulling weeds, the sound of a thousand bicycle wheels, the invisible fountain that strikes up from the ground when the sun hits the surface of the ocean. Yes, I want it all. And in the silent sometimes waking hours, I want to be with those of you who know worthless things or else alone.

San Francisco, California

LOMBARD STREET, JULY 1999

BY CHARLIE KOMANOFF

You San Franciscans are certainly expert at [demonstrating that cycling is fun]. I can still feel the lift to my spirit from the November 1992 and February 1996 Critical Mass rides. Now I have another indelible moment to take home: three thousand of us streaming down Lombard Street like falling water.

I have a confession. On a previous trip to San Francisco I cycled to the top

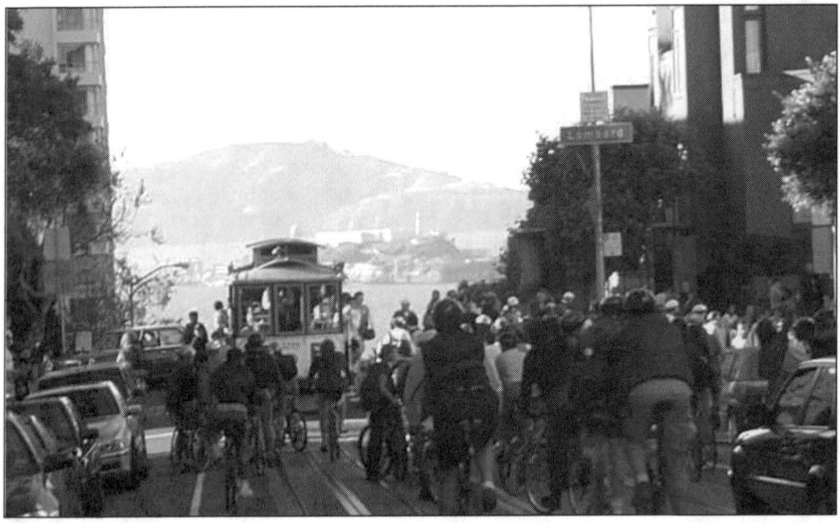

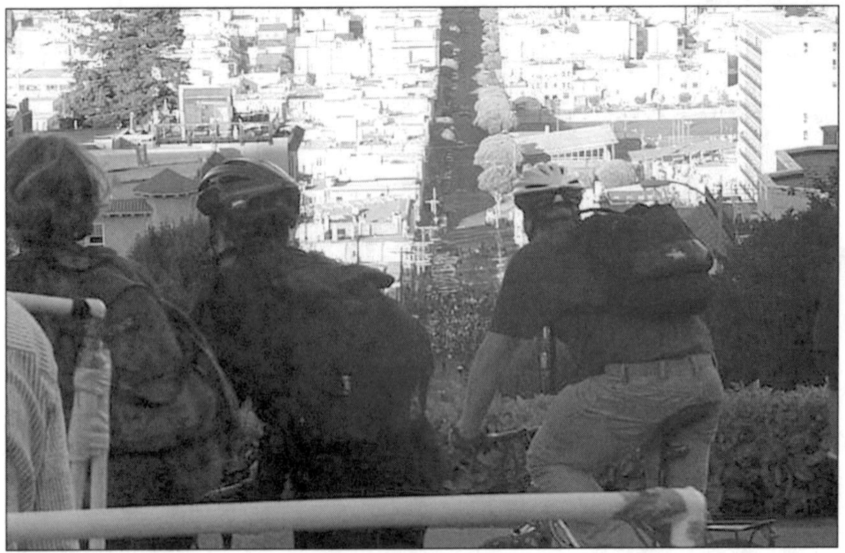

PHOTOS BY DANIEL KOPALD, JULY 1999

of Lombard, stared down that steep and twisting road, and froze. The grade was frightening, the bricks looked slippery, and the line of cars behind me was scary. So I walked down! But on Friday, in true Critical Mass spirit I took courage from everyone around me and plunged ahead. Riding was easy, of course, and wild, and beautiful.

As I neared the final turn, I saw hundreds of cyclists at the foot of the street applauding us—me! What a feeling! At the landing, as I joined in cheering the riders coming down, their bikes and bodies and faces blended into one long silky liquid motion, like a river winding down a mountainside.

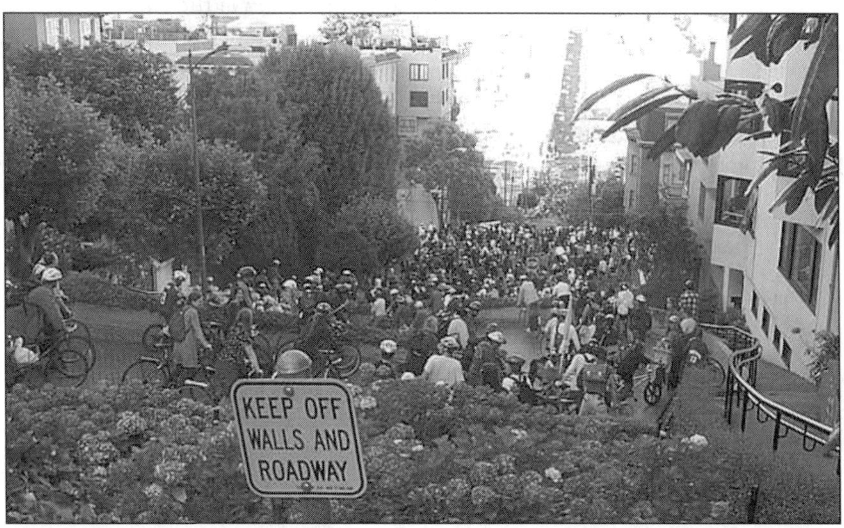

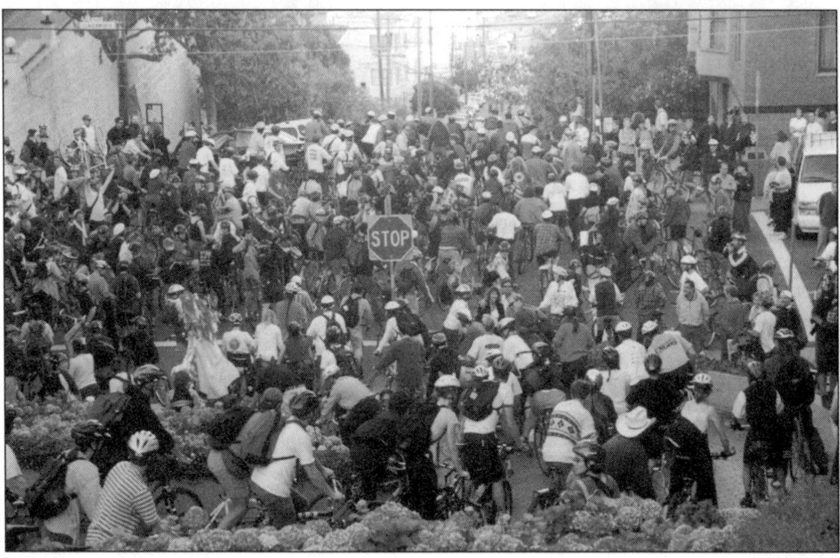

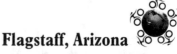

Flagstaff, Arizona

MAYBE YOU SHOULD READ THE STATUTE AND CONSIDER WHAT'S REASONABLE

BY JEFF FERRELL

This chapter is adapted from Jeff Ferrell's book, *Tearing Down the Streets: Adventures in Urban Anarchy* (New York: Palgrave/St. Martin's, 2001).

During the 1990s, Critical Mass rides migrated from their Bay Area origins to Flagstaff, Arizona, just as they did to hundreds of large and small cities around the United States and the world. In many of the larger cities, the rides quickly began to attract participants, with hundreds of riders regularly coming out for the event. By 1996, even Flagstaff's Critical Mass, though based in a city of only 50,000 people, had drawn enough interest and attention to force a confrontation between a hundred participants bent on taking back Flagstaff's streets from automobile traffic and, ironically, local bicycle-mounted police officers intent on keeping such traffic flowing—even to the point of arresting a number of Critical Mass riders. What with Flagstaff's often inclement winter weather, though, and the coming and going of students from the local university, Critical Mass rides themselves came and went over the next few years.

Then, in the spring of 2000, the rides began to re-form. As with earlier Flagstaff rides, participant numbers even at their best were no match for the thousands of riders in the Bay Area. Yet the numbers were sufficient to achieve a critical mass, a collective experience of spatial reclamation and celebration; to ignite within this experience the usual dynamics of direct action and do-it-yourself resistance; and, like all Critical Masses, to set in motion the possibility of some other explosion.

My involvement in this resurgence begins in late February of that year when I discover and then reproduce a flier promoting a ride scheduled for the usual Critical Mass date: the last Friday of the month. Bicycling up to the designated meeting spot that Friday—some picnic tables across the street from Macyy's, a popular alternative coffeehouse—I notice two signs: "Seating for Macyy's Customers ONLY. No Loitering, #13-2905," and a larger "No Loitering" notice posted on a nearby building. With nothing on me but six bucks, a pocket knife, and a microcassette recorder, and no Macyy's coffee in hand, I sit down and proceed to loiter. After awhile a young woman bicycles up.

"Is this where we're meeting for Critical Mass?"

"Um, I think so."

"Well, maybe I'll swing back by in a while to check if the ride goes." She does; it doesn't. And some time later, after it's clear that indeed a critical mass won't be achieved today, a young guy walks over from Macyy's. It's Clayton, writer of Critical Mass fliers and local anarchist agitator, a guy I've been meaning to meet. Along with discussing fliers and xerocracy, we talk about his and others' attempts to launch an underground radio station, his work with the local Food Not Bombs chapter, and other forms of activism past and present. All the while he sips from his mug, filled with strong Macyy's coffee and pasted over with

Wobbly stickers, including "An Injury to One is an Injury to All."

Clayton's comments remind me of the ways in which the anarchic, do-it-yourself dis-organization of Critical Mass and like undertakings provides threads of activism and community, but no ties that bind. Fliers get made and posted, *sans* membership list or map grid; Clayton and I and others meet, interact, learn, but with no one in charge of the meeting. And Clayton, like other street activists, stretches his web of anarchist sensibilities across Critical Mass, Food Not Bombs, underground radio, and other sorts of activism, not because they're all coordinated under the same organization, but because, after all, an injury to one is an injury to all.

Sitting in the cold after Clayton leaves, getting ready to ride home, I think about Bakunin, too, and the multitude of ways in which destruction is creation; failure, success. Today the Critical Mass ride didn't come off; despite our fliers and our on-the-spot convergence, we failed. But in not happening, it seems to me, the ride exists as an accomplished anarchist event, preferable in its shambling failure to whatever success might be brought about by bylaws, committees, and a designated event coordinator.

A month later, bicycling uphill and against a cold wind to our gathering spot, I almost turn back, sure that nobody's as crazy as I am, and that we'll fail again. As I arrive, though, Clayton comes over from Macyy's and, gesturing to a motley crew across the street, tells me that this time we've reached Critical Mass, albeit a small one even by Flagstaff standards. So, the nine of us set off down the street—eight guys and one girl, most all in their teens and twenties, sporting a collection of ragged pants and shorts, longjohns, and anarchy patches, astride a hodgepodge of mountain, touring, and BMX bikes. Despite the fact that we're occupying only one of two southbound lanes, horns are honking within thirty seconds, and a tough boy is leaning out of an SUV and yelling. "Single file, assholes." We smile and wave. Over the next hour and a half I lose count of the number of middle fingers shot at us from behind the rolled-up windows of cars and SUVs, though I do remain aware of an ongoing, angry horn cacophony. Unfortunately, no one's remembered the "Honk If You Like Bikes" signs.

From the first, the Mass emerges as an exercise in fluid, on-the-fly cooperation, collectively negotiating the next twist or turn in what is largely an unplanned route anyway. Rolling around corners, changing lanes with a flurry of hand traffic signals, the Mass moves like some multiwheeled amoeba, riders ebbing and flowing from front to back. Early on, a young kid coming toward us on a skateboard smiles, yells "Hey, Critical Mass!" and reverses his course to skate along with us for a few blocks. A few minutes later, we decide to circle back toward Macyy's, hoping to pick up a couple of riders we seem to have left behind—and there they are, two kids just passing through Flagstaff, in from Vegas, veterans of Critical Mass there. Ready to resume the ride, we decide to wait until a train has finished crossing the street north of us, so that we can pull out in front of a nice tight group of overheated motorists. And, aware that our gender balance seems a bit askew today, I'm pleased to see that Lyndsay, the lone woman in the ride, takes an active role in this and other decisions.

As the ride moves along, we're amazed by the power of our direct action—by the ability of nine dis-organized bicyclists to directly and effectively interrupt the usual, taken-for-granted flow of automotive traffic. We manage to shut down one or more lanes on major thoroughfares, to completely block downtown streets, and to pile up some one hundred cars behind us while we climb Humphreys Street, a two-lane road rising from downtown to the northern suburbs—all the while smiling and waving at those caught around and behind us. Indeed, we joke and laugh all the way to the top, riding into the wind and now-falling snow—Clayton's joke is, "This isn't Critical Mass, it's Critical Masochists!" As we ease back down the hill, another long line of cars forms behind us, and finally an SUV driver has had enough. Whipping around in front of us, he stops his vehicle dead in the street—we appreciate the help in blocking traffic—and jumps out. "What do you think you're doing?" he screams back at us. As we ride up to him, someone in the group simply smiles and says, "We're riding bicycles." "Um, ok," and he gets back in the SUV, apparently a bit braver behind the wheel than in the street.

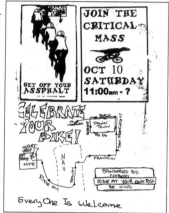

Just as Beth Verdekal and Jim Swanson would predict, the ride also emerges as a "social space," a street space where people can "converse and interact."[1] By riding slowly and in a relatively tight formation so as to more effectively interrupt auto traffic, we also set a leisurely pace for ourselves, and facilitate bike-to-bike conversation. Putting ourselves and our bicycles on the line, confronting automotive dominance through direct action, we invent the impossible: an island of safety, calm, and conversation in the middle of a busy street. And, in fine reflexive fashion, we inhabit this island with talk of Critical Mass rides in other cities, strategies for surviving encounters with motorists, sabotage in the workplace, anarchist history, and other subversions. As we hook a collectively illegal U-turn in the middle of one car-choked street, Clayton leans over to me and says, "No manmade law governs my bicycle."

Later, I'm telling my friend Barry, a fiddler and street busker, about the ride, the rolling blockade of car traffic, the pissed-off motorists, the pleasure of it all. A veteran bicycle racer and bicycle mechanic himself, I figure Barry might want to join us for the next ride. "That's punk rock, man! That's punk rock! Hell yes!" he says as I recall the ride. And indeed it is—punk rock on two wheels. Johnny Rotten and The Sex Pistols would understand, I think—understand anarchy in the Flagstaff streets just like anarchy in the streets of the U.K.

When the next ride comes around at the end of April, Barry does indeed join in the anarchy. The weather's better, and it's obvious early on that this will be a larger and even more energetic ride than the last one; twenty or so riders have pulled up across from Macyy's, and everyone's talking and laughing in preparation for getting underway. It's obvious also that this time we have a gender mix more in keeping with the tradition of Critical Mass, as an equal number of women and men head off down the street. By the time we get to Milton Avenue, a major North/South thoroughfare near the university, we've picked up a few more cyclists, and we now have enough bikes to effectively block both southbound lanes. Hundreds of cars are backing up behind us amid the usual soundscape of horns and shouts; some accelerate through the left turn lane and blow by us, with one car cutting fast a foot or two in front of the lead bikes as its driver and passenger yell obscenities out the windows. Surprisingly, though, we're seeing "thumbs up" gestures mixed in with the middle fingers, and hearing almost as many shouts of "Alright!" from motorists and pedestrians as we are curses. I ride up alongside a couple of first-time Critical Mass participants; they're grinning, and one says, "Wow, this is amazing; this feels great!"

As we swing a U-turn though a strip mall parking lot and head back up Milton, with both lanes of northbound traffic now slowed behind us, I'm feeling great, too, high on the adrenalin of the ride and the reactions to it. Then I notice the cops. Intercepting us from the north are two Flagstaff officers in a patrol car, the driver shouting out his window for us to pull over into an adjacent parking lot. We all glide over into the parking lot, but while some roll slowly through it, others accelerate, splitting off and scattering along various frantic trajectories. Ten of us keep the mass together, and as we coast out of the parking lot and onto the university campus, the patrol car catches up to us, lights on, the driver demanding over his loudspeaker that we pull over—now. We do.

By the time he's out of his patrol car, he's already yelling. "How many people here think that's the stupidest thing they've ever seen, riding like that down the middle of Milton?" Judging from the lack of response, the answer is two: himself and the officer riding with him. Within a couple of minutes, automotive reinforcements arrive—another Flagstaff police officer in a second patrol car, and a university police supervisor driving a large, official SUV—and the lengthy process of identification and ticketing begins. We're informed that we're being charged with violation of Arizona Revised Statute 28-704A, that is, proceeding "at such a slow speed as to impede or block the normal and reasonable movement of traffic." Invoking Critical Mass's essential concept, we of course immediately counter that we weren't blocking traffic, we were traffic—and the officers just as quickly dismiss the notion. During this process, the university police supervisor also begins to ask whether everyone involved is a student at the university. Everyone (except me) is—which is lucky since, as some in the group recount from previous run-ins with university police, his question is actually one of

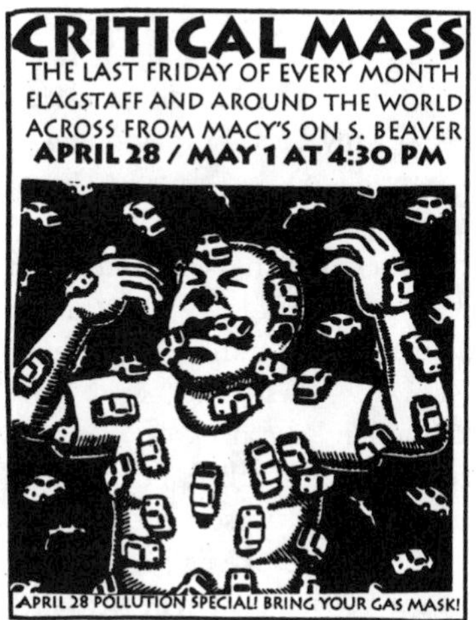
CRITICAL MASS
THE LAST FRIDAY OF EVERY MONTH
FLAGSTAFF AND AROUND THE WORLD
ACROSS FROM MACY'S ON S. BEAVER
APRIL 28 / MAY 1 AT 4:30 PM
APRIL 28 POLLUTION SPECIAL! BRING YOUR GAS MASK!

spatial control: trespass charges can be filed against anyone found on campus who is not a student or otherwise involved in official university business. And just as these interactions evidence a certain disagreement regarding the nature of traffic and the control of cultural space, an off-and-on civics lesson that the cops deliver while writing tickets seems designed to emphasize the desirability of representational democracy over direct action.

"There's a reasonable way to go about" achieving better bicycling conditions, they tell us. "There's an easy way to do it . . . you know how to go about doing that, instead of driving in the middle of the street? Go to the city council . . . easy way to do it, right next to the courthouse . . . then what are you doing out here causing problems? Go to city hall . . . if you have a problem, you need to go to city council . . . that's the way you should take care of it. . . . If you guys didn't know, in May, the next election's coming up, there's some initiatives on there to get more bike paths."

Just like back in high school civics class, I don't pay much attention, instead passing the time in a reverie of direct action and free association. Our ticket for impeding the "normal and reasonable" movement of traffic reminds me of the old "move on" laws enforced during Wobbly free speech fights, and reminds me of an image I'd seen in a recent Critical Mass video. It's a big Critical Mass ride in Austin, Texas, and a patrol car rolls alongside the riders, an officer wagging his finger out the window and warning them:

"If you don't pick up the pace you'll be issued a citation for impeding traffic; you better move on. You better move on!"

"I'm moving."

"You're not fast enough, you better move on!"[1]

The ongoing tension between the civics-teacher officers and the members of our group produces a more violent confluence of images as well. After thirty minutes or so of ticket writing, as all three police vehicles continue to idle within a few feet of us, Clayton asks the nearest officer, "Can you turn your cars off?" "My car's always running," he says, and elaborates: "Next time when you're getting your ass kicked over here, and I have to take the time to turn my car on to get to you to help you, you'll wonder why my car's always running, ok? When you're bleeding and sitting on the ground and need help right away, that's why my car's always running. . . . I can let you sit there and bleed for as long as I want, I'll do that for you. That's why my car runs all the time." Hearing this, I can't help but wonder who's doing the ass-kicking, and who wants to let it bleed—and can't help but think of a previous ass-kicking image involving a police officer and a Critical Mass rider. Widely circulated in the bike activist underground, the photo comes from Willie Brown's July 1997 crackdown on San Francisco's Critical Mass. It shows a helmeted San Francisco cop, his right arm locked in a chokehold around the neck of a female Critical Mass rider, his left hand, partially hidden behind his police motorcycle, grabbing at her around the waist.[2] Once she's released, I think to myself, perhaps she should report the incident to the city council, or vote for more bike paths.

Once we're released, the ten of us cycle over to some benches to sit,

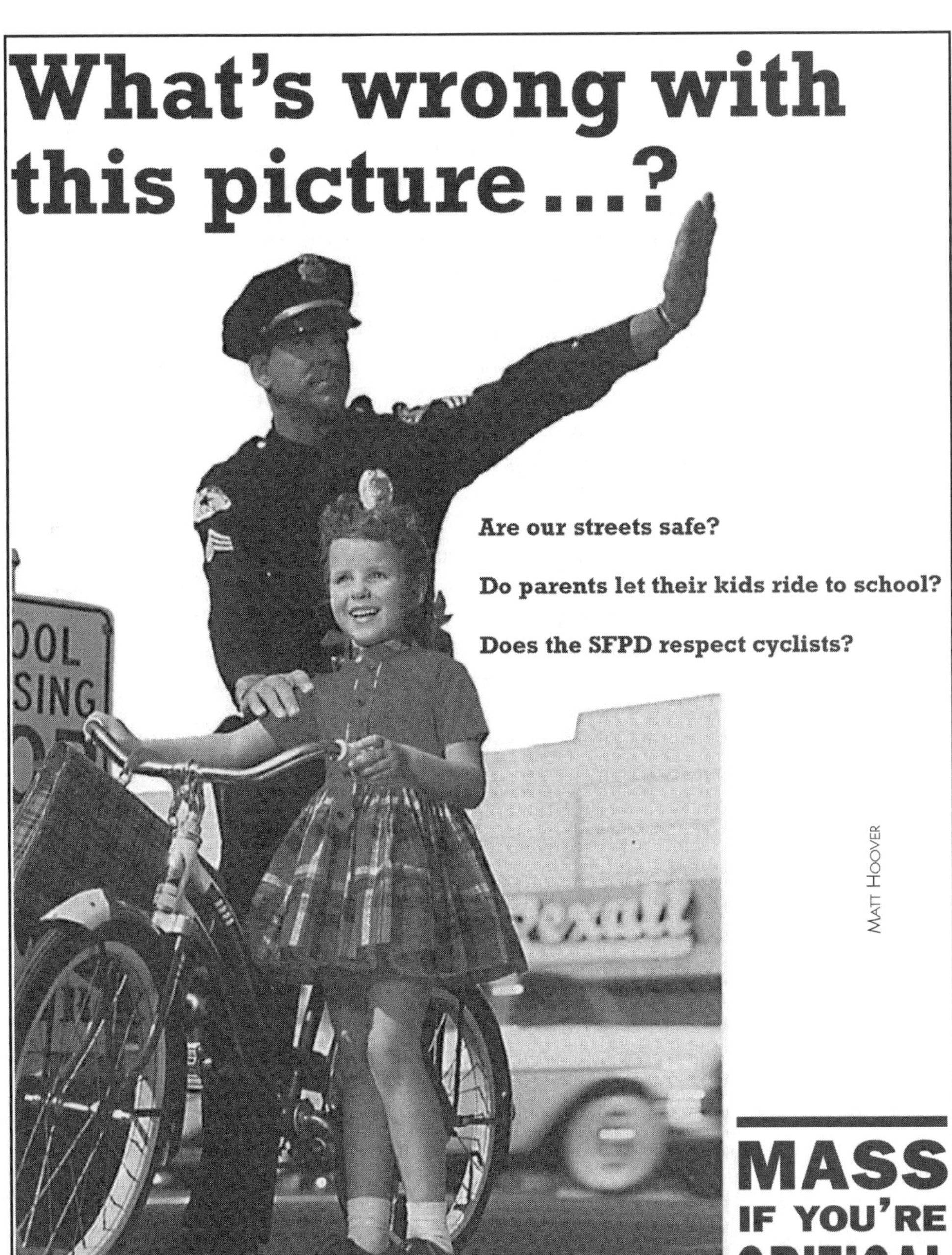
What's wrong with this picture...?
Are our streets safe?
Do parents let their kids ride to school?
Does the SFPD respect cyclists?
MATT HOOVER
MASS
IF YOU'RE
CRITICAL

exchange phone numbers and email addresses, and begin the process of planning a court challenge to the tickets. Riding away from this impromptu meeting, Barry laughs and says, "Nice of the cops to get us organized like that." But Clayton is less amused. Clayton says that today's events in a way bring his own politics full circle, that it was just this sort of street dynamic—being harassed by the police when, at age twelve, he was riding his skateboard in the streets of his neighborhood—that radicalized him in the first place.

A month later, eight of us appear in court. The arresting officer testifies that while he had probable cause for charging us with both obstructing a public thoroughfare and unlawful assembly, and could have "arrested and taken [us] to jail," he found it "in the best interest of the City of Flagstaff to issue a civil citation." Though the judge finds the first two riders "not responsible" on a legal technicality regarding the officer's identification of them, she finds the next four guilty; and then it's my turn. Putting the officer on the stand, I decide to try a new approach. Questioning him about the incident, I argue that the motorists' cell phone calls that brought him to the scene may have reflected nothing more than anticycling bias on their part; that the bicyclists were part of a heavy rush hour traffic jam, not demonstrably the cause of it; and that, in any case, the officer's dealings with us were evidence more of interpersonal hostility than competent police work. The judge seems persuaded, addressing probing follow-up questions to the officer, asking me for clarification and elaboration, consulting the statute in her law books. Then, after more consideration, comes the verdict. "No, no," she says, seeming to stop herself just short of reversing her prior decisions. "This was intentional. Guilty."

Returning to my seat in the gallery, I'm reminded of a comment the arresting officer made during the ticketing process, upon discovering that unlike the rest of the group he had apprehended, I wasn't a student but a faculty member. "Professor," he said, wrapping his suggestion in a full metal jacket of derision, "maybe you should read the statute and consider what's reasonable." I'm not sure I've gotten around to doing that, or that the judge got around to it that day in court; but someone else has. The senior police officer in the first 1996 police confrontation with Flagstaff Critical Mass riders—an officer who at the time made the decision to arrest and handcuff one of the riders in order to "clear the road of cyclists and allow cars to proceed"—later enrolled in our graduate program, and decided to write about his experience. Looking back on what he had seen then as "a simple traffic jam," he now argued that "Critical Mass riders attack the meta-narratives of current culture by challenging taken-for-granted notions of car-culture and transportation issues." But beyond this, he suggested that, for cops as much as for Critical Mass riders, what at first seems reasonable might not be what's right: "Bicyclists taking over roadways established and dedicated to motor vehicles interrupt and confuse, and therefore threaten. Police arrive and attempt to establish order out of apparent chaos. . . . Police, agents of social control, are at times 'agents of the status quo,' even if it is not recognized at first glance."[3]

Notes

1. In Ted White, *We Aren't Blocking Traffic, We Are Traffic!* (video), 1999.
2. See Bikesummer Editorial Collective, "Bike Summer," 1999, page 12.
3. Matt Pavich, "Critical Mass," unpublished paper, December 1997.

MASSIVE CRITIQUE

BY HUGH D'ANDRADE

So much of our lives we are forced to accept situations which we have not chosen for ourselves. As consumers, as voters, as employees, we allow crucial decisions about our lives to be made by other, more powerful people. How sad it is then—and yet how predictable—that our movements for social change are so often cursed with this same problem. When we join a political party, or sign a petition, or take part in a rally, more often than not we are simply accepting someone else's opinion, chanting slogans we did not create, and endorsing laws we do not understand.

Critical Mass is, or should be, something different . . . A space where people do not have ideas or actions imposed on them, where people can take an active, rather than passive role in building a livable future, in however small a way.

Because no one is in charge on our monthly ride, and no specific ideology is set forth, participants are free to invent their own reasons for being here. The lively Xerocracy that has sprung up, the preponderance of flags and hand-painted signs—not to mention the fact that Critical Mass is spreading to other cities—these things are all signs that we are doing something right.

Unfortunately, not everyone sees things this way.

The Horse and the Rider

There are those who enjoy Critical Mass and regularly participate, but who criticize the ride for its formlessness and what is called its "apolitical" nature. For these people, the task at hand is to politicize the ride by setting up some sort of steering committee, complete with chants, bullhorns and official security (in day-glo jackets, no doubt). If you listen carefully, you can hear talk of "pulling in the reins," "harnessing" the energy of Critical Mass in order to attain some worthy, though predetermined, political goal.

But who is the rider here? And who the proverbial horse? Not only are such

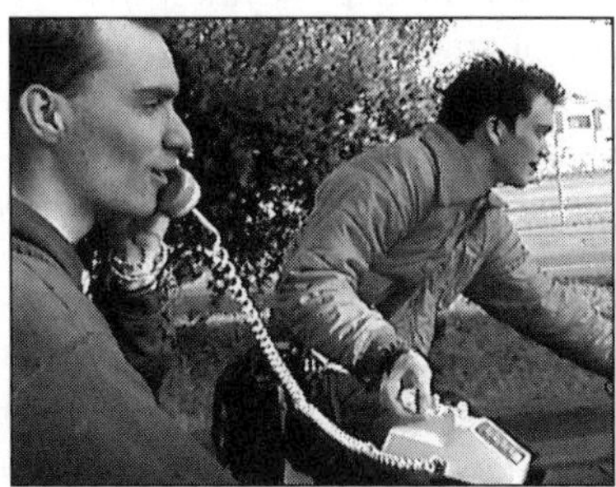

The CELL PHONE RIDE responded to an anti-bike conservative councilmember from the wealthy Berkeley Hills who had proposed a Cell Phone Ban for bicyclists ONLY (despite the major studies showing that motorists using cell phones are as dangerous as drunk drivers, and no statistics about danger with regards to bicyclists). Major media uproar erupts, which we made the most of while having fun with it. Biker-X brought a boxfull of home-made fake cell phones for the ride. News helicopters above, we played phone games rolling through the streets! These riders supplied a Sex Information Line during the ride.

analogies absurd and repulsive, but the approach is counter-productive, as those who have been to or heard of the over-organized but sparsely attended Santa Cruz ride can attest.

Tyranny of the Minority

Another group who would seek to impose the stamp of their political ambitions on Critical Mass, and who have been to some extent more successful, are those who advocate an aggressive, antagonistic stance for the ride. Tactics along these lines have included surrounding and harrassing motorists who inch toward the Mass, baiting the police, and pedaling up to the front of the ride and abruptly turning off the agreed route in an attempt to "hijack" the ride.

The purpose is presumably to "radicalize" Critical Mass by pushing it in a more confrontational, even violent direction, an idea that recalls Chomsky's comment that tactics, in and of themselves, do not amount to radicalism.

What both of these approaches share is an impatience with the slow, painstaking task of educating others and organizing toward a future worth living. A truly radical approach to the social problems we face would be to build community and to offer an alternative—a fact that apparently eludes those who believe people have to be tricked or stampeded into creating a better world.

❄Welcome to the Berkeley Streets❄

The streets of Berkeley are provided free of charge to all citizens, regardless of race, gender, or sub-culture, as a public service. While they are specifically designed to facilitate transportation from one place of economic activity to another, the streets may also be used for purposes unrelated to productivity.

There are, however, some general principles concerning the use of public space that must be obeyed. Though vague and often unenforcable, these social norms are nonetheless imperative to the effective operation of government in a democracy. For your own safety, please obey them all:

- City streets are not to be used as arenas for loitering, relaxing, story-telling, or any form of unproductive social interaction. Use of public space for such purposes typically leads to instability and economic flabbiness.
- All forms of transportation are tolerated, however, the streets are specifically designed for use by motorized traffic. The city cannot accept responsibility for any discomfort or dismemberment experienced by citizens not transporting themselves encased in steel and rubber.
- Harmless political groups with mild reformist demands may use the streets for political "protest", as long as participants remain orderly and uncreative, and their analysis remains unappealing to the vast majoritiy of the population. Spontaneous theatrical actions are strongly discouraged.

Please enjoy your access to Berkeley's streets. As long as the above principles remain dutifully obeyed and only dimly understood, we can expect the dominant social order to continue unabated.

Note: The above rules are do not apply in cases of natural disaster or social upheaval

Obviously, no one should be barred from expressing themselves or sharing their thoughts or opinions. We all want to see Critical Mass be a space where diverse political strategies can be debated and experimented with. The point is that if you want to see Critical Mass go in this or that direction, make copies of your ideas and pass them around. Only cowards and authoritarians shrink from the challenge of persuasion!

It could be that all we're doing is riding from HERE to THERE on bikes. But what is so amazing is that in attempting such a simple task, so many important and provocative questions come up. For a moment, a window is opened onto a possible future: a future where no one is in charge and most people ride a bike!

PUBLIC LIFE ENDS WHERE THE STREETS BEGIN

THE BICYCLE TERRORIST

Lampooning the status quo projection of cyclist banditry.

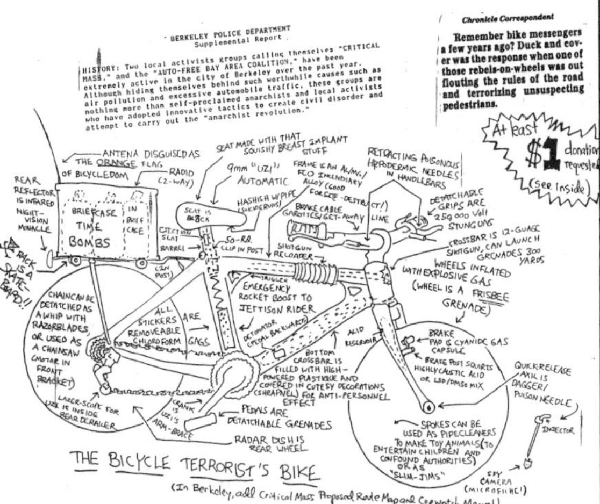

BERKELEY POLICE DEPARTMENT
Supplemental Report

HISTORY: Two local activists groups calling themselves "CRITICAL MASS," and the "AUTO-FREE BAY AREA COALITION," have been extremely active in the city of Berkeley over the past year. Although hiding themselves behind such worthwhile causes such as air pollution and excessive automobile traffic, these groups are nothing more than self-proclaimed anarchists and local activists who have adopted innovative tactics to create civil disorder and attempt to carry out the "anarchist revolution."

Chronicle Correspondent

Remember bike messengers a few years ago? Duck and cover was the response when one of those rebels-on-wheels was out flouting the rules of the road and terrorizing unsuspecting pedestrians.

Berkeley, California

Critical Mass took the I-80 freeway on July 9, 1993, which helped produce a dynamic of criminalization on the East Bay ride. One answer was the publication (left) of *The Bicycle Terrorist*. Later East Bay bicycling radicals led an aggressive attempt to open the Bay Bridge to bicycles (bottom left and right).

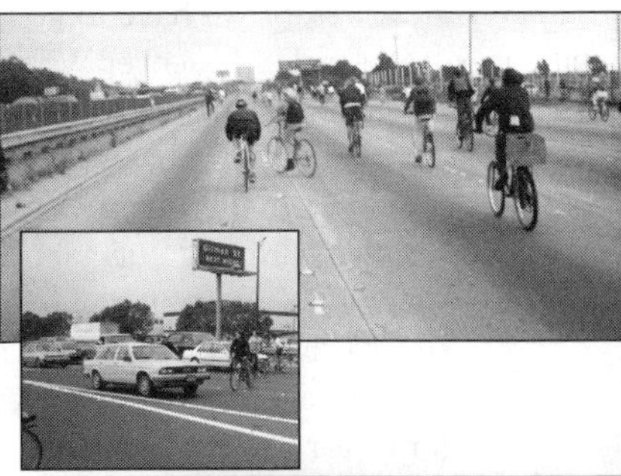

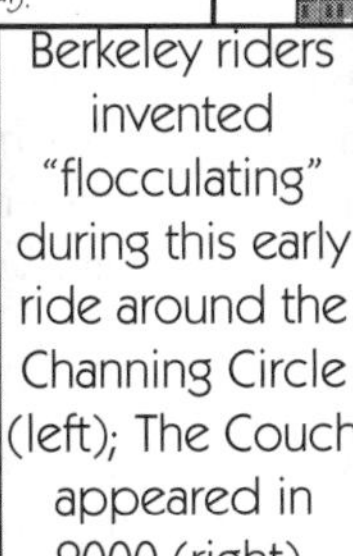

Berkeley riders invented "flocculating" during this early ride around the Channing Circle (left); The Couch appeared in 2000 (right).

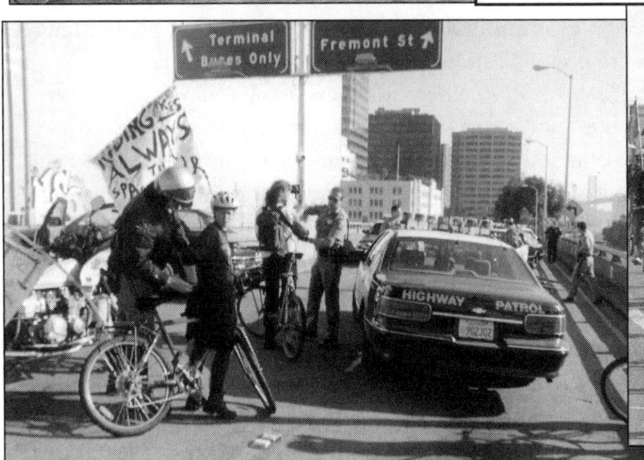

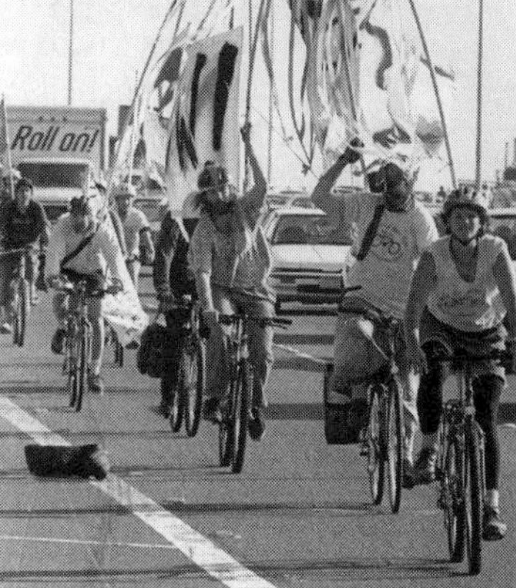

CRITICAL MASS MARCH MADNESS! HALE BOPP! HAIL BOP!

BY HOWARD WILLIAMS, REVISED FROM *VOICE OF DA* #5, SPRING 1997

The 55th San Francisco Critical Mass held on March 28, 1997 will be remembered as one of the most exciting CMs ever. But to know the whole story, we have to go back to August 1996. Most of us who worked on the 1996 Cycle Messenger World Championships (CMWC) can't recall what we had for breakfast this morning but we all remember the Critical Mass of August 30. That was the kickoff event for what many still consider the greatest CMWC of All Time but at the time most CMWC "organizers" (or whatever we were) were all sleepless, drugged out, jabbering idiots who were saved from being reduced to a state of Pure Zombiehood only by intense nervous anxiety. There were a few who steadfastly refused to be drugged out. Many objective observers believe these people were even worse. In any case, many of us CMWC volunteers had been this way for a year. In short we were people you wouldn't want to invite to opera opening nights, the Black & White Ball . . . or mosh pits.

And what happened in the days preceding the CMWC ? Into our lives came the self-styled "Owner" of Critical Mass who shall remain nameless (Christian Johannes Lackner—oops must be a typo) who informed us that the August Critical Mass "traditionally" went to Sutro Beach (two times—wow, what a tradition) and that we should not try to present a different route. He wrote his route, we wrote ours and we all wondered what the outcome would be. In situations where there are 2 or more routes presented before each Mass, the Massers choose the route by voice vote. The SFPD then announce the result. So we prepared accordingly.

Critical Mass was started by the late Marcus Cook and other messengers and cyclists in September 1992 as a way for bike riders to travel safely for one lousy hour in a month. The police were never at the first Masses and most of us feel we can still do it ourselves. We certainly don't want a situation that enables an Owner to tell us where we're going 12 months ahead of time.

So what happened August 30, 1996 when 5,000 cyclists gathered at JHP for Critical Mass ? Well, to make a long and ugly story short, while we were working the crowd for the vote, somebody told the cops that we had accepted a "compromise" route that was exactly like the Owner's. The cops announced this while we were deep in the crowd and it would have taken at least five minutes to get to the cops to tell them there was no such deal. So reluctantly, we accepted this *fait accompli* but many of us vowed that if anybody ever tried to overthrow the Owner at a future Mass we would support the freedom-loving rebels. It wasn't so much that the Owner had a different route; it was the deceitful and cowardly way our plan was stabbed in the back.

Which brings us to March 28, 1997. There had been talk about proposing an alternate route to the Owner's Nob Hill destination. Many wanted to go to

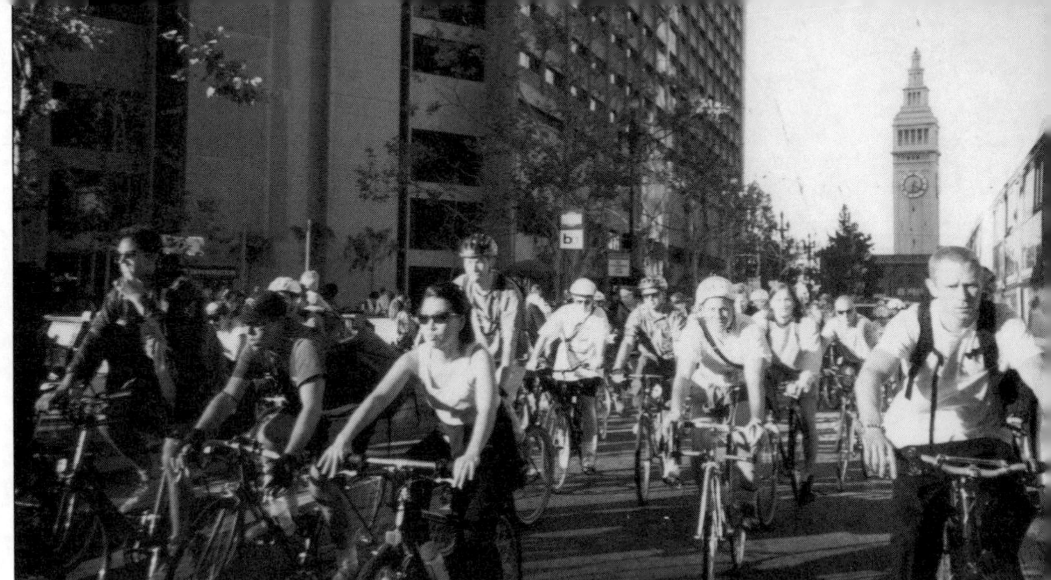

San Francisco, summer 1998

Alta Plaza for a view of the Hale Bopp Comet. The ancients believed that comets are harbingers of big changes. But I didn't hear of any specific challenges to the Owner and one friend politely dismissed my route plan. So I was feeling depressed on the afternoon of March 28. My girlfriend Omi was working late and would miss the Mass and I was probably going to work late myself. Both the *Bay Guardian* and the *Chronicle* had reported that the Mass would go to Nob Hill. Someone had sent the Owner's route to the media, probably to tip the balance in his favor. Then around 3 pm, while riding in the belly of the beast (i.e. the Financial District), I saw Dave Powers, a worthy foe of the Owner. He handed me a few fliers showing his route—one which included the Wall and Herb Caen Way and finished at Alta Plaza for a prime view of Hale Bopp. Instantly a basic, primeval human feeling shot into my soul. Revenge! . . . I mean: Justice! Justice!

Suddenly I knew what to do. I called my dispatcher. He gave me a run ending in my neighborhood. Everything was falling into place but I barely had enough time. Isn't it always like that?

At my apartment I got my mini-box and my Charlie Parker cassette. If you Hale Bopp you should also Hail Bop! At a grocery store I got some salt peanuts—the Official Legume of Hale Bopp in honor of the late great jazz musician Dizzy Gillespie (composer of the Bop classic "Salt Peanuts"). Down to 1095 Market—the Grant Building—where I began copying hundreds of fliers. The clock ticked past 5. Out the door and into the street where people were riding to the Mass. As I rode with them I began handing out fliers. When I rode onto Justin Hermann Plaza I saw the Owner's few allies talking to the police. I handed a couple fliers to the officers. "Here's the route gentlemen. Don't believe everything you read in the *Chronicle*."

"Somehow this doesn't surprise me," one cop replied.

I worked the crowd like a shameless advance man for a crooked politician. Except that this was for a good cause of course.

"I have a route map," people would say.

"That's the *Chronicle* Ride. This is the Comet Ride," I replied.

"The Comet Ride? What's that?"

"Tonight," I replied, brimming with fake confidence.

"Go for the Comet Ride not the *Chronicle* Ride. It's up to us." This confused some folks. "What do you mean, it's up to us?" some asked. It was sad that I had to explain this original Critical Mass concept to so many people but such was the success of the Owner. Still, people usually like the idea of democracy when you explain it.

A few riders made applesauce and vodka jokes, referring to the Southern California mass suicide a few days earlier. Still I got the sense that the Comet Ride was gaining support. Yet I couldn't hand out fliers to everybody. I had a few hundred fliers but there were thousands of riders. I looked for messengers but most were still work-bound. And where was Dave Powers? He was the bum who'd got me in this mess! I handed out another flier.

"I've already got one for the Comet Ride."

All right! Dave *was* there with his fliers. A few more people said they'd received his fliers. For them I changed tactics.

"Well then take the cute flier." The cute flier (mine) was a way to add a humorous touch to our argument. Now it was 6:00, the usual getaway time.

I was too nervous to mount the garbage can to call for the vote so I conned Lx to do it. He called for the vote but there was too much noise. Then a cop got on the police bullhorn. His amplified voice helped still the crowd and he called for the voice vote. The crowd delivered an awesome roar for the Comet Ride, bounding off the highrises and making their windows shudder, sending flocks of pigeons flying. The response to the Owner's route was a pathetic scattering of groans and sarcastic bleatings.

It was a landslide. We stood silent for a moment not quite sure of our deed. Then, even before the police announced the obvious results, I was slapping high

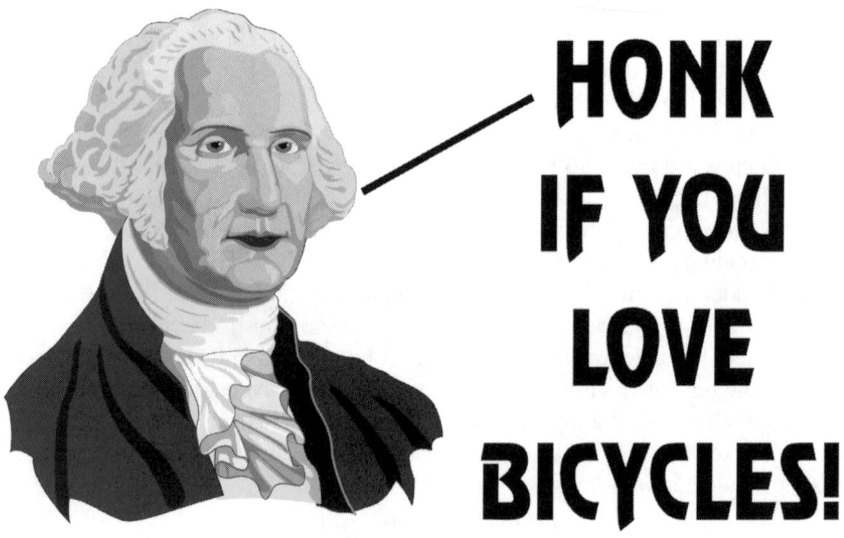
HONK
IF YOU
LOVE
BICYCLES!

5's with Lx and Eric Scudder. We had done it! We had battled the Owner in a fair fight and squashed him like a bug!

When I saw the Owner a few minutes later he was jabbering frantically about the riders who wanted to go to Nob Hill and now wouldn't be able to. Why? Did the vote make it illegal to go there?

Then he spouted some ridiculous prediction that the century's brightest comet would be invisible from Alta Plaza. And when he said to Eric "This just goes to show—" I interrupted him—a difficult task—and snapped, "This just goes to show that you don't mess with messengers!"

But I really didn't feel like arguing so I set up my mini-box and popped in my Charlie Parker tape. The energetic opening notes of "Now's the Time" announced the start of the 55th Critical Mass.

"Hale Bopp! Hail Bop!" I yelled euphorically. "Bird lives! Diz lives! Monk, Miles, Prez . . . Mingus! They all live! Just listen!" I cranked the volume.

"I subscribe to that theory," Beth declared as she glided by on her one speed.

From there the ride itself was almost anti-climactic. We rode past the Wall at 6:30, empty now except for the ghosts of too many long gone messengers. A few blocks up Sansome we turned right to boogaloo down Broadway. From funky Broadway we turned onto the Embarcadero. Near Herb Caen Way we broke up an altercation between a Masser and a ped. I was still so dizzy with euphoria that I couldn't feel any anger toward any of my fellow creatures. Maybe H.G. Wells was right. Maybe the comet would bring The Change.

I discussed bop music with a musician who was a former criminal psychotic. When "President" Lester Young began his driving tenor sax solo on his great tune "Lester Leaps In" we listened silently not because the Prez is dead but because the Prez lives! Some of us helped Lx fix his flat in front of Slim's and then caught up with the Mass on Polk Street. As we rode north our eyes scanned the northwestern sky. Still no comet. Could the Owner be right? But as we rode onto Alta Plaza it appeared above us. Soon I was eating salt peanuts, listening to "Now's the Time" again and viewing Hale Bopp with my binoculars which I shared with others.

Then, perhaps seeking revenge, the Owner approached me and started talking to me. But he was foiled by my beloved Omi who arrived from work on her bike. I snubbed the hapless Owner and walked over to embrace my favorite pastry chef.

The alternate Critical Mass arrived. Another group of riders had started at a different location and had taken their own route to Alta Plaza. They were also glad to hear that we'd thwarted the nefarious plots of the Owner. And so the 55th Critical Mass ended under the celestial wink of the bright comet which had inspired a motley gang of cyclists to recapture the original spirit of Critical Mass. Hale Bopp! Hail Bop!

UPDATE 2002: Many changes did occur that year. We almost lost Critical Mass as it endured its greatest crisis that summer of 1997. But CM emerged stronger than ever as the riders regained control of the Mass from politicians as well as the Owner. That was also the year San Francisco bike messengers began our collective quest for greater job rights and union power.

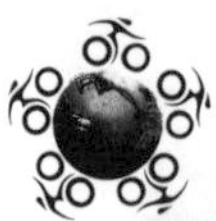

U.S. Gallery

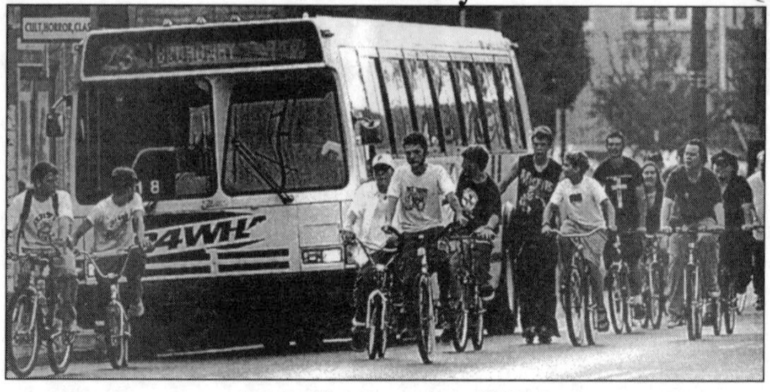

Louisville, Kentucky, 1997

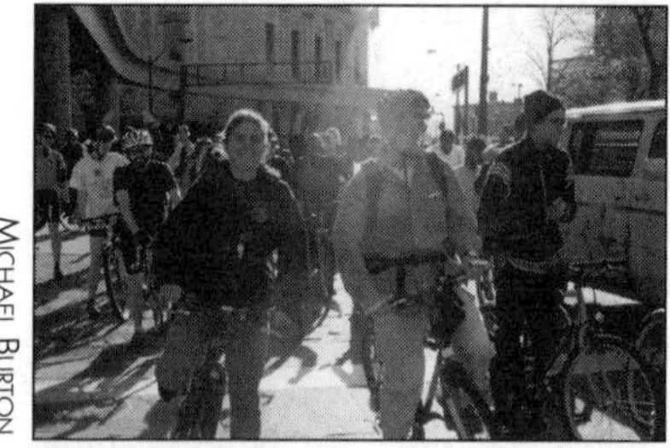

MICHAEL BURTON

Detroit, Michigan, 2001

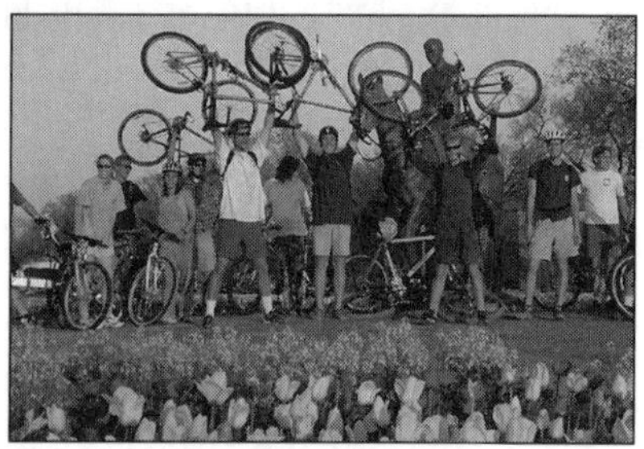

Lubbock, Texas

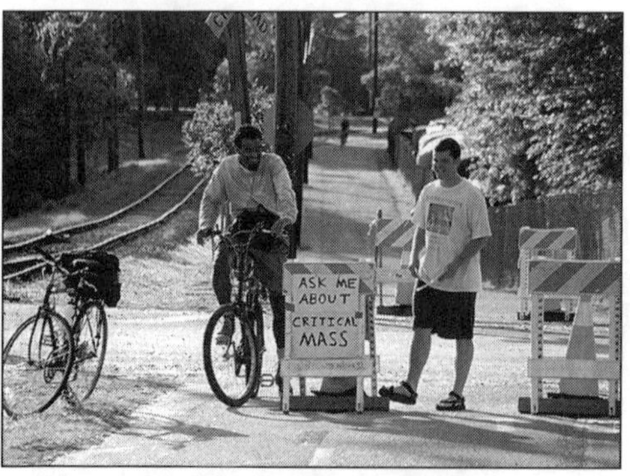

ASK ME
ABOUT
CRITICAL
MASS

Chapel Hill, North Carolina

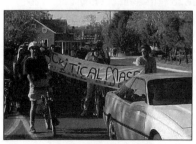

CRITICAL MASS

Santa Fe, New Mexico

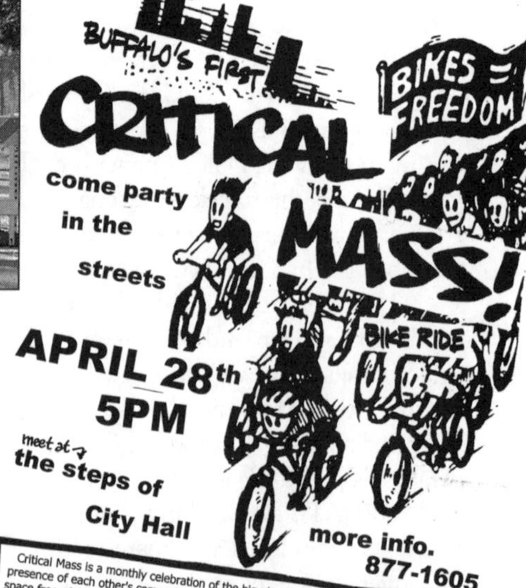

BUFFALO'S FIRST
CRITICAL
MASS!
BIKES = FREEDOM
BIKE RIDE
come party
in the
streets
APRIL 28th
5PM
meet at the steps of
City Hall
more info.
877-1605
Critical Mass is a monthly celebration of the bicycle. It's main purpose is to enjoy the presence of each other's company as we ride home together. It's about creating a public space free of transactions, free of buying, supplying, and selling--an alternative approach to urban life. There are no organizers or sponsors, just people wanting to make the streets a little safer for bicyclists...

Buffalo, New York

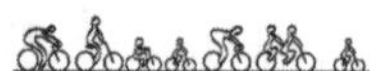

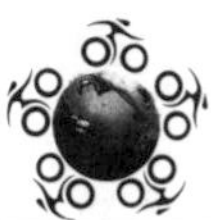

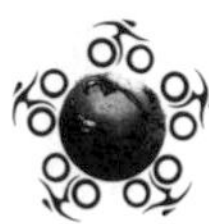

U.S. Gallery

I Ride A Bike
Because
I Can't Afford A Car

I cant afford to pollute my city,

I cant afford to support the domination of the oil and insurance industries,

I cant afford to ~~put~~ risk others' lives,

I cant afford to get commuter stress,

I can't afford to miss...

CRITICAL MASS

That one time each month when I get together with all my friends who ride bikes and ride as if we didn't have to be scared for our very lives, as if auto-domination was a thing of the past, as if our community was people-scaled.

Last Friday of Each Month
July 25th 5^15 ← not the price
City Hall Park
all non-motorized transport encouraged to attend.

: The CRANK, Burlington VT

Burlington, Vermont

Critical Mass

friday, june 29 at 5:00 pm
after that, the last friday of every month.
Critical Mass is pure, simple, spontaneous fun, a group bike ride to increase visibility for bicyclers and bicycle rights. we are not blocking traffic, we are traffic. meet at cannon park, downtown at rutledge and calhoun.
www.charlestoncriticalmass.com

Charleston, South Carolina

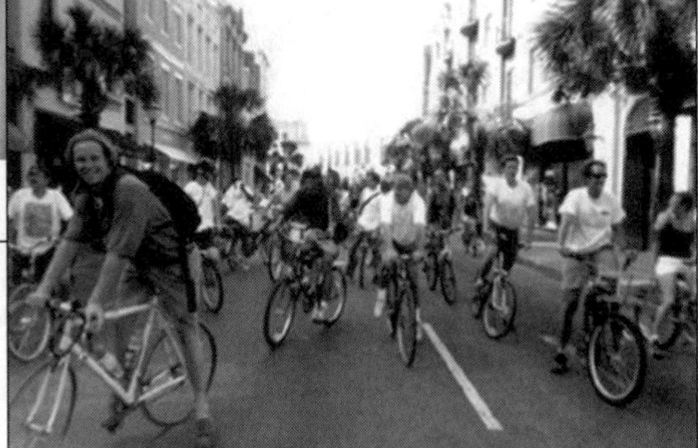

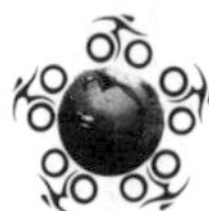

U.S. Gallery

Santa Rosa, California

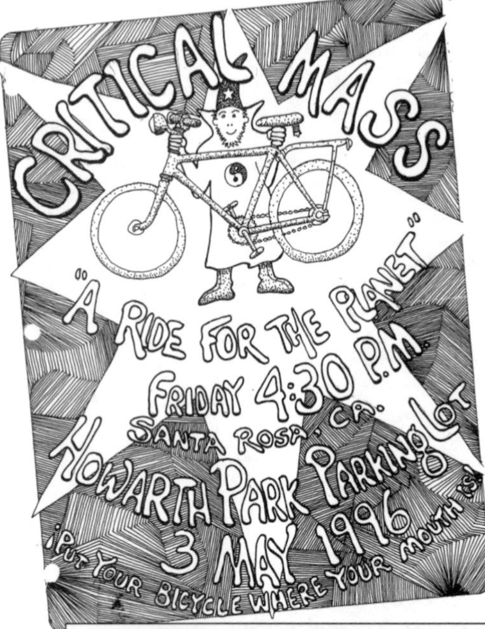
CRITICAL MASS
"A RIDE FOR THE PLANET"
FRIDAY 4:30 P.M.
SANTA ROSA, CA.
HOWARTH PARK PARKING LOT
3 MAY 1996
¡PUT YOUR BICYCLE WHERE YOUR MOUTH IS!

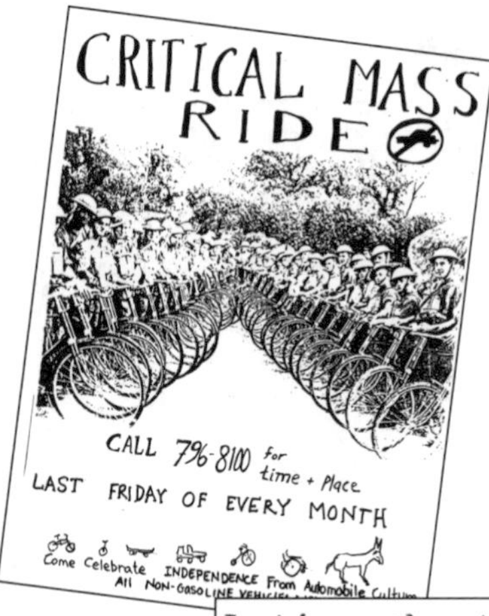

Portland, Oregon

let's make the streets of Champaign-Urbana safer...

FOR BIKES

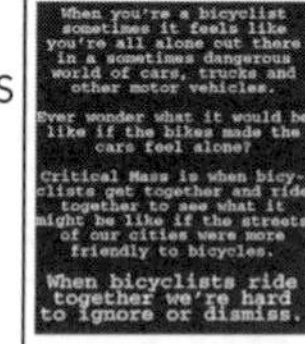

When you're a bicyclist sometimes it feels like you're all alone out there in a sometimes dangerous world of cars, trucks and other motor vehicles.

Ever wonder what it would be like if the bikes made the cars feel alone?

Critical Mass is when bicyclists get together and ride together to see what it might be like if the streets of our cities were more friendly to bicycles.

When bicyclists ride together we're hard to ignore or dismiss.

Ride with Champaign-Urbana Critical Mass the last Friday of every Month 5:00 PM at The Alma Mater

CMI Critical Mass
http://critical-mass.groogroo.com

Champaign-Urbana, Illinois

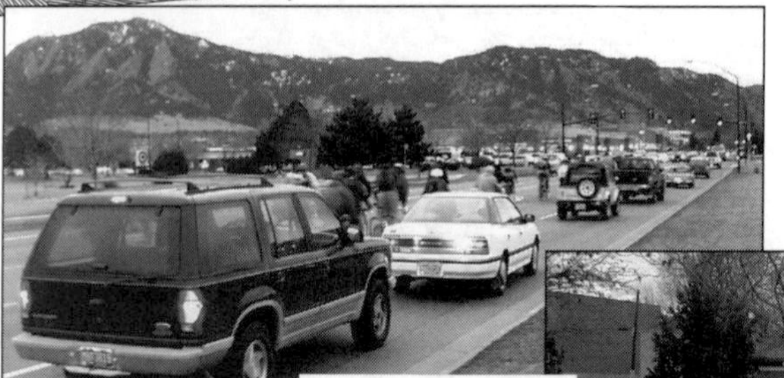

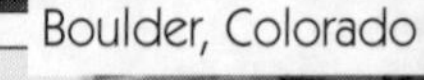

Boulder, Colorado

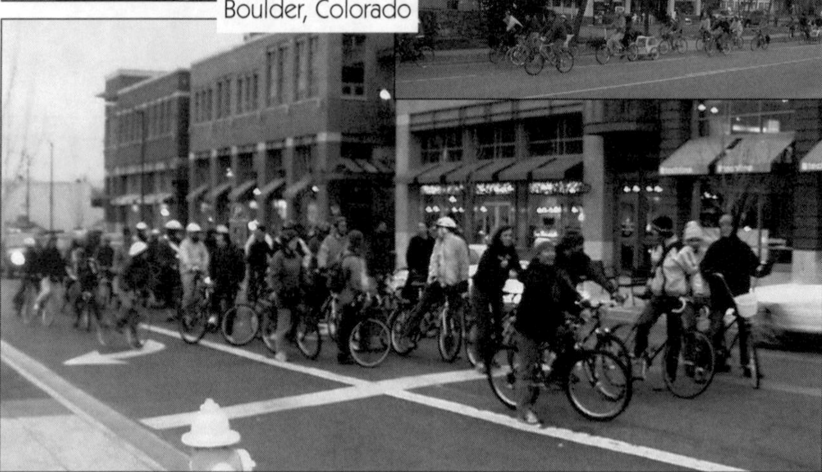

MAKING MEDIA, MAKING HISTORY

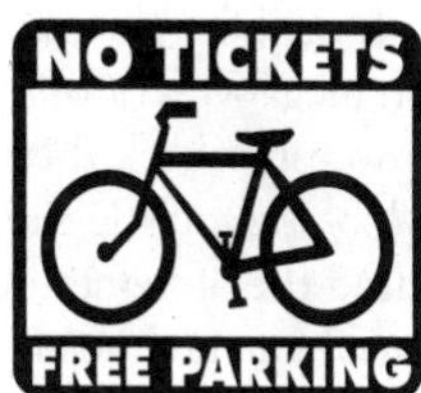

THE VELORUTION WILL NOT BE DIGITIZED

BY JYM DYER

It's April 9th, 1993, and I'm pedaling furiously through the streets of Berkeley, California, trying to find the Critical Mass ride. Berkeley's first CM had taken place a month earlier, but I didn't find out about it until afterwards, from a ride report I saw on the Internet. I didn't want to miss the second one, but I was running late, for reasons that also had something to do with the Internet.

You see, earlier that day I was at work and didn't know when and where the ride was starting, so I went online, looking for this simple information. Instead I chanced into the middle of a heated argument about Critical Mass. Apparently, according to one contributor, having 100 or so bicyclists on the streets was going to bring the entire city to a standstill, and thousands of pissed-off motorists (always "pissed-off," never "angered" or even "PO'ed") were going to respond by running us cyclists off the road. Yes, even right-thinking cyclists like myself, who were well-versed in the law-abiding techniques of vehicular cycling. Oh, and the bad publicity was going to set the cause of bicycle advocacy back a few centuries.

And so on. There I was, with my bike gloves already on, sitting in my cubicle and impatiently slogging through megabytes of this sort of thing. The Internet didn't have search engines or even websites back then, and it was slow going. By the time I finally found what I was looking for, the ride had already started. No problem, I thought, I'll just have to find the aforementioned apocalyptic traffic jam, or merely some signs of a wave of mayhem, and head for the epicenter.

Except that I found no such thing. I went all over the city as fast as I could, while timidly conforming to every law on the books or even imagined to be, so as not to draw the ire of those pissed-off legions. Eventually I realized that drivers weren't acting any worse than usual. I stopped now and then to ask people whether they'd seen a traffic jam or even just a bunch of bicyclists. Most of them had noticed nothing, but twice somebody pointed me to where the bikes had gone, which led me to, well, nothing unusual. Until I found a discarded flier with the route

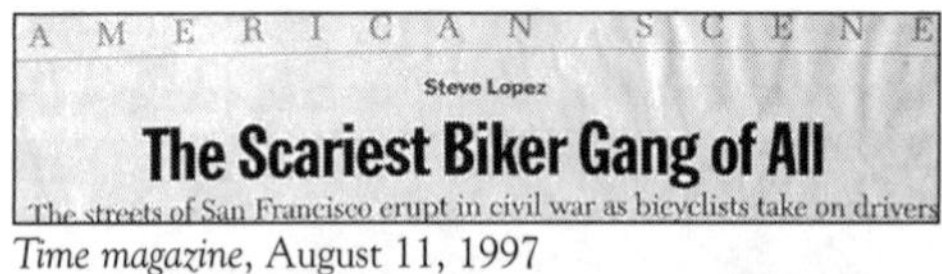
AMERICAN SCENE

Steve Lopez

The Scariest Biker Gang of All

The streets of San Francisco erupt in civil war as bicyclists take on drivers

Time magazine, August 11, 1997

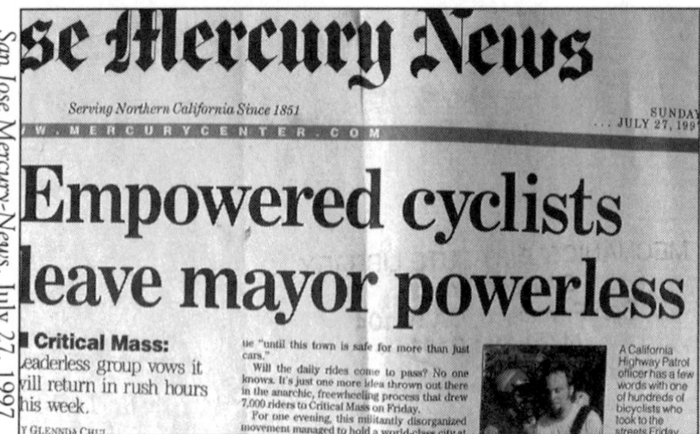
se Mercury News

Serving Northern California Since 1851

SUNDAY ... JULY 27, 199

W.MERCURYCENTER.COM

Empowered cyclists leave mayor powerless

Critical Mass: Leaderless group vows it will return in rush hours this week.

Y GLENNDA CHUI

ue "until this town is safe for more than just cars."

Will the daily rides come to pass? No one knows. It's just one more idea thrown out there in the anarchic, freewheeling process that drew 7,000 riders to Critical Mass on Friday.

For one evening, this militantly disorganized movement managed to hold a world-class city at

A California Highway Patrol officer has a few words with one of hundreds of bicyclists who took to the streets Friday

San Jose Mercury-News, July 27, 1997

drawn onto it, and followed it and found, well, not much of anything.

I gave up and went home. And, of course, went online to report what I'd seen. It didn't seem to have much impact.

A month later I showed up on time and counted 150 cyclists there. I didn't know any of them, but after talking to a few people I matched one face to an email address. Everyone started ringing their bicycle bells and the ride took to the streets.

The first thing I noticed was exhilaration. This was a rolling street party, a celebration, and the feeling was in the air like electricity. The sheer physicality of it was something like a charity bike race, but even more like a dance floor. Many of us were everyday bicyclists with environmental leanings, and we'd been wondering where all the others were, and here we all were, dancing with each other. A new culture was growing right under our wheels.

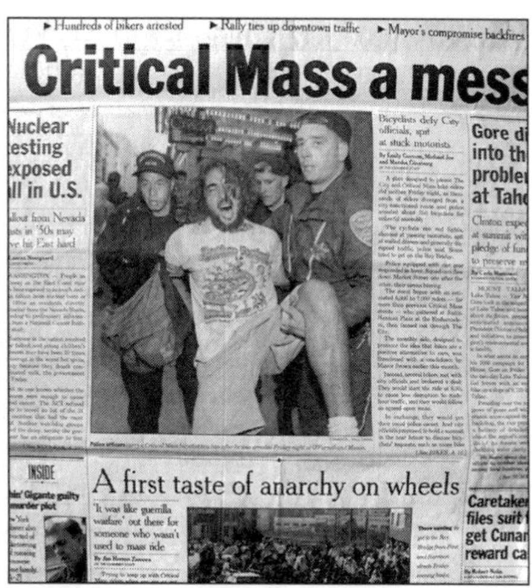
▸ Hundreds of bikers arrested ▸ Rally ties up downtown traffic ▸ Mayor's compromise backfires

Critical Mass a mess

Nuclear testing exposed all in U.S.

Fallout from Nevada tests in '50s may have hit East hard

Bicyclists defy City officials, spit at stuck motorists

Gore dives into the problem at Tahoe

Clinton expected at summit with pledge of funds to preserve

INSIDE

A first taste of anarchy on wheels

'It was like guerrilla warfare' out there for someone who wasn't used to mass ride

Caretaker files suit to get Cunanan reward cash

San Francisco Examiner, July 26, 1997

The second thing I noticed was more exhilaration, the freedom of being right out there on the street without having to constantly defend our right to do so, one on one against a heavily-armed aggressor. . . A freedom some of us hadn't felt since childhood, if ever. All told, this ride was the social event of the year for me, and if it was a demonstration, it was a new and a very much improved form of it.

I took a look at the motorists we encountered, and indeed a few of them did seem angry, so there was a germ of truth in *that* assertion. Yet it didn't seem that there were any more angry motorists than normal, and most of them just had the same bored look you usually see on people in cars. I was surprised, in fact astonished, to see how many of them were delighted to see us. Some were giggling in their seats with unconcealable glee. This was a minority of the car-dwellers, but a pretty large minority, and it included just about all of the children. A lot of pedestrians, too, stood by and cheered us along.

I didn't like everything about the ride. There was a small contingent I dubbed the Young Obnoxious White Males, who spent their time berating everyone in sight. There was also a "Two Wheels Good, Four Wheels Bad" chant, which is sort of funny in an ironic way, but the people I talked to had never read George Orwell's *Animal Farm*, which made me uneasy.

That stuff aside, the actual real-life experience of the ride made me the newest, biggest fan of Critical Mass. I gushed about it to everyone I knew. I rounded up friends and brought them on the next ride, and the ride after that. I made new friends in the ride and even in the cars stopped by the ride. Of course, I also went online and wrote up a glowing report, but I wrote it warts and all, like a good journalist. It didn't seem to have much impact.

In the months and years to follow, I started going on these rides every month, then twice a month, then every week. While elements of that first ride—the exhilaration and the warts—have been constant, Critical Mass was ever-changing. It evolved in ways that nobody could predict, with a full-fledged culture blooming all around it. It's spread to 300 cities so far, on every continent but one—Antarctica is the stubborn holdout.

The Internet also changed, and I found it a useful tool for creating and maintaining a list of every Critical Mass ride I can find. Naturally, I keep the list on a website:

http://www.critical-mass.org/

As my enthusiasm grew, I started to plan vacations so that I'd be in certain cities on the last (or whichever) Friday of the month, to go on the ride and meet the local Massers in person. Every locale has its own unique style and culture.

On the Internet, though, I kept running into an alternate reality Critical Mass, one that's the same in every city and never seems to change. Online, the ride is forever creating traffic jams, undermining the authority of STOP signs, and setting back the cause of vehicular cycling.

To some people, this is the only reality of Critical Mass. Eight years after slogging through that first heated argument, I met a friendly bicyclist while riding through Atlanta, Georgia. We talked about a few things, and eventually conversation turned to the Atlanta CM, which was starting to come into its own. "Oh, I'd never go on that," he said, "It just pisses off the drivers." Or so he'd read on the Internet.

Additional online forums have popped up, though, with contributors who have actually participated in the ride and who write from that experience. In a 1997 *Wired* article, Ashley Craddock wrote that "the Net offers a communications forum that almost perfectly mirrors the ride's structure—or lack thereof." This refers to the leaderless nature of most of the rides, and that is indeed mirrored by unmoderated forums which are open to all, but these forums also tend to feature many nonparticipants who spend a lot of time talking about the alternate reality Critical Mass.

Structural similarities notwithstanding, online forums can never hope to really reflect the immediate experience of the ride. Pedalling and moving puts your body and mind in a very different state than sitting in front of a screen, and talking to someone in person involves many channels of communication that simply cannot be digitized.

Since CM and the Net made a big splash at about the same time, there are those who blur the two realities together, to the point where some spend more time dealing with these online forums than on the ride itself. Part of this is dealing with factions and would-be leaders or owners of the ride, part with the neverending heated argument, and part with the inevitable communications glitches that come with the medium's limitations. Craddock did note that, at one point, the discourse in San Francisco's online forums got so out of hand that it had to be resolved with a face-to-face meeting.

A friend of mine found a very moving account of a Critical Mass ride online and reposted it to seven bicycle-oriented email lists, not knowing that this would touch off The Great Flamewar of 1999 (as we've come to call it). For some reason, and I think January cabin fever was involved, this attracted a lot of comment, and comments about the comment. The discussion spread to other email lists, and soon there were hundreds of messages, some of them pretty nasty.

It turned into a showdown between Critical Mass participants and the alternate reality CM. Tempers flared, mailboxes overflowed, and a number of the email lists became moderated forums with closed memberships. When the smoke cleared, I combed through the smoldering embers and discovered a number of original insights. They didn't seem to have much impact. (Some of them were dusted off and published in a magazine named *Bike Culture Quarterly*, though.)

A more familiar alternate reality started showing up when the news media discovered Critical Mass. Orwell once said that no event is ever correctly reported, and coverage of the ride has borne him out.

The media predictably oversimplifies Critical Mass. Usually this has taken the form of seeking out a leader or spokesperson for the ride, somebody who could summarize everything in a soundbite, or a few column-inches, depending. Yet in city after city, reporters walk away scratching their heads because nobody can name such a person.

Those of us who participate in the ride can see that it's not something anyone could "lead" in any meaningful sense of the word. As for spokespeople, ask three participants what the ride is about and their answers may contradict each other. This is easy to understand when you experience the ride directly, but not something most reporters have been able to convey.

Media coverage of demonstrations was turned into a formula not long after the 1960s wound down: Explain the reason for the demonstration in as few words as possible, but not so many words that the reader or viewer could understand why. Show only portions of the crowd, never the whole thing, and always quote an authority's underestimate of the turnout, dismissively reducing the event to its "body count." If there's any conflict, find an authority to blame it on the demonstrators and, if it comes to that, overestimate the number of arrests.

These have all been applied to Critical Mass, sometimes with the usual humdrum result, but at other times in very amusing ways. I've seen a TV anchor announcing that the ride's purpose was to win bike lanes, while behind her people rolled by with signs demanding rail transit and the banning of car alarms. I've seen footage of smiling cyclists riding through traffic, while the anchor tries to convince viewers angry protesters are causing gridlock.

The media has an online presence these days, which leads to a compound alternate reality effect: doubly-mediated discourse based on inaccurate news stories. Online forums do provide the opportunity to make unedited rebuttals, but there are still plenty of people who still trust the "unbiased" authority of the media over the "biased" accounts of actual participants.

The media, by the way, never says "pissed off." However, they eventually do manage to get around to announcing that some ride or other turned out to be a

"... [pause for effect] ... Critical Mess."

Since Critical Mass usually only takes place once a month, people in most locales only know about it from the news media, if they've heard of it at all. They're often very surprised when they encounter it in real life and see a rolling celebration instead of an angry protest, and they can even learn something about us, when somebody hands them a flier.

One thing that's pretty consistent with CMs all over the world is the use of a classic solution to a deeply flawed news media: creating media of your own. A "xerocracy" of fliers and zines have been part of the ride from its inception, and since then the ride and the culture that's grown from it has expressed itself in publications, posters, and documentaries, and some of the expression has made the leap from media to art.

There are also online self-created media efforts, notably Indymedia, but these have not been entirely immune from trouble. I once went on the Vancouver CM with a local activist who wore a wonderful heart-shaped "Reclaim the Streets for People" sign on her back. Later I looked at the Vancouver Indymedia website and discovered that somebody had downloaded a photo of her with her sign, and digitally altered it so that the sign displayed a racist message.

Naturally, this led to a heated online discussion that careened into an alternate reality. It is to the credit of the Indymedia concept that the creator of the bogus photo was not perceived as a media authority, but those of us who'd seen the original sign with our own eyes had to upload some of our own photos to really convince people that the altered photo was a hoax.

The self-made media is a fine form of outreach, but at its best, can only show part of the picture. It's a fine accessory to the ride, but no substitute.

Critical Mass is so important because it is a direct, unmediated experience. In our culture, vast numbers of people experience much of their lives though mass media. They may even know that the spectacle on the TV is all lies, but it still has their eyes and ears, so it also has some of their minds.

We were not meant to live our lives separated from reality by a pane of glass. Mediated experience through a television or computer screen—or for that matter, a car's windshield—keeps us distanced from what is real, and from each other. Critical Mass helps us take back our streets, but we're also taking back our lives. And that's something that has a lot of impact.

Nine-time championship race car driver and heir to a vast family oil fortune, Jym Dyer was driving one of his stretch limo SUVs on the road to Damascus when he saw a great light coming from the heavens — which turned out to be one of his family's refineries going up in flames. He traded in the limo for a bicycle and never looked back.

REELS ON WHEELS

BY TED WHITE

Movers and Shakers

My life in bicycle culture and politics started in 1990. It was the 20th anniversary of Earth Day and some people had organized a bike ride to celebrate bicycling and challenge car-dependence. The flyers announced "Bicycles Aren't in the Way, They Are the Way!" When I look back on it now, the foreshadowing of Critical Mass is amazing: the Critical Mass rallying cry of "We Aren't Blocking Traffic, We Are Traffic!" is essentially the same motto.

As I anticipated the 1990 Earth Day ride I got more and more excited. I realized that the bicycle movement was my movement, the thing I'd been waiting for. It was fresh and fun and feisty. The vibe around other political causes totally depressed me. They seemed whiny and embittered, and centered on issues which were happening in other countries. I felt we should deal with our own shit first, and in America, car-dependence is our shit. This Earth Day bike ride seemed to have a similar spirit to the punk rock scene which had been a real important thing to me in my younger days. I liked the combination of joyfulness and rebellion which appeared to be the essence of this fledgling bike movement.

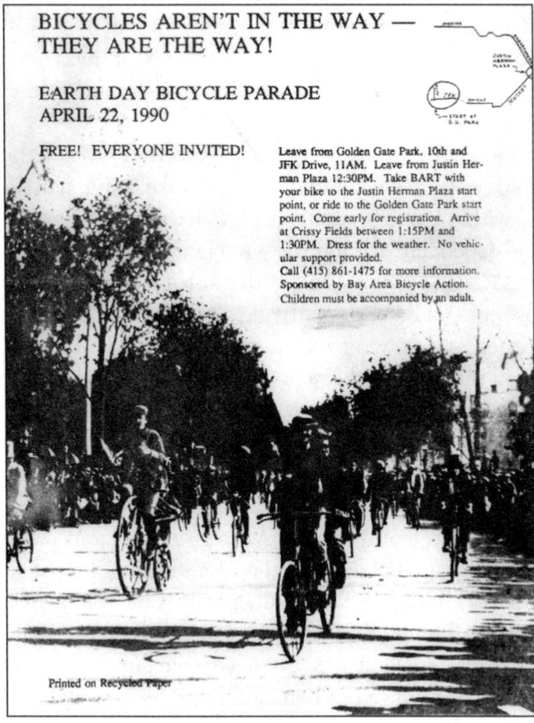
BICYCLES AREN'T IN THE WAY —
THEY ARE THE WAY!
EARTH DAY BICYCLE PARADE
APRIL 22, 1990
FREE! EVERYONE INVITED!
Leave from Golden Gate Park, 10th and JFK Drive, 11AM. Leave from Justin Herman Plaza 12:30PM. Take BART with your bike to the Justin Herman Plaza start point, or ride to the Golden Gate Park start point. Come early for registration. Arrive at Crissy Fields between 1:15PM and 1:30PM. Dress for the weather. No vehicular support provided.
Call (415) 861-1475 for more information.
Sponsored by Bay Area Bicycle Action.
Children must be accompanied by an adult.
Printed on Recycled Paper

The political bike movement had a new vocabulary and rules. It was almost completely pro-active. If you didn't ride a bike, well then you weren't part of the movement, were you? You couldn't just learn the jargon, get a t-shirt and be a bike radical. There was no established bike movement infrastructure back then either, it was all just being created, and by hand at that. It was a political and cultural frontier.

There were already a few bike activists out there but you could count 'em on one hand. One key figure was John Dowlin in Philadelphia, who published perhaps the first bike activist 'zine in the eighties: *Network*

News. It was like an *Utne Reader* for bike issues. He'd cut and paste articles and graphics from newspapers and magazines all around the world. He compiled all this stuff about bicycling, and related urban development and health issues and created a new context. It was all about bikes as transportation (and even transformation), not racing and sportsy-type biking, so reading it, you got a sense that bike advocacy was a new issue rising up on the global agenda. Since I was a filmmaker, John's *Network News* really inspired me to give the bike movement some more of its own imagery, stories and commentary.

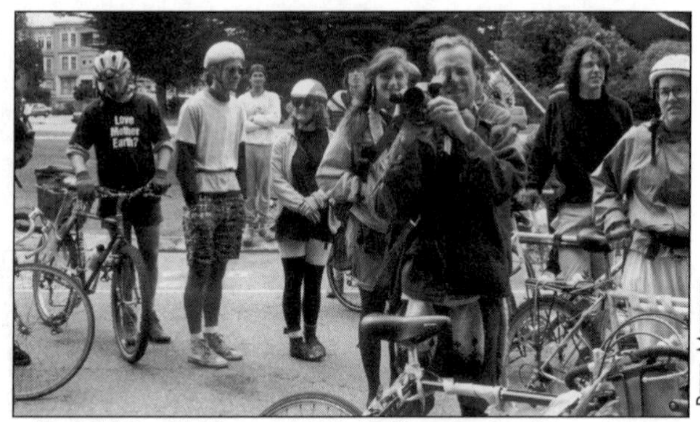

Ted White filming at 1991 SF Bicycle Coalition Auto-Free Golden Gate Park rally.

Charlie Komanoff, John Orcutt, and Cindy Arlinsky were doing great bike work with the group Transportation Alternatives, a serious political organization fighting New York City bureaucrats over bike policies and infrastructure. Around Boston, Mira Brown and Carl Kurz were doing cool work with Bikes Not Bombs locally and in Central America. Bikes Not Bombs began more or less as a recycling and relief effort sending fixed-up bikes from the U.S. to the poor in Central America. They were all pioneers. However, their work hadn't quite found "Mass" appeal yet, so to speak.

Before long though, the hundredth monkey dynamic started. Through the grapevine I heard that a lot of hip people were coming onto this bike thing more or less simultaneously. For anybody with a liberalish political conscious, it became clear that car culture and our fossil-fuel dependent economy was to blame for myriad environmental, economic, and even social problems. You'd better at least start questioning cars and considering the possibility of bikes or be the biggest lame-ass hypocrite.

The Earth Day ride happened and it was even more fun than I had hoped for. There was a surprisingly good turnout. In the years since, I've pretended that there were about two hundred people on the ride, which can't possibly be true, but I'm sure there were at least fifty. Anyway, it felt like a lot. I don't think I knew one person, but as we rode through the city I felt a lot of camaraderie, like I was part of a really fun gang.

I took my super 8 camera to the ride and shot a few rolls. Aside from being excited about the whole bike thing it was also a real turn-on for me as a filmmaker. I rode my single-speed cruiser with one hand on the handlebar and one holding the camera. The footage came back all bumpy and chaotic, but sort of beautifully insane. To quote—I think—a cigarette jingle, it was "alive with pleasure." I did get a lot of horrible, unwatchable, dizzying footage but here and there I got some flowing, elegant stuff. The subject matter was pretty interesting too: imagery of adults having fun together on bicycles. It was obviously not a sports event. The bicyclists were too diverse and weren't wearing bike racing clothes. They were short, fat, tall, skinny and were wearing overalls, wide brimmed hats, sun dresses, plaid sport coats, bow ties, you name it... so somehow it had more of an eccentric picnic-on-wheels feel—it was just irresistible. As I reviewed this footage, I became dazzled with the possibilities of filming from a bike and impassioned with the sense that I had found a political cause that really "spoke" to me (pun intended).

Soon after, I began working on my first real bike movie or "bikeumentary": *Return of the Scorcher*. Around this same time, I had seen a slide show on bike history presented by author and professor Iain Boal [see his "The World of the Bicycle" elsewhere in this volume], in which he described the whole legacy of bike radicalism, suffragettes in bloomers, bikers fighting for better roads a hundred years ago. It was fascinating. In *Scorcher* I wanted to combine radical bike history with the emerging bike renaissance and the surrounding environmental and social crises. Fortunately, I discovered George Bliss: a New York City bike tinkerer, designer, and visionary. He became the star of *Return of the Scorcher* and was a wonderful inspiration to many new bike activists, including myself. He is very articulate, fun, inventive and kind of offhandedly handsome. He looks more like a disheveled gym-teacher than another dredlocked tree-sitter type. People were ready for a new look and style of activist and he was a good example. He was not a policy wonk, not an academic (he's a college dropout), not a scruffy hippie freak, nor an embittered politico. His message about the power of bikes had a real warmth and sincerity.

In *Return of the Scorcher* I wanted to show societies which had fully integrated bicycling into the culture, like China and the Netherlands, and then ask why we weren't following a similar path. George Bliss and I went to China to check out the bike scene there and do some shooting. In the film George described the flow of bike and car traffic in China's cities as "a kind of Critical Mass thing" in which "the bikes come up to an intersection and wait till they have enough numbers to push through the cars and make them stop, and vice versa."

Scorcher came out at the right time and place (Summer of 1992, San Francisco, a few months before Critical Mass debuted) and with the right people watching. Chris Carlsson and Jim Swanson saw it the very first time it played publicly. Dave Snyder, Donald Francis, Bogart McAvoy, Travis Moraché, Sarah Winarski, Markus Fur and

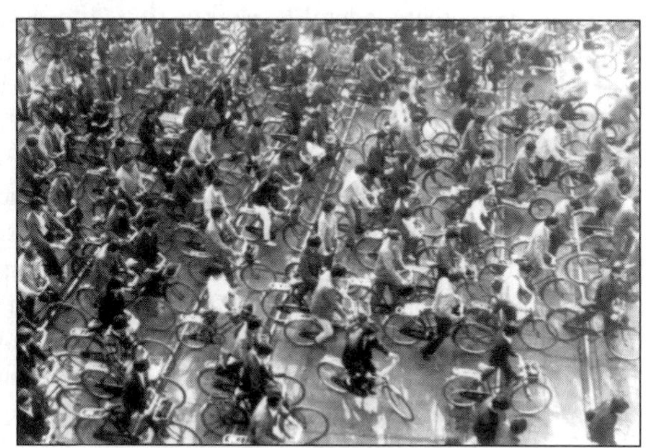

Normal bicycle traffic in China, c. 1990.

other early CM enthusiasts saw it right away too. That "Critical Mass" scene in China really struck a chord with people and within a couple months what had begun as the "Commute Clot" was being called "Critical Mass." So for the record, it was George Bliss who inadvertently named it "Critical Mass." I had no clue that my little film would accidentally help lend a name and some inspiration to an incredible new movement but I'm totally pleased that it turned out that way. As an independent filmmmaker you get used to not having enormous expectations, so this was wonderfully encouraging to me. I felt that George Bliss and I had contributed a little gem to the great continuous unfolding of folk culture.

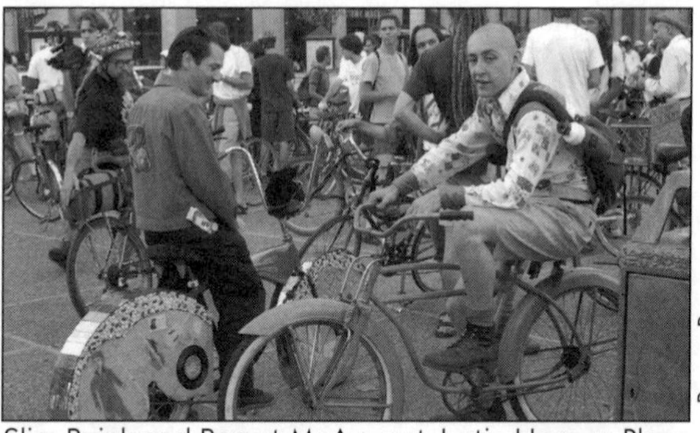

Pamela Palma

Slim Buick and Bogart McAvoy at Justin Herman Plaza as Critical Mass gathers sometime in early 1993.

Critical Mass is Born and Blossoms

When Critical Mass really got going it was exhilarating. It was fun and scary and had the thrill of seeming like a rebellious act, which it was, but it also had the feel-good element of promoting bikes, fun and sociality. Most of the Critical Mass riders would smile and wave at people on the sidewalks and on buses or even in cars. It felt really good to be nice to all the strangers who you normally just pass by but who are actually your fellow man. Within the Mass itself, the camaraderie was palpable; when everyone would go "whoooooop!!!" together it was completely joyous.

Obviously though, not everybody thought Critical Mass was so cool. I was really surprised to learn that some bike activists were strongly opposed to Critical Mass. Clearly, Critical Mass fulfilled so many of the elements lacking in "typical" bike activism: spontaneity, refusal to work within "the system," inclusivity, joyfulness, unapologetic creativity. But some long-time bike advocates felt that Critical Mass was too audacious and that there'd be a backlash against cyclists, setting their work back years. Many of these people formed strong opinions before ever going on a Critical Mass ride, and some never got around to going on one at all.

Frankly, I think Critical Mass gave the bike advocacy movement a bigger boost than anything had since maybe the suffragettes wearing "bloomers" in the late 1890's. Standard bike politics can be incredibly boring, tedious, and disempowering—a contrast to bicycling itself. Critical Mass (as with Food Not Bombs and Earth First!) has really breathed life into the issues it confronts by acting so directly and powerfully. Critical Mass shoved right through the quagmire of polite bike politics and asked huge questions and demanded, at the very least, attention (if not answers). Then, suddenly, everyone who was interested in bike politics—whether they hated or loved Critical Mass—had a much bigger audience. I remember seeing a front page story on the cover of *USA Today* about bicyclists becoming a powerful political force, and thinking "I guess we're having an impact now." So in the big sense I think all bike advocates benefitted from the attention that Critical Mass attracted.

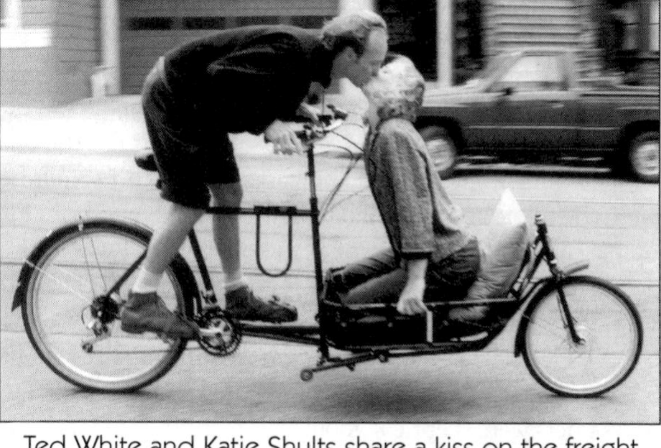

Ted White and Katie Shults share a kiss on the freight bike from which *We Are Traffic* was partly filmed.

As Critical Mass began to grow and expand and spring up in cities all around the globe I decided I should make a new bikeumentary: a sequel to *Scorcher* and a portrait of Critical Mass called *(We aren't blocking traffic,) We Are Traffic!* The making of *We Are Traffic!* was a real challenge, because to try and define Critical Mass seemed nearly impossible. It is so many different things to different people. It defies defining. Some people think it's about promoting bike lanes, others think it's about freeing ourselves from a dehumanizing, corporate-controlled, car-obessed world. Some people think Critical Mass should be well-behaved and others think it should be very flamboyant and full of piss and vinegar. All in all, it is the antithesis of a predictable, carefully controlled, sanctioned public event. It's totally about "what if?" All this made it a bit daunting to attempt to capture or portray CM in a movie.

The ownership of Critical Mass is collective and though several people collaborated with me on the film* (helped shoot, edit, etc.), ultimately it was a subjective presentation (but hey, that's personal expression for ya!). In fact, all informational media is subjective, and most mainstream media carries an insultingly simplistic, jingoist, exploitive message. In my films I try to lend a voice to the underheard, to achieve a better balance of perspectives. In this case, the big newspapers and TV news had represented Critical Mass pretty poorly so making this documentary was a chance for some of us who were really involved in Critical Mass to make our own movie. We had watched ourselves condescendingly portrayed in 10 second sound bites, and it was time for a rebuttal.

In 1996 I began shooting at most San Francisco Critical Masses. In the early years, I had gone on almost every ride but I hardly ever filmed. I just wanted to be there and enjoy it like everyone else. I didn't want to be documenting it and worrying about camera angles and all that. One time I towed a local musician, French accordionist Odile Levault in a trailer behind my bike during Critical Mass. It was like a live boom-box—people dug it, and that was fun. Then at a certain point, when I really decided to make the new film, I became the docu-

* Caitlin Manning cinematographer, Bill Daniel, Sharon Johnson, Katie Shults, Rock Ross, Julie Searle.

mentarian again, compelled to go out and shoot at every ride I could and try to capture enough moments to convey the feelings, stories, and spirit of the ride.

For a lot of my shooting, I used a special cargo-bicycle built by my friend Jan VanderTuin of Eugene, Oregon. It's a long wheel-base delivery bicycle which can carry two hundred pounds. One person would pilot the bike, and the camera person (usually me) would ride in the cargo rack. Bill Daniel, Erik Zo and my wife Katie were the pilots and they had to be both butch and brilliant because they had to ride up big hills and keep control of the bike while I was squirming around trying to get good shots. The bike was great for filming and also acted as an ice breaker when I wanted to interact with other riders in the Mass. It looked so unusual and was such a clever design that most people who saw it smiled or shouted "cool bike!" That created a friendliness and trust between me and the people I was filming. Many Critical Mass riders were skeptical about talking to the "media" because they knew that they were likely to be misrepresented. With my little camcorder and weird bike I think most people could tell I wasn't the big bad corporate media and that being in my film was probably an OK thing. One Halloween ride, I wore a skeleton mask the whole time I filmed and had some great interactions with people who didn't even know who I was or whether I was even human!

I shot footage here and there from early 1993 to 1996, but the main production was from 1997-1999, during which I also got video makers from various other cities to send me scenes of their rides. Through the Freedom of Information Act, I also got some footage shot by the Austin Texas Police Department which was very self-incriminating.

At last, after a couple years' focused work, *We Are Traffic!* premiered at the first BikeSummer gathering (July 1999) and has shown around quite a lot since then. It's been screened on PBS stations, on Belgian Televison and on FreeSpeech TV (a national cable network for activist videos). There have been tons of screenings at independent movie theaters, galleries, universities, bike events, and museums. It's shown at quite a few film festivals and been rejected from a few too. A lot of people have bought copies and had their own screenings; people in all parts of the U.S. and Europe.

I often get e-mails or letters back saying how the film provoked a good discussion, or sometimes even helped instigate a Critical Mass in that town. I think most people who saw it were at least temporarily inspired to ride a bike, and some became truly impassioned bikers. When I showed it in Chicago at the "Bike Winter" festival it was March and had been snowing for days but after the screening we all got out anyway and rode around all night sliding around in the ice and snow and having a blast. Both my bikeumentaries have played the "Bike-In" (not "Drive-In") movie night in Portland OR, which is a free show held outside under the stars. And interestingly, several people from different parts of the U.S. have contacted me to get the film for research because they were doing their college theses on Critical Mass.

Generally, the distribution has been very grassroots which seems appropriate to me. I distribute through my own website and via three other small distributors. Somebody told me I should sell it through Amazon.com. I thought about increased exposure versus collaborating with a ruthless corporation—it just felt weird to me, so I didn't do it. I did sell National Geographic Television some footage and I think they did a pretty good job with it. I didn't feel sleazy about that.

The most satisfying thing about making *We Are Traffic!* is that I've gotten to present it to so many people who previously knew nothing about Critical Mass or had only heard negative things. Almost everyone who sees the film realizes that there are wonderful aspects to Critical Mass. I recently showed excerpts to government officials and urban planners in Sacramento, California—some of whom were fairly straight-laced bureaucrats. After the screening, they were much more open to the strengths, creativity and independent spirit of Critical Mass. It's exciting to witness that sort of thoughtfulness and consideration as people open up. The scene that always gets people is the corking scene where the "Thanks for Waiting" sign flips to the "Honk if You Love Bicycles" sign. Most audiences find that strategy of sincere diplomacy sprinkled with mischevious humor to be irresistible.

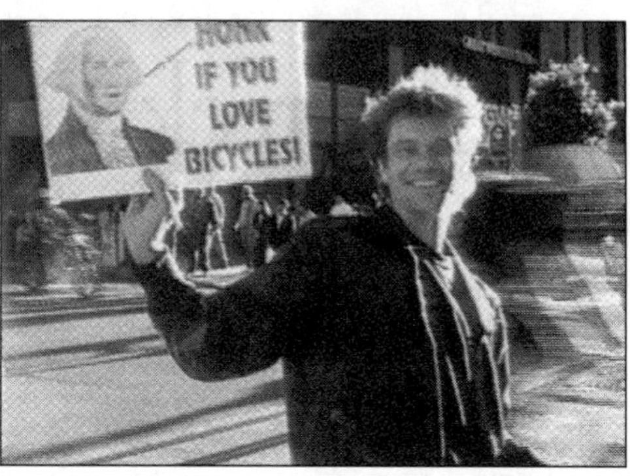

FROM *WE ARE TRAFFIC!*

Both Sides Now

Ironically, a few years after making the film, I became the Executive Director of the Sonoma County Bicycle Coalition, doing traditional bike advocacy. I have always been averse to this kind of work. Having to beg and plead with some really pathetic bureaucrats just to put in a bike lane or put up a few "Share the Road" signs is not empowering. Instead, we create our own programs and put on our own events. Most mainstream bike advocates find themselves going to endless meetings with politicians and trying to fit into their agendas. The idea of being on the offensive, of taking the lead and not just groveling for a little so-called respect is something I've tried to borrow from Critical Mass.

Our local bicycle coalition has been co-sponsoring a fundraising ride. It is ironic how much time, effort, promotion, insurance, route mapping, rest stops and support vehicles go into a ride that will probably have about 300-400 riders (about a third of the riders that come to a typical San Francisco Critical Mass). The beauty of Critical Mass is that it is so experiential, and as a friend once said, "its means is its ends." However Critical Mass doesn't directly result in more bike parking racks or bike access to trains, etc., so old-school political bike advocacy certainly still has its place too. I just wish that more bike advocates would realize that it doesn't all boil down simply to infrastructural changes. We can get all the new bike lanes we want, but we also have to be excited and personally motivated to get out there and actually ride. You can't just design and install new attitudes and lifestyles for people, they have to develop and flourish organically.

There are so many people who have a genuine interest, a passion even, for all kinds of civic, social and environmental causes. Unfortunately, many of them don't see how they can participate. There seem to be two choices. Run for elective office and go to meetings and be on committees, take bribes, do favors and all that. Or, alternatively, to be some sign-wielding, angry, protester nut-case. It's tragic that a nation that was practically founded on activist principles now suffers from such ambivalence, apathy, and passivity. In general, I would say that for most middle-American folks, both politics and activism are exceedingly uncool these days (except maybe waving a United We Stand flag against "terrorism").

That's why Critical Mass as a new model for activism and social change is so interesting. It enables many people to participate because there's no entry fee, no sign-up, no election, no paperwork, no insurance waiver, no membership card, no expectations. It's a context that invites anyone: the artist, the intellectual, the jock, the homeless person, the yuppie. This mix of people is stimulating, bizarre and wonderful. Critical Mass doesn't defer to "experts" for governance and that's also very appealing to many people. I think many people yearn for activities which are less controlled from above but they are afraid that "anti-authoritarian" has to mean chaos, immaturity, and destructiveness. So they end up feeling stuck.

To me, Critical Mass is akin to block parties, or potlucks or dressing up for Halloween or having a neighborhood clean-up. It's in the same tradition of street artists and musicians freely expressing themselves in public. These things are less organized and more organic, where the infrastructure and red tape don't overwhelm the simple good spirit which people want to bring to the event. All the bureaucracy and complexity that we've created (and now have to wade through to do much of what we do) is a real drag, a spirit-killer.

Personally, I don't believe in "top-down" change. I think change occurs best when it sprouts up in a small intimate arena and then it spreads to other intimate arenas and communities. Of course, in the process of spreading, ideas get tweaked and reshaped and rethought, which keeps it fun and stimulating for people. Then, as with Critical Mass, changes happen in a folk-movement style. I think government and official agencies should be the last to get on board with social change. For example, with recycling it took a generation of dedicated hippies to start funky little recycling centers in parking lots and educate people and get kids out there having fun smashing aluminum cans. Now, a few decades later we've got curbside recycling. Let government in when it's all set up for a slam dunk. They should follow, not lead. We'll be the hearts and minds of this velorution, and they are welcome to assist us.

As an independent media producer, working in the huge and constant shadow of mainstream media, trying to make one's voice heard through small, low-budget independent channels can sometimes appear improbable, even pathetic. Fortunately, I've been happily shocked at how much hope Critical Mass has given me for what can be done on a small scale yet still have a far-reaching impact on society. Into gloomy and oppresive urban environments Critical Mass has brought magic and I feel very lucky to have been able to document and disseminate some of that magic.

Madison, Wisconsin

"IF YOU DON'T MOVE, I'LL RUN YOU DOWN!"

BY JESSICA BECKER

Madison, Wisconsin has historically been called an activist town. I had been exposed to different incarnations of Critical Mass while living in DC and Austin and, when planning to move back to Madison after several years away, looked forward to finding an active Critical Mass community. While bike trails run through much of the downtown area, bike commuters are highly visible, and "Share the road with bikes" bumper stickers are common on local cars, I was disappointed to find only a few references to a Madison Critical Mass-style ride in 1995. It was not until I had been in town for a few months that I saw a flyer for a showing of the film *We are Traffic* at a local coffeehouse's independent film night.

It was difficult to find bike parking that night—-all the signposts, trees and fences were already crowded with bikes when I rode up. The event was sold out, but I managed to squeeze in. The first film was a locally made documentary called *Pedalphiles*, produced by Brian Standing, about a group of Madison anarchists who scavenge parts and build bikes. *We are Traffic*, Ted White's now classic documentary of the origins of the Critical Mass rides, followed.

After the movie was over, someone in the crowd yelled "So, when's the ride?" The call fell on dead silence. Being new to town, I was emboldened by my anonymity and took up the call. I made some posters inviting people to meet on the last Friday of the month and put them up all around town.

The first of what are now regular monthly rides was in April of 2001. I had optimistically envisioned a modest beginning, so was thrilled as the group of about 50 riders gathered. The energy was palpable as I walked amongst the crowd passing out maps of a suggested route. *En masse* we charged full force down West Washington, the main boulevard in town. Bikers spread across the wide artery casually, yet full of steam. The ride meandered, sticking loosely to the route, shifting as the mood and leaderless decision-making process dictated. We relaxed into the beautiful groove of Critical Mass: leisurely travel, quiet streets, friendly conversation.

About 30 minutes into the ride, the group turned onto a three-lane, one-way artery that carries

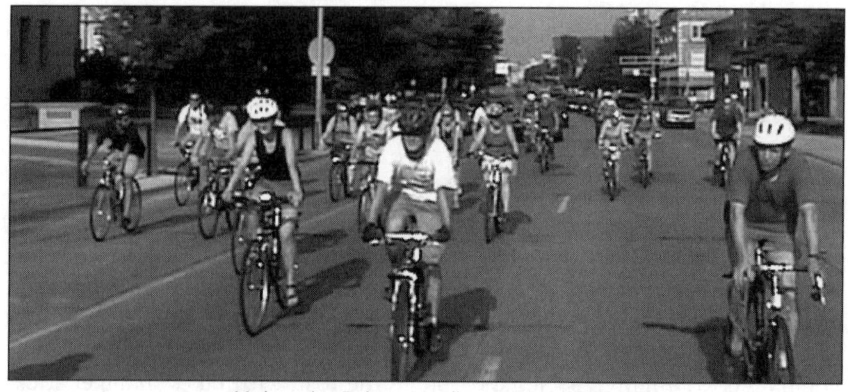

Matt Logan

University Drive, Madison, May 2001

rush-hour traffic out of Madison. Traffic behind us backed up, probably for miles. I understood that not all the honking was for the love of bikes. The car driver immediately on our tail yelled "If you don't move, I'll run you down."

And then he did.

He hit a cyclist named Kurt. He used his car as a weapon. He also made what had been slowly progressing traffic into a completely congested accident scene. For the next two hours, the rush-hour crowd inched by the details of a bike "accident." Unfortunately, most of those drivers probably don't realize that approximately three bikers are hit every day in Madison, a town of 200,000 people (Only about one hundred of these bike/car collisions are actually reported every year. National studies done in the 1980's found only about 10-20 % of hospital emergency room admissions for bicycle-related injuries had been documented in police reports. Presumably, the number of actual bike/car collisions annually in Madison is over 1,000). Passing drivers also couldn't have known that the police did not give the car driver a ticket.

For some people, their first Critical Mass ride may have been their last. Luckily, Kurt was not too seriously hurt, but the incident brought home concerns about safety. I'd guess that some people went away from the ride questioning the effectiveness of Critical Mass for dealing with traffic, belligerent drivers, or any of the other challenges a biker faces on the streets of America. Likewise, the interaction with the police worried some people not interested in testing police tolerance for Critical Mass.

But a lot of people came back in May, and others who had heard about the previous ride came out to show support for Kurt, to protest, to get involved, or whatever reasons motivate people to ride with Critical Mass. Since that first ride, I've given more thought to why I ride. I've been asked, "Does Madison really need a Critical Mass?" I've lived and commuted by bike in other, less bike friendly cities. I do acknowledge and appreciate the many accommodations and concessions given bikers throughout the city.

So, why do I ride? For me, Critical Mass is just one piece of the picture. For me, it is part of the revolution—a personal resistance against a culture that worships automobiles and concrete, against big oil companies that have their claws dug into every inch of society, against a government that has paved over the earth to exploit its people and resources. Critical Mass is not an answer to these evils, but it is an opportunity for cyclists to exercise our rights, celebrate our way of life, and shake things up a little. What confuses those who have not yet experienced Critical Mass is that it does not proselytize one message or forward one agenda. People come for their own reasons, make their own meaning, and go off to further their own visions of a better world.

Critical Mass brings together creative energy, it inspires activism, and it celebrates resistance to dominant culture. Because of Critical Mass rides, I have met activists, honed my organizing skills, learned my rights as a biker, challenged police authority, communicated with my legislators, and talked to many people about the virtues of biking. The listserv dialogue, local website, written materials, films, planning meetings, and social interactions that have come out of the rides are a testament to the potential such a forum has to energize and activate people. At its best, Critical Mass is dynamic, interactive, and more fun than any meeting, teach-in, or panel discussion I've ever been to. The bike is a revolutionary vehicle and Critical Mass further empowers the revolutionaries who ride in them.

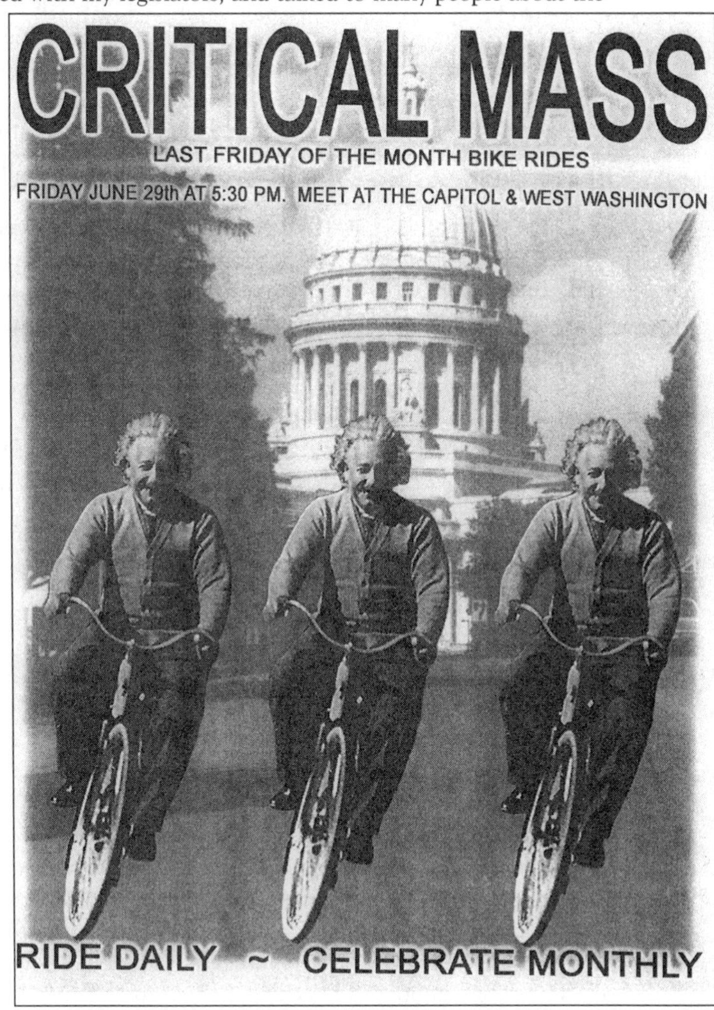
CRITICAL MASS
LAST FRIDAY OF THE MONTH BIKE RIDES
FRIDAY JUNE 29th AT 5:30 PM. MEET AT THE CAPITOL & WEST WASHINGTON
RIDE DAILY ~ CELEBRATE MONTHLY

The monthly rides in Madison continue to meet at the Capitol at 5:30 on the last Friday of the month.

Videotaping: Theory and Practice at Critical Mass

"A WELL-CAMERA'D SOCIETY IS A POLITE SOCIETY"

BY JASON MEGGS

Depending on what city, what part of town, and with whom you ride, Critical Mass can go from being a beautiful safe space to a terrifying war zone, usually thanks to the actions of motorists and police. How can we protect ourselves? How can we prevent these abuses? Knowing our rights and gathering our own evidence are two very powerful tools.

When we are organized and prepared, the dirty tricks that police use become liabilities to them and begin to lose their appeal. Showing that you know and are prepared to defend your rights is not only empowering and a deterrent to police abuses, but it helps break down the wall preventing communication between ourselves—the rollers—and they, the coppers. Once that wall is dismantled, and assuming they are not under orders to abuse our rights, they are much less likely to attack.

KNOW YOUR RIGHTS. Simply knowing the Vehicle Code (VC) and basic citizens' rights puts you in good position. In California, the VC is available for $3 from the DMV. Groups like CopWatch hold trainings and have publications to familiarize yourself with how to deal with police abuses. This type of information is online, such as the "Bike Rights Survival Package" found at www.xinet.com/bike/. In California, you have a right to observe from a "safe distance." Don't let the police intimidate you away.

A USEFUL RIGHT TO BE AWARE OF: You don't have to show ID unless detained in regard to some crime that the officer knows has happened or thinks is happening.

—OFFICER: "SHOW ME SOME ID!"
—YOU: "AM I BEING DETAINED?"
—OFFICER: "YES".
—YOU: "With regards to what crime?"

If the officer can't answer this, you are being harassed.

But all the righteous posturing in the world can't prove that you've been abused. Fortunately, the availability of cheap, quality camcorders has given the citizen activist enormous protection and recourse. "A well-camera'd society is a polite society."

Video evidence has been used again and again to show in court, on the television news, and to Citizens Complaints departments what really goes on with the police. There's just no substitute. Good video shows people what happened and moves them emotionally. Good video can be carefully analyzed for details and provide an order-of-events analysis that could never be obtained through eyewitness testimony. Video can get the cops off your backs. In Austin, Texas, after police arrests at the first Critical Mass there made the news, the ride tripled. Eventually, the police's own video was used against them and so embarrassed them that they "disappeared forever" from the rides. The footage of the recent police riot in San Francisco has been aired on all the local television stations and has been submitted to the Office of Citizens' Complaints (OCC). The flip side of this is that any crime you record on camera can be used in court. Your tape can be subpoenaed and even used against your own friends. Keep this in mind.

"But," you protest, "don't they just want to nail the person with the camera?"

Never fear. You are well protected if you're in a group, you know your rights and use your camera well. The fact that you are recording means that everything that happens to you is recorded—at least in audio. And if the police turn off your camera, that will look very bad for them in court: as suppressing or destroying evidence. This leads us to the golden rule: NEVER TURN OFF YOUR CAMERA! The police may order you to turn it off—but if it doesn't interfere with their duties, there's no justification for their order. If necessary, put the running camera out of sight. Even if you are in cuffs, the audio is important.

STAY LEGAL. It is important that you stay legal when you record. Your bike should be up to code, and you should not be violating even the smallest law. You need to be verbal when accosted by police. Assert your rights, and be very clear if you are being roughed up or otherwise violated. "Hey, that hurts, why are you pushing me." It is critically important that you maintain a professional demeanor. To be best protected, you need to act as a Legal Observer. A legal observer does not get involved in conflicts, confrontations, fights, shouting matches, escalations, name calling, or any law breaking no matter how minor, if at all possible. Legal observers tend to get special consideration in court.

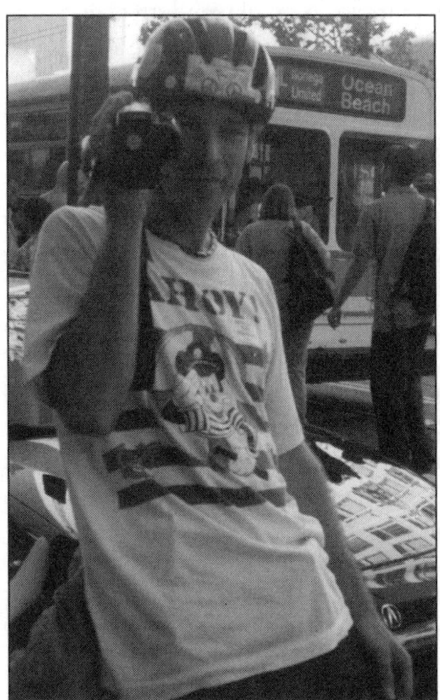

Jason Meggs, the Bay Area's most prolific Critical Mass videographer

"CAN I RECORD THIS?" Yes. If it's in public, you can record it—although you need permission to record an interview. Police have no reasonable expectation of privacy in California. In some states things are more repressive and you may at least need to inform them that you are recording.

These rules go for audiotape as well. Phone calls are another story.

BUDDY SYSTEM. It's very helpful to have a buddy. Your buddy watches your bike and your back, has spare batteries and tapes, calls out license plates and badge numbers, etc. Because the police tend to cuff camerapeople first if they are making arrests (e.g., the Bay Bridge 6), make sure your buddy is prepared to take the camera off your neck and keep recording. Do so smoothly and on the up-and-up, but as quickly and subtly as possible. Also note that your tape may go into custody for months if they confiscate it. If it's clear you won't be able to record any more, or if you've been surrounded by police and have a chance, switch tapes and give your most recent tape to someone you trust who has no camera to protect (always demand a property receipt whenever a cop takes something from you).

FIVE SECOND RULE. Hold that camera steady. "Firehosing" is when you wave the camera every which way. This can sometimes be helpful for detailed analysis but not for watching by actual people. Hold your shots for at least five seconds.

PRACTICE. Crazy things happen to you during violent situations. Cameras get turned off, the picture goes crazy, you may start babbling useless information that destroys the audio or even destroys your credibility as a witness/legal observer. Practice in tense situations. Practice biking with the camera. Role play. One game that works well for us is playing a pin-the-tail game where people are trying to get a red felt tail off a velcro belt, then pin it on themselves and run. Your job is to keep up and get a clear picture of who "stole" the tail each time, even while running.

WATCH YOUR FOOTAGE RIGHT AWAY. You learn the most from feedback, lessons that can save you in the future.

IF AN INCIDENT OCCURS: Go into high-gear record mode. Where are you exactly and what time is it? (Always catch public clocks on film and street and store signs). Who was there? Get the names of witnesses on film. Exchange names and numbers with whoever else was recording or photographing (we've been doing that at SFCM before the start of the ride, too). While the incident is occurring, do not speak unless absolutely necessary. Get the widest view possible. Try to hold the camera steady on the action. If it's a free-for all, brace the camera with two hands or against a pole on the main action and look from side to side for any other incidents of abuse. In the Market and Powell police riot, you see a wave of cops swinging batons rush past the cameraperson, but the cameraperson didn't notice.

TRY NOT TO ZOOM. Zooming is generally a bad idea because you can miss a lot while you're waiting to un-zoom. Zooming on badge numbers often doesn't work. Try to get a buddy to call out badge numbers.

DEBRIEF. After an incident, write down EVERYTHING you can remember in painstaking detail. Ask everyone else to do the same. Offer to interview them on tape. Remember, get their name and number so they aren't lost. Sad to say, in this society, people just wander away and drop all responsibility. Someone's life and freedom may depend on their testimony. Be forward, don't delay.

GET IT TO THE MEDIA. You can call the newsrooms of the local networks. If you capture police abuse or other violent incidents, they may actually buy a copy of your tape. You can demand that they not take it out of context but describe it as what it is. A bad public image can do wonders in reforming your local police.

Video is fun, it's empowering, and it helps protect our rights to peaceful assembly. It's worth it.

CROSSING THE POND UNDERGROUND

By Victor Veysey

In the fall of 1992 I somehow wound up at Critical Mass SF, being a bike messenger and vague proponent of bikes. I remember how Joel Pomerantz used to excitedly count us off as we would pass him on a corner, and as each ride grew so did the kaleidoscope of people and bicycles that came. In 1994 I was in England for the 2nd Cycle Messenger World Championships and participated in an incredibly confident and controlled Mass of international messengers from the Docklands into central London.

Due to love and a pair of handcuffs, I spent the next three years participating very regularly in London Critical Masses, which were quite a contrast to their San Francisco counterparts. There were four masses: Main, meeting under the Waterloo Bridge, had hundreds of participants, over a thousand at times, and usually broke up into segments pretty fast due the choppy geography of London. South was much smaller, as was East, and met on different days. Most mythical of all was West, where you could show up and find just a couple of folks, but there was some action, miniature as it was.

The Main London Mass went off on the last Friday just as in San Francisco, but the rules of etiquette and engagement with cars and society were different. Preconceptions of how to behave during 'demonstrations' and 'protests' understandably were brought to Mass, and there was quite a bit of 'correcting' of the behaviors and messages communicated at Mass by those who thought themselves

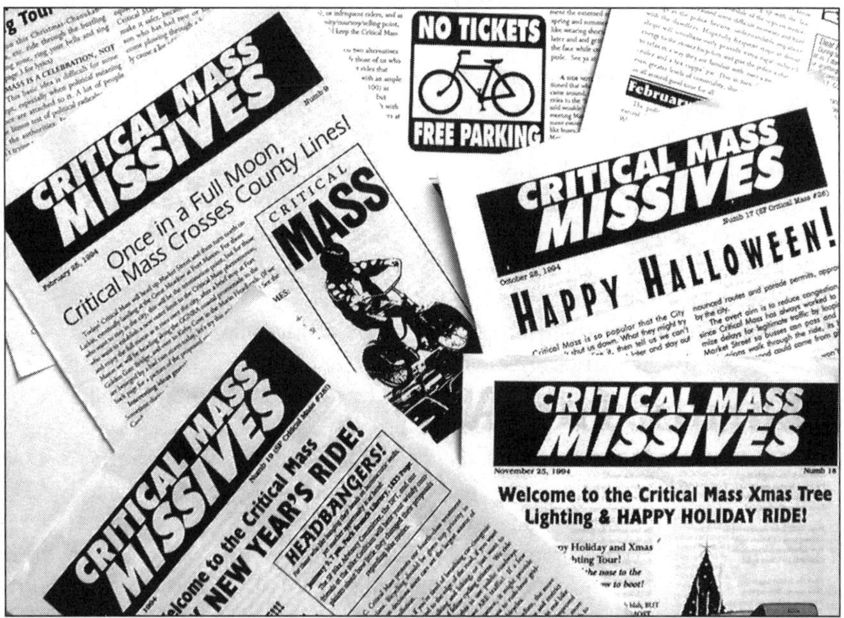

suited to do so. As in America, the struggle for control of what is by nature an anarchistic and uncontrollable act of spontaneous mobile bicycle society by any one segment is doomed to failure. As in America, people bent on proselytizing their own agenda will attempt to take over anyway, and drive a lot of peaceful folks away. The grand difference, if I may hazard such a wide categorization, is that in London the Controllers were yelling that Mass was about More Bike Lanes, whereas in SF the shouting at each other was mostly about Where to Go or How to Deal with the Cops. Not to say that both didn't share the same experience of multifarious discord, only that the tenor was different in each arena.

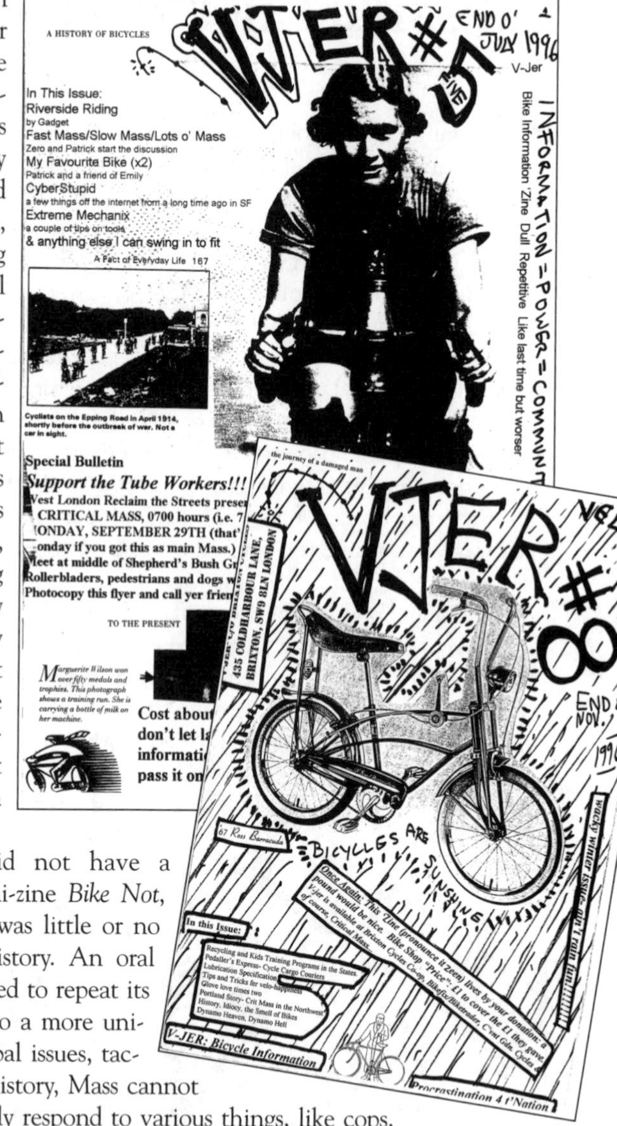

London, however, did not have a Xerocracy. Besides the mini-zine *Bike Not*, put out by X-Chris, there was little or no written Mass culture or history. An oral society is more easily inclined to repeat its mistakes and not progress to a more universal understanding of global issues, tactics, and history. Without history, Mass cannot learn how to most effectively respond to various things, like cops, cars, and obnoxious participants, all of which are going to occur anywhere Mass does. With that in mind, in February of 1996 I set out to write a zine to address the lack of historical and global knowledge of London Massers. *V-jer* grew to become a regular assault on the British Mentality of Doing Nothing, and I had to endure some seriously misguided attempts to "correct" me, but it flourished and was effective. My target audience was Massers and general London cyclists, and by issue five I was up to several hundred copies at twenty pages each. I had a variety of original writing and photos, mostly by friends but some international. I also had respectful reprints of great pieces of writing about bikes, from Dervla Murphy's shooting a wolf off of her arm as she rides a one-speed from Ireland to India to techie things I admired, mechanical tips, and historical documents. Accounts of Masses in a wide variety of locales and circumstances were also a regular feature. By Issue Ten, in 1997, I was back in the US, still owing myself two issues, which will come out when I have the writing mood and some contributors.

One of the most important, fragile, and overlooked aspects of Mass is how dense a society it is. Each act of spontaneous congregation creates hundreds of interactions and environments, and each individual comes away with impressions of hugely different aspects of the same event. I have seen violence in both London and SF, and yet often just twenty yards away there are people oblivious, engaged in discussion, peaceful and unaware. We all experience different versions of Mass, and often a Mass of any size breaks into different groups with differing routes. Recognizing the primacy of the individual is the first Freedom of Mass, to me; you can always just ride away or take some people and split off, metaphorically or physically, from the ride.

As an individual I was also able to intervene in the escalating tensions in SF between police and Massers. By summer of 1993 the police had started calling for a "representative" to be responsible for Mass, and wanted to issue a parade permit. This was percieved as an unwarranted intrusion on Massers' right to assemble, and led to a very anti-police attitude amongst many riders. Continually restating that I did not represent anyone other than myself, I interviewed the cops and put out *Coptalk*, a dense one-page mini-zine. Just having someone talk to them seemed to please the cops, and as Massers read the transcription of the meeting they seemed to relax. As usual, a little understanding goes a long way, and this rare mo-

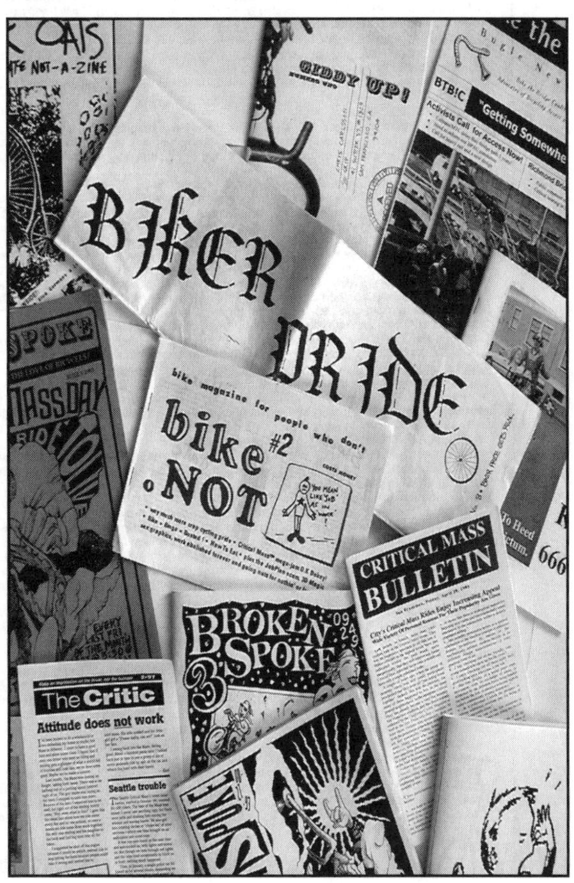

ment of diffusion reinforced my sense that publication yields notable social results.

In contrast to mainstream media sources, this was reporting that Massers could identify with. The lack of comprehension of the Critical Mass social phenomenon in the mainstream media was frustrating for many riders, and it was refreshing to finally hear our own voices. As a writer I found it heartening to have people recognize my efforts. As a reader it was great to see the efforts of others and to learn about Masses in other cities. SF zines like *Broken Spoke* & *Critical Mass Missives* gave us a real sense of continuity to Mass. 'Zines like *Bike Not*, *V-jer*, and many others helped to spread the word and solidify local scenes. In contrast to the commodified horror of bicycles as leisure device, self-published 'zines let the growing grassroots movement—both around Critical Mass and bikes in general—find a voice. I feel honored to have been a part of it.

Coptalk

issue number one **An interview conducted with Captain Michael Yalon, Lieutenant Barry Johnson and Officer Tom Mandelke (a dedicated bike cop), at the Southern Police Station, Wednesday 11-17-93, 3.15 pm,**

Ok, Ok, so I heard that the police were looking for someone(s) to talk to RE Critical Mass and finally took it upon myself to dust off the interview skills and approach them AS A PRIVATE INDIVIDUAL NOT "REPRESENTING" CRITICAL MASS IN ANY WAY and see what their views were. And I am happy to say that things look good for Critical Mass. But don't ask me- read for yerself– so sez
Victor Veysey pager 698-4226 home 861-8942 Mail: 692 Oak St. SF 94117

On the subject of using bike officers to patrol Crit Mass:

Captain Yalon: "In fact we did have some bicycle officers at the last Critical Mass but we need to be more mobile than the bicycle officers can be so what we do is utilize motorcycles and Hondas to skip ahead." They total four bike cops at the last Crit Mass.

On permits, etc.:

Captain Yalon: "When a group gets together, and by getting together all that's required is that they come together, somewhere and they move on the streets for more than a block, they are a parade...a parade needs a permit....and the reason for that is so that it can be coordinated with other events and with traffic and other things going on."

At this point I went on at length about the globular, destructured nature of CM.

Captain Yolan: "We have to be with Critical Mass. We would like to figure out a way even if you can't get anyone to come forward with a permit, we'd be willing to try a cooperative effort even without a permit of facilitating your event. We'd be willing to move you along through the streets. We just want to work with you to get this thing done. You want to get from Point A to point B, we need to know what way we're going so that we can stop traffic to get you there, and we would be willing to stop traffic except in those few places where it isn't safe to do so in order to get you through. We would be willing to give you an entire half of the street on most of the streets where you go through. And especially as it becomes dark earlier now, we want to make sure that your people, our people and pedestrians can all get safely through the streets at the same time. That's our concern is a public safety concern in addition to this permit issue. ....and if you guys want to act crazy within the law en route there's no problem. The vast majority of people involved with this event are pretty much on line with that. We know that any group of any size has a few people that want to push the envelope but we don't want it to get to the point where it's an Us and Them fight because there are so many other things we have to do."

What they think of Critical Mass in General:

Captain Yalon: "...your event is basically a good event. It's got a good cause. Many of our officers, especially our bicycle officers agree with you. We wish there were bike paths out there. We wish that some of our bigger streets had areas designated where people could safely bicycle... so we would rather not be put in a position where we would have to stop it. But we know on the other hand that... there have been incidents. I can remember one assault incident where a guy was pulled out of a car- the people with Critical Mass or at least a few of them were involved- alleged the he cut them off- and he alleged that they cut him off, but nevertheless people in Critical Mass pulled this guy out of the car, broke the car windows, and beat the guy up. And that was one block after our officers pulled off because it had been a peaceful event."

On Earlier Masses in Relation to that Mass:

"...it was a much smaller event then, but it had a positive image. We'd be at a demonstration on Market St. on the four hundred block and see a bunch of bike riders coming through and people would say 'Hey you got a bunch of people coming to create a problem for you' and we'd get on the radio and say 'No, this is that last Friday ride'- it think it was called at that time When You Ride Alone You Ride With Hitler [a WW II carpooling poster someone appropriated]**-'It's just a group who come through every last Friday, don't worry about it.' Well, that changed with that event because we realized that we could no longer not worry about it because this has the potential for people to get hurt.."**

Officer Mandelke: "One of the problems is that many bike people feel that it's us against them with the motorists, with the motor vehicle community in general. That's one of the reasons that we should have police facilitate it makes it safer because otherwise you have confrontations in just the normal course of riding a bike down Market Street. Motor traffic don't really give bikes a whole lot of respect because they don't consider them to be equal partners on the street. So that's one of the reasons that I think it 's really critical for Critical Mass to have police participation in it, to make it safer. Because it wouldn't take but one person who has had two or three too many drinks to come plowing through a bunch of bicyclists and really cause a lot of havoc."

On the last Critical Mass:

Hey, they appreciated getting a route map given to them before the ride. And oh, the You May Be Cited For Violations etc. Speech Lieutenant Johnson gave was done in part to limit police liability for accidents.

Lieutenant Johnson (head cop at last Mass) on just what happened:

"So, your people came down the street and my bike officers said when they saw the police [at the Pacific Stock Exchange] **they thought we were trying to block your folk in. It got confused. These other guys had nothing to do [with Critical Mass] at all." "We had our police bicyclists up front just to make sure that everything was going ok and they observed some things that shouldn't have taken place- the guy with the watergun squirting people...**

Nov. 1993

London, England

CRITICAL (BIKE-NOT) SNACK

BY X-CHRIS

This piece is from *bike.not,* a London Critical Mass 'zine in 1994-95.

Yep! Just like all bottom feeders Friday evenings snacks ... you go in one and out the other and Critical Mass is just another bottom feeder. Sucks us in and shits us out. Oh my, how times change. I still [heart] (the idea of) Critical Mass, but sometimes you have to bail out, sensing you're losing ground. Maybe I always just took the Critical bit more seriously than the Mass part. I've still been riding in the odd Mass but it doesn't really make me come anymore.

I gave up "organizing" ("flyering" for Crit.Mass after the (then) biggest ride of all, the October 1994 jobbie, the Anarchy in the UK swell ride. It probably had 300 riders on it and that satisfied me and my numbers craze. We also got to make love to our bikes in the middle of Whitehall, 200 yards from Downing Street. Emily, Jason, Tom and me (sex starved heroes for a day!) stopped as the other 294 riders rode past ignoring the pre-arranged time we flyered (Bike Love-in—7 pm) to get down and prove how sexy we Massers are. You lot, you're so English! As the others rode around us, some urging us to get up, we humped our bikes, finally throwing them and us together for a bike orgy completely with high-pitched orgasm sounds. It was great fun. The Mass itself continued through all that Winter '94 rain and cold stuff dipping to about 30 riders in Dec. and Jan. and surviving a serious drive-thru car frenzy that threw a few people (extra air-conditioning was added to the attacker's car via swift and vengeful D-lock action) but I waited for a little sun and inspiration again.

The March 31st 1994 ride, with a Hardcore 'Cars Are Terrain' Cycle Crew, was a victorious Critical Mass replete with tons of riders and a bike Invasion of McDonalds (as support for Dave and Helen, the Mclibel 2 currently on trial for 'libel' against McD's). Then some hooligans went and chained shut the heavy gates on Admiralty Arch blocking the flow of car traffic into the Mall. Ho! Ho!

April, the CM one year anniversary, was just a fucking super-jam of cycle/car mingle chaos. Very slow and dense and funny despite a ridiculously crap attempt at an "action" consisting of stopping the Mass at Park Lane and rolling a toilet roll across the road to symbolise "erecting our own cycle crossing." A bunch of us took the "cars-only" Strand Underpass which was fun AND scary as the place was re-painted with witty and not-so witty anti-car slogans. The sound of three hundred tons of racing cars and lorries behind us was getting louder and louder throu the tunnel and making us inches and seconds away from a big smoosh. We finished up and scrammed as the first car bullet left the tunnel chamber. Close but no ambulance necessary thank you. For the anniversary, maybe something that actually we could all have taken part in would have been more smile worthy. The toilet roll caper was noticed by about 20 people on the ride, those at the back remained confused. Alongside this was the hilarious leaflet from the organisers stating "be composed, witty and articulate when being interviewed on telly (if you can)" and "don't piss drivers off by cycling in ones and twos in front of them" Huh? Like who's life is it anyway? OK enough carping (for) now. I guess you get the point that I think Critical Mass can be much better, more fun, much more liberating etc. We flyered every Mass with ideas, leaflets about solidarity, dealing with cops and arrest, getting skateboarders to come, fun things to do, etc., but not much ever changes. The picnic after the June ride was cool and the ride was massive (1000+) and fucking so messy and slow and wonderful, infuriating, offensive, pissed off, gnarly, loud, glorious etc. Car drivers were given no quarter —the ride was IN THEIR FACE big time. Then I stopped going on the Mass because, well maybe I mentioned it somewhere else!!

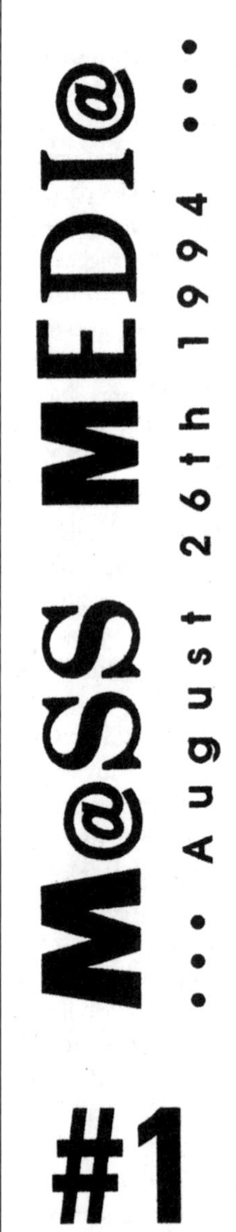

Another London Critical Mass 'zine.

The excellent Martika quite rightly sums up Crit. Mass on her classic first album, *'it's not what you're doing but what you're not doing, baby'*... That sums up my attitude, too. We (my critical cohorts and myself) tried endlessly to kick it out further, because, well, how much fun is it repeating a slow ride through London, bouncing cars off our back wheels, having the cops increasingly since June '94 telling us what to do, having the ride diverted off to the latest political cause, listening to people who like to think of the ride as "people power" informing us of the route, destination, end time, this road and that road, do this, NO, NOT THAT WAY!! If it seems like I'm just never satisfied, then that's right because I'm not. Crit. Mass ain't my monthly tranquilizer. Riding in the midst of a Massquerade of genuine community ain't my Xanax to keep me happy and jolly and out of wankers' faces whether they're cops, dangerous drivers, angry pedestrians OR people on bikes costing what I live on in any one year. Just because we ride bikes, dudes, it doesn't make me part of your protest club. I'm gonna say it (LOW SLUNG INVECTIVE AHEAD): a lot of Mass (London) participants are just a bunch of privileged fucks with some stake in how things are currently run, i.e. they aren't interested in freedom from poverty and shit lives for people like me. They want the freedom to cycle about a place in peace and with good air. That's cool! I want that too but I want freedom for everyone on this planet to live a decent life from rules and people telling us what and what not to do. Worse than being privileged is that they can't even be Tories or Libertarians with it but nothing else than a bunch of liberals (excellent definition > people who don't see the influence of class, sex, and eth-

bike magazine for people who don't

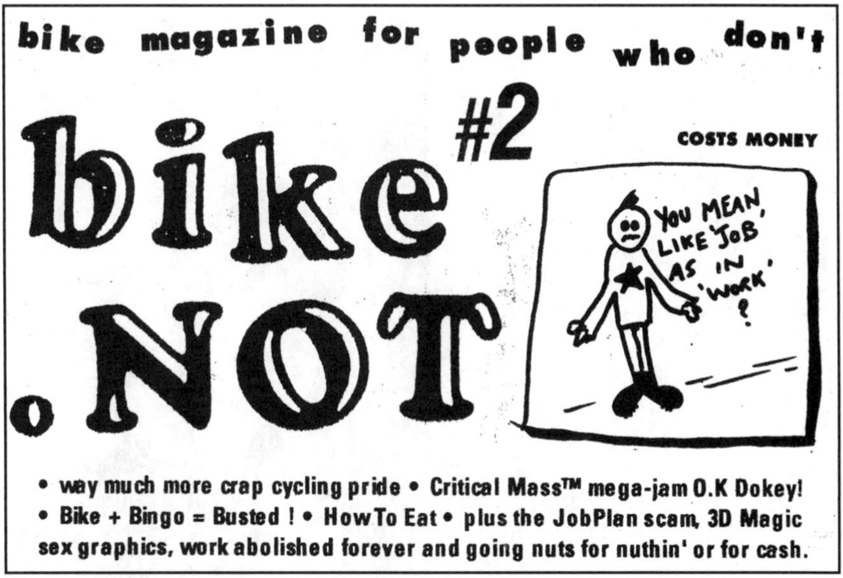

bike.NOT #2

COSTS MONEY

YOU MEAN, LIKE 'JOB' AS IN 'WORK'?

• way much more crap cycling pride • Critical Mass™ mega-jam O.K Dokey! • Bike + Bingo = Busted ! • HowTo Eat • plus the JobPlan scam, 3D Magic sex graphics, work abolished forever and going nuts for nuthin' or for cash.

nic relations on power and subordination, who assume we have a freedom to interact with each other in any way we choose). Ever thought about how we have things set up right now—wage slavery, consumer frenzies, economic wars—we choose to perpetuate this shit too. And more! What price cycle lanes, cycle power? What price eh?

So anyway, so much for my illusion that I rode the Mass as part of a "spontaneous coincidence," without leaders and without rules. It was contradicted in the small print all along. Yet I know that my version of reality is just the reverse of their version of reality. Nobody is really right in the end but I just can't quit that politics stuff, you know. Stuff like how inspiring the early c/Masses were to me, all that novelty and seemingly new way of trying to change things, new community etc. I don't believe that spirit has been lost, it's just a few liberals thought they'd better keep it clean and organised just in case it got in the way of their plans. Yeah, a thousand Massers can live with that but I can't. Sorry I really just want to state that feeling of mine. I hate to leave my own radical subjectivity (whatever that means) so unqualified because I just sound like a hysterical flat-Earther, stamping my foot on the ground and screaming a lot. Who cares eh? I don't.

So, my own Crit Mass death knell (you know 100% on the Disillusion-o-meter) must have been the sight of a lone and obviously confused Socialist Worker paper seller on the start of the August ride. Confused because a) he assumed that this assembling crowd, just like any crowd of more than three people gathering together for a cause, is a target audience for his wares and b) being a SWP paper seller is about as dangerous to capitalism as lifting your Cannondale repeatedly over your head as a protest about how nasty everything is.

An Unknown and Unexpected Prehistory....

CRITICAL MASS RAMSGATE

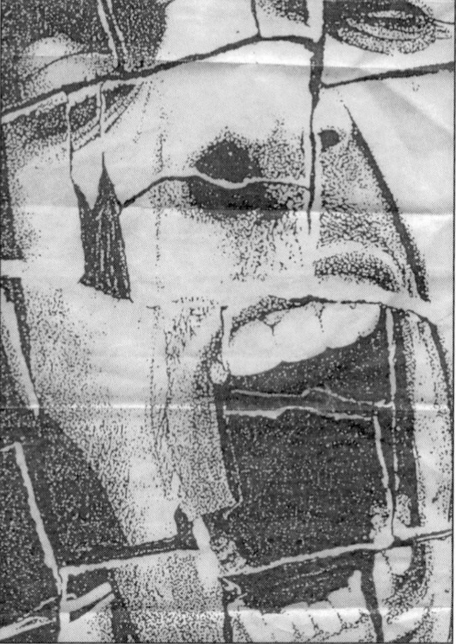

During the period of 1984 to 1986 I made several visits to the seaside town of Ramsgate in Kent, England, where I became acquainted with a group of people who could be described as both progressive and bohemian, earnestly campaigning for environmental issues. From that group of friends, in either 1984 or 1985 emerged Critical Mass, co-founded by Fadra, a mystic and avant-garde artist I had known for some years.

Ramsgate Critical Massers, as I remember, were enthusiastic campaigners for environmental and social issues, and soon became well known in the East Kent area, even appearing on the local TV news. Equipped with printing facilities, Critical Mass members produced leaflets, badges and t-shirts. Their emblem was a somewhat striking monochrome shouting face shattered into shards as if viewed in a broken mirror.

In 1986 Critical Mass members were planning a mass bicycle ride through Ramsgate as I recall. However, I lived a little over 100 miles from Ramsgate during the mid-1980s, and subsequently lost contact with the group around that time.

—Arch, England, March 2002

Greetings, and salutations,

I am contacting you because my good friend ARCH mentioned your new CRITICAL MASS project. I was the Secretary of the Ramsgate Flat Earth Society and Critical Mass from 1983/7. We publically promoted networking to generate an interest in all environmental issues, and matters of a political nature such as homelessness and poverty.

Our efforts were quite parochial at first but gained a lot of publicity nationally, appearing on the BBC. Our membership was informal, and tended to be composed of anarchists and reformers—quite an explosive mix. CM was an open forum for debate and action, supporting the travelling communities, free festival organisers and the green movement. I am convinced that our network, which moved to London to spread into Europe, seems to have survived in the new mass which you are a part of.

YOURS AUBI FADRA 1st. Sec. C/M.
(fester@chaosmagic.com)

THE WORLD OF THE BICYCLE

BY IAIN A. BOAL

I.

The field of bicycle history remains complacently oblivious of the critical ferment produced by the social and revolutionary movements of the second half of the twentieth century. Honorable exceptions exist, to be sure—Andrew Ritchie's biography of Major Taylor, an exemplary act of historical retrieval from the amnesia of a racist society, comes to mind. Still, the historiography of the bicycle is, it must be said, overwhelmingly Eurocentric, both in its themes and unspoken commitments.

To compound the matter, bicycle history is cripplingly essentialist. Essentialism leads to, or perhaps springs from, a fetishizing of the artifact. This is hardly surprising in a world dedicated to the production and celebration of commodities, but passionate attachment to bicycles—sheer love of the machine—particularly for those historians who begin as collectors or enthusiasts, carries a price. It results in the *déformation* of the historian of technology, namely the risk of attributing to the object of study a magical essence and agency, which is often smuggled into historical explanation.

To those familiar with the history of science and technology as a discipline, these traits are quite characteristic of the field in general. The explanation is not hard to find. Science and its technical applications are, in the self-understanding of the West, the very hallmark and guarantee of European exceptionalism. The job of the historian has been to write what one might call "palace" history, which turns out, predictably enough, to be a triumphalist story of progress and improvement, based on (male) reason. The traditional historian of science and technology (often a retired scientist, out to pasture) has typically functioned as the spaniel of science—running at the heel, with tail wagging—whose role has been to endorse the inventive heroes of the past and to ratify the present. Although a cohort of critical historians, emerging in the crucible of the social movements of the 1960s, declined to genuflect any longer before the altar of science and technology, still most historical writing remains in the grip of these tacit assumptions.[1]

This picture first became clear to me when I was commissioned in the early eighties to write a review essay for *Industrial Design* about the socio-technical history of the bicycle.[2] Especially striking was, firstly, the Darwinian framework informing many accounts of bicycle design history, which acts to naturalize the evolution of forms, and which my own narrative by no means escaped; secondly, the compulsive search for origins, the moment of invention.[3] The origin myths continue to be reworked obsessively, in part because of evolutionary assumptions, in part because of national or local chauvinism, but also because of the diffusionism built into Eurocentric ideology, which in principle favored diffusion over independent invention.[4] The logic of diffusion needs an origin point, whether it be the German forests for the *draisienne*, a Scottish forge for MacMillan's machine, or Mount Tamalpais in the case of the mountain bike. These charter myths, with their narratives of Promethean inventors in quintessentially Romantic settings—forest, Celtic fringe and sacred mountain—tend to systematically obscure, respectively, the environment of Heidelberg as a center of innovation, the industrial dynamic of the Scottish lowlands, and California's aero-space complex.[5]

Soon afterwards, in 1984, I remarked to the science and technology editor at Princeton University Press that there was no general history of the bicycle from a global, polycentric perspective. He told me, with a straight face, to produce one myself and then he would publish it. The project was impossibly large, premature, and stillborn. A cursory survey two years before, at the time of my inquiry into design history, had revealed how little there was, at least in the English, German and French literature, about cycle history in Africa, South America and Asia, the places where now the majority of the world's cyclists live. I had absorbed, however, the lesson of Joseph Needham's *Science and Civilization in China*, that Western histories of science and technology were seriously distorted by ethnocentric and orientalist assumptions.[6] If the work of Needham was anything to go by, then we might expect a non-Eurocentric cycle history to overturn a number of Western assumptions about the transmission direction of scientific and technical knowledge between metropolitan and "peripheral" societies.[7] Needham himself notoriously showed that Francis Bacon's pantheon of Western scientific inventions— gunpowder, the compass and the printing press—all probably had a Chinese provenance.[8]

In the intervening years, valuable work has been done, though much of it within quite traditional frameworks and assumptions. Still strikingly unusual, therefore, is Hans-Erhard Lessing's genealogical speculation, drawing explicitly on Needham, that there may a direct connection between Karl von Drais's machines and a wheelbarrow in the Heidelberg collection designed on ancient Chinese principles, with a wheel below the center of gravity. He notes that Drais claimed that his Driving Machine Two was "intended not only for the transport of humans, but also small loads" which could be "moved more advantageously than…a wheelbarrow."[9] The point, however, is not necessarily to reverse the arrow of cultural and technological transmission—a move that, in any case, remains inside the logic of diffusionism and some originary site—but to aim for a radical opening up of research methods, angles of approach, and dimensions of causal agency. For example, in recent years, owing to the apocalyptic threat of global warming and nuclear winter, "nature" is making a comeback as a historical agent, after the discrediting of Victorian environmental and geographic determinism. Again, Lessing introduces global climate as a material actor in the development of the bicycle, specifically the effect of an 1816 volcanic eruption in Asia on grain harvests and the cost of horse fodder in Europe. Lessing hypothesizes that the global weather change produced by the eruption stimulated Karl von Drais to develop alternatives to horse-drawn vehicles in Europe.[10]

Besides the recent critical sociology of science and technics, cycle historians should be drawing substantially from cultural studies, "history from below," post-colonial and subaltern studies, and the legacies of the feminist, environmentalist, and third world struggles. Here is a list that is intended merely to illustrate the range of themes that invite deeper and sustained investigation:

• histories of the bicycle as "beast of burden" (taxi, portage, etc); a comparative sociology of the bicycle as tool versus toy.

• the role of the bicycle in third world movements and anti-imperialist struggles.

• the history of "off-road" modifications in bicycle design in the global South.

• the bicycle as a gendered artifact, e.g., patriarchal sanctions against its use by women in different societies.

• the comparative impact of the bicycle on patterns of household work and leisure, land use, and travel, cross-culturally.

• the urban sociology of the bicycle, and its possibilities and limits in ecological city planning.

• the history of "Critical Mass" bike rides and their global spread.[11]

• comparative histories of the bicycle industry worldwide, and of particular firms in colonial and post-colonial contexts.

• histories of cycle advertising in imperial, national and cross-cultural perspective.

• the history of pedal power (energy generation, pumps, saws, etc.), and improvised uses of the bicycle in the global South.

• the relation of bicycle history to railway history globally.

A "world history" perspective would necessarily pay as little respect to local, regional and national boundaries as officers, factors and agents of the colonial powers did in their search either for the commodities that went into the making of bicycles or for the labor that extracted them. The mythos of Dunlop, the solicitous father and inventor of pneumatic cushioning for his son's bicycle, needs to be articulated with the global history of rubber, and the extraordinary human costs of its production. The rise of metropolitan cities like Belfast and Edinburgh depended on colonial plantation economies and the brutal recomposition of labor, from petty extraction to industrial monoculture, mediated in the case of rubber by the Royal Botanic Garden at Kew. Seeds of Brazilian rubber, *Hevea Brasiliensis*, were exported illegally via Kew to British colonies in Asia; the expropriating of natural resources was justified, grotesquely enough, as a hedge against overexploitation by native peoples.[12] The race to capitalize on the rubber boom, caused in part by the success of Dunlop's invention, led to slave labor on a vast scale and the deaths of between five and eight million Congolese in a barbaric genocide between roughly 1890 and 1910. King Leopold understood that there were staggering profits to be realized by the extraction of rubber from scattered wild Landolphia vines in the equatorial rain forest of the Belgian Congo, but they would drop as soon as the plantations of rubber trees in the Britain's Asian territories were mature.[13] Later, fear of a bottleneck in the supply of rubber led Henry Ford to purchase a million-acre estate in Brazil for a rubber plantation. "Fordlandia" was one of the great fiascos of economic botany.

II.

I would like to demonstrate the proposed method by way of an example from a still earlier episode in cycle history, and to illustrate the heuristic for a non-Eurocentic historiography by focusing on the landmark year in bicycle history 1869-70, but at a "marginal" location, namely, Japan at the Meiji restoration. The Meiji period (1868-1912), that followed the demise of the Tokugawa shogunate, was a time of crash modernization. In 1859, trade agreements with the US, Russia, the Netherlands, England and France opened Japan to the West, and led to the rapid development of commercial cities and ports like Yokohama and Nagasaki. Japanese publishers found a huge market for woodblock prints, catering to the demand for an inexpensive artform among the mass of new city dwellers, who as a class were intensely curious about all things foreign. As a result many of the woodblocks were commentaries on the process of modernization and the anxieties it induced.

A print made about 1873 by Utagawa Yoshifugi, *Imported and Japanese Goods: Comic Picture of a Playful Contest of Utensils*, portrays a world where things have come to life (Figure 1). Yoshifugi's print seems to be a humorous gloss on Charles Marx's comment that, under commodity capitalism, artifacts dance. The battle of the goods is led by two generals, traditional at upper left, and at upper right a modern one, equipped with whisky, a book with Roman script, a brick, and a chair. In all the prints with this subject matter the modern commodities generally defeat the old-fashioned articles—in the center of the Yoshifugi woodcut an ancient Japanese letter box is retreating before a modern Western model, introduced in 1870 by an American postal expert, Samuel Bryan.[14] To its left can be seen the only winner on the Japanese side: native rice overthrows the foreign import.

Further to the left, the new-fangled rickshaw is chasing off the traditional *kago* (palanquin basket-chair). For the historian of the bicycle and human-powered vehicles, the Meiji restoration of 1868 is of peculiar interest, because it coincides precisely with the moment of the boneshaker and the rickshaw, which is why both of them came to be viewed as icons of the modern. The rickshaw, which is etymologically a borrowing from the Japanese *jinrikisha* (literally, "man-powered vehicle"), seems to have emerged from the workshop of Izumi Yosuke at the foot of Nihombashi ("Japan Bridge") in Tokyo some time in 1869, apparently inspired by the Western, wheeled, horse-drawn carriage. When Izumi Yosuke applied to the Tokyo authorities for licensing rights, he described his contraption as "a little seat in the Western style, mounted on wheels so that it can be pulled about."[15] It was an immediate and enormous success; by 1871 there were 25,000 rickshaws in Tokyo, according to a contemporary account.[16]

The "triumph" of *jinrikisha*, that is, of human-drawn over horse-drawn carriages as a mode of urban transportation may be partly a function of the equestrian and martial history in Japan. Because of the cultural identification of the horse as an instrument of war, its appearance on the streets of Tokyo and Yokohama would have had some of the impact that a tank might have today.[17] By 1880 *jinrikisha* had reached India and Singapore, and they were soon ubiquitous across Asia, though later challenged by buses, taxis and the three- wheeled cycle-rickshaw.

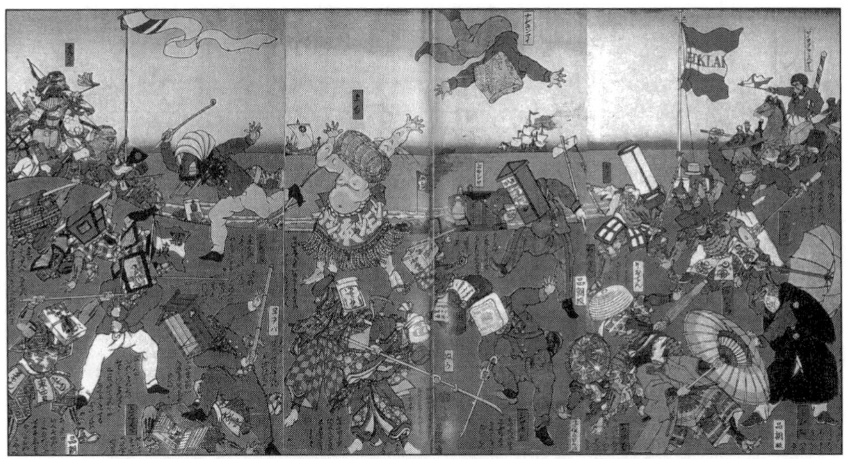

Figure 1: Imported and Japanese Goods: Comic Picture of a Playful Contest of Utensils by Utagawa Yoshifugi.

After the Second World War, hand-pulled rickshaws became an embarrassment to modernizing urban elites in the Third World, and were widely banned, in part because they were symbolic, not of modernity, but of a feudal world of openly marked class distinctions. Perhaps the seated rickshaw passenger is too close to the back of the laboring driver, who, besides, is metaphorically a draught animal harnessed between shafts. More importantly, rickshaw pullers and drivers, constituting as much as a fifth of the working population, were able to bring cities to a halt by strike action. In 1897 the Singapore authorities declared martial law to end a four-day rickshawmen's strike.[18]

The collective power of cyclists was not historically confined to laboring rickshaw drivers of colonial cities in the global South. In Weimar Germany the workers' cycling association, Solidarity, could mobilize thousands of members riding under the red banner of socialism. In its heyday Solidarity's membership numbered close to three hundred thousand. The immense throngs of proletarians on wheels caused the word "cyclist" to be spoken as a term of bourgeois abuse in the 1920s. Perhaps the last red stragglers of Solidarity, now reduced to a tiny remnant, might feel scant affinity with "black" cycling, with the critical masses who ride beneath the flag of anarchy. Nevertheless, they might agree that, though socialism did not arrive on a bicycle, a better world, if it is won, will mean reclaiming the streets from the tyranny of automobilism.

It is the task of critical historians of the bicycle to help recover the real history of the complex material relations between the bicycle, the automobile and the roads they share. It is necessary, for instance, not to flinch from the fact that the Good Roads Movement in the US in the late 19th century was instigated and led by bicyclists, nor from the reality that there was, and is, massive continuity and overlap between the cultures of the bicycle and the motor car. Bicycle purists, who imagine that they are somehow unambiguously an antithesis to motorists, need to rethink this fantasy. Perhaps if motorists also understand their historical debt to the bicycle, the hostility and carnage on city streets will be reduced.

Vehicles on the Streets of Tokyo (Figure 2) is a woodcut print made in 1870 by the artist Utagawa Yoshitora. Its subject matter—the forms modernity was taking in the streets of the capital—is in considerable tension with its own form, which, as it were, resists the barrage of the new. Yoshitora has not, for instance, imported three-point perspective in the modern fashion; the mode of representation remains traditional. And it does so, I think, for good reason. It is a celebration of the wheel in two dimensions, specifically of modernity on wheels; although the tricolor undercoat vaguely suggests back-, middle-, and foreground, the impression is of a depthless array of floating, wheeled vehicles, displayed side-on (save for one orthogonal rickshaw at the left edge), and filling the entire triptych, as crowded as a Tokyo street. We survey a dense jam of new-fangled vehicles: there are more than a dozen rickshaws, which had only arrived on the streets of Tokyo earlier in the year—some of them liveried and highly lacquered; a large steam engine at top center, and to its left three vessels driven by paddles—a small ferry, a larger steamship, and a barge of sorts; a horse-drawn carriage on the left, and at right a two-horse vehicle, looking like an omnibus. A traditional dray loaded with rice is exiting bottom left, drawn and pushed by four half-naked men; following them, at bottom center, is a man on a boneshaker, which can have only recently arrived in Tokyo. A woman in a passing rickshaw is twisting sideways, perhaps to catch the strange new sight, hardly less strange in 1870 in London, Paris or San Francisco.[19] If she were to look the other way, she would see another odd vehicle, a hand-cranked five-wheeled carriage for two people, steered at the front and driven from the rear.

If we take seriously the category *jinrikisha*, four kinds of vehicle in Yoshitora's woodcut qualify; it has the effect of rendering narrow the Western taxonomy, which makes a fetish of cranking with the feet off the ground; all else is consigned either to the pre-history of the bicycle, or to some quite different category—hobbyhorses, scooters, skateboards, Chinese wheelbarrows, and so forth.

The Japanese sociologist Maeda Ai believes that the reception of the

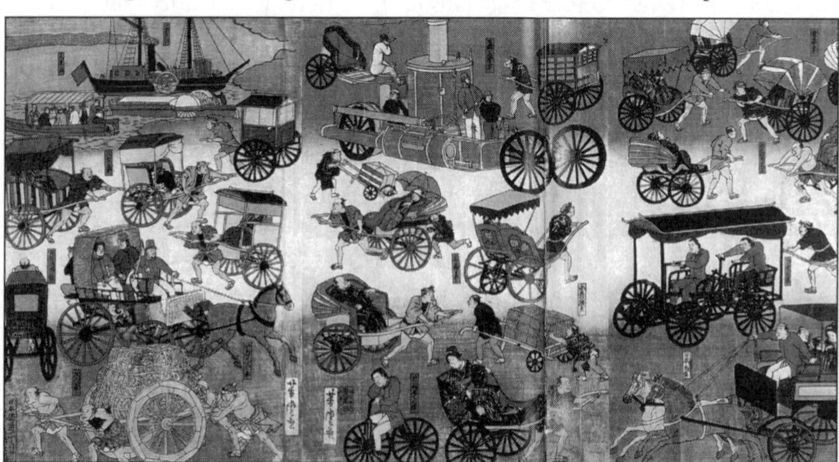

Figure 2: Vehicles on the Streets of Tokyo by Utagawa Yoshitora.

Boneshaker, the Ordinary and the Safety in Japan was a function of their being perceived as types of this much older category, *jinrikisha*.[20] For what it is worth, Thomas Stevens' account of his ride through Japan in 1886, on the last leg of his round- the-world tour on a high-wheeler, contains no descriptions of "mobs" of inquisitive onlookers that fill his travelogue earlier.[21]

In conclusion, the bicycle in world culture is a strangely ambiguous, contradictory object. It is seen in certain contexts as an instrument of liberation ("Socialism will arrive on a bicycle," rational dress for women, unchaperoned mobility for children), in others as a sign of poverty and backwardness. It is a quintessentially Victorian object (the canonical bicycle *qua* logo is still the high-wheeler) and at the same time a utopian machine of the future. It is thought of as a green mode of transportation, yet it is intimately linked to the history and culture of automobilism and to the development of ecologically destructive roads. It is both a cause of exploitation (rubber slavery) and a means of open-air pleasure, providing us with the lovely word "freewheeling."

These contradictions need to be explored honestly. Northern proselytizers for the bicycle over the motorcar are in no position to preach to inhabitants of the global South. Historians too will have to be conscious of their own positionality. "World history" can be just another ruse by Eurocentric scholars to claim universality for a particularist view.

Most of all, what is needed is to open up a space for dialogue, using old and new means of connection, with freewheeling historians and cyclists worldwide—in India, Africa, Indonesia, China, Brazil, wherever people use human energy for transportation, which is to say, everywhere.

Acknowledgements: For their comradely help, thanks to John O'Brian, Andrew Ritchie, and Kaz Koike, scholar-cyclists one and all. An earlier version of this essay was delivered at the 11th International Cycling History Conference in Osaka, Japan, in August 2000.

Footnotes

1. See, e.g., the critical scholarship of Hilary Rose, Robert Proctor, Ludmilla Jordanova, and Donna Haraway; journals such as *Social Studies of Science* and *Science as Culture* have been congenial forums for critical studies in science and technics. All are working in the long shadow of Lewis Mumford.
2. "The bicycle," *Industrial Design*, July/August, 1983, 34-41.
3. The "growth" of the ordinary in the 1870s tends to be either interpreted in biological-developmental terms (often reinforced by a photographic series)—a paradigmatic case of genetic explanation—or else explained in terms of the "natural" desire to gear up for more speed. Either way, the socially embedded contingency of the bicycle, as of all human artifacts, is occluded. At the same time, of course, the high-wheeler is taken to be a poignant example of an evolutionary cul-de-sac—the "dinosaur" of the technological bestiary, large and safely extinct. For a "de-naturalizing" social constructionist account of the bicycle's development (containing a number of factual errors which do not however vitiate the general approach), see Trevor Pinch and Wiebe Bijker, "The social construction of facts and artifacts: Or how the sociology of science and the sociology of technology might benefit each other" in *The Social Construction of Technological Systems*, W. Bijker, T.P. Hughes & T. Pinch, eds, MIT Press, 1987, pp.17-50.

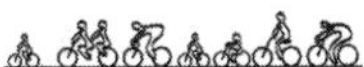

4. This is in no way to deny the phenomenon of diffusion, but to notice how it works as ideology. It is an empirical question whether in any particular case the presence of some technology or other is to be explained by diffusion, or independent development, or some amalgam. For a general discussion of Eurocentrism and its relation to diffusionism, see James M. Blaut, *The Colonizer's Model of the World: Geographical Diffusionism and Eurocentric History*, New York: Guilford Press, 1993.
5. See Hans-Erhard Lessing, "Aspects of the early invention of the bicycle," Cycle History 11: Proceedings of the 11th International Cycling History Conference, Van der Plas Publications, San Francisco, 2001, 28-36. An adequate account of this very complex subject would have to tackle also the cult of Lockean individualism, its relation to capitalist regimes of property, in particular the patent system, and the way they operate to deny (in order to privatize) the social nature of knowledge production, not least the informal and vernacular artisanal traditions that have always been central to bicycle culture. See, for example, Joseph Corn, "Object Lessons/Object Myths: What Historians of Technology Learn from Things," in David Kingery, ed., *Learning from Things*, (Washington, D.C.: Smithsonian Institution Press, 1996), 35-54.
6. J. Needham, *Science and Civilization in China*, multi-volume series, Cambridge University Press, Cambridge, 1954- ; see also his *The Grand Titration: Science and Society in East and West*, Toronto: University of Toronto Press, 1969.
7. J. Needham, *Science and Civilization in China*, multi-volume series, Cambridge University Press, Cambridge, 1954- ; see also his *The Grand Titration: Science and Society in East and West*, Toronto: University of Toronto Press, 1969.
8. Bacon was the English prophet of industrialism, and patron saint of the Royal Society, the first modern scientific society. His technocratic utopia *New Atlantis* was a kind of 17th century R&D park.
9. See Lessing, op.cit.
10. For an extended argument for nature's agency in 19th century colonial and political history, see Mike Davis, *Late Victorian Holocausts*, Verso, London, 2000.
11. When I first issued this challenge, at an international gathering of cycle historians in Osaka, Japan, in August 2000, I did not know of Chris Carlsson's plans for this book on Critical Mass cycling, though it was adumbrated in Chris Carlsson, *Shaping San Francisco*, CD-ROM and website (www.shapingsf.org), 1995- ; see also the video documentary, *Return of the Scorcher*, by Ted White. Critical Mass and its relation to bike messengers now needs to be compared and contrasted with earlier histories of rickshawmen's agitation.
12. Richard Drayton, *Nature's Government: Science, Imperial Britain, and the 'Improvement' of the World*, Yale University Press, 2000, Ch.7.
13. Adam Hochschild, *King Leopold's Ghost*, Houghton Mifflin, Boston, 1998, pp.158ff.
14. Julia Meech-Pekarik, *The World of the Meiji Print: Impressions of a New Civilization*, Weatherhill Press, New York, 1986, p.99.
15. Quoted in Meech-Pekarik, p. 84.
16. The Far East, March 16, 1872.
17. I thank Kaz Koike for this insight, and for his help in interpreting the Utagawa Yoshitora print, *Vehicles on the Streets of Tokyo*.
18. Tony Wheeler and Richard I'Anson, *Chasing Rickshaws*, Lonely Planet, Melbourne, 1998, p.181. See also, from the perspective of labor history, R. Gallagher, *The Rickshaws of Bangladesh*, University Press, Dhaka, 1992, and James Warren, *Rickshaw Coolie: A People's History of Singapore, 1880-1940*, Oxford University Press, 1986.
19. Assuming Yoshitora is picturing a velocipede he had seen in Tokyo. According to Meech-Pekarik, he could not have seen the steam engine until two years later.
20. I thank Mark Driscoll for this information. The late Maeda Ai's work on the bicycle has not yet been translated; a large collection of his manuscripts is now deposited with Cornell University.
21. Thomas Stevens, *Around the World on a Bicycle, Volume 2, From Teheran to Yokohama*, New York, Scribner's, 1888.

THE GREAT BICYCLE PROTEST OF 1896

ED. NOTE: The 1890s popular movement for Good Roads, pushed most ardently by bicyclists, is of note for several reasons. Primarily the fight for better conditions for bicycling unknowingly set the stage for the rise of the private automobile. Within a decade of the big demonstrations detailed here, better roads and improved tire technology combined with breakthroughs in internal combustion to launch the car industry. Obviously the private automobile has played a pivotal role in transferring the cost of transportation to the individual (thereby intensifying financial needs, summed up in the absurd conundrum of "driving to work to make money to pay for my car to drive to work"). It has also been central to the speeding up of daily life, especially in the sprawl of the post-World War II era. (Of course if you're stuck in a traffic jam during every commute, you may question how "speeded up" the car has made your life.) In any case, the colorful popular demonstrations that filled San Francisco's decrepit streets in the 1890s find a contemporary echo in the monthly Critical Mass bike rides that started in San Francisco in 1992 and spread across the world. The unintended consequences of the 19th century popular mobilization for Good Roads provide important food for thought as we engage in political movements of resistance and imagination.

—C.C.

BY HANK CHAPOT

In the lase decades of the 1800s, the bicycle became an object of pleasure and symbol of progress to Americans. Enthusiasts hailed it as "a democratizing force for good, the silent steed of steel, the modern horse." The Gilded Age was the Bicycle Age. Millions of new bicyclists demanded good roads to accompany their embrace of this newfound means of transportation.

San Francisco, though third wealthiest city in the nation, was an aging boomtown. Streets were muddy, cobbled, unpaved and increasingly crisscrossed with streetcar tracks and cable slots—an unpredictable, hazardous riding surface. The city's old dirt roads and cobblestone thoroughfares, originally laid for a village of 40,000, now served a metropolis of 360,000.

On Saturday night, July 25th of 1896, after months of organizing by cyclists and good roads advocates, residents cycled the streets in San Francisco, inspired by the possibilities of the bicycle.

Enjoyed by perhaps 100,000 spectators, the parade ended in unanimous resolutions in favor of good roads and a near riot at Kearny and Market. The next day's headlines in the *S. F. Call* captured the rally's success: "A Most Novel And Magnificent Wheel Pageant Did Light Up Folsom Street" and "San Francisco Bicycle Riders—Disciples Of Progress."

Since the 1880's, riders across the country agitated for access and safer urban streets. Increasingly organized, their mission was political and social as cycling became a way of life. Bicyclists demonstrated in large American cities like Chicago, where wheelmen and wheelwomen held riding exhibitions and mass meetings, eventually forcing the city to withdraw a rail franchise for a West End boulevard.

The bicycle's popularity exploded with the Safety Bicycle in 1885 which eliminated the danger of riding the giant "high wheelers." The invention of the pneumatic tire in 1889 cushioned the ride. Bicycle ownership exploded in the 1890's among all classes, shop owners purchased delivery bikes and businesses purchased fleets. Riders worked in organized "wheel clubs" that in addition to political activism, promoted social events, elected officers, ran competitions, sponsored dances and country rides. Many had clubhouses in the city and ran "wheel hotels" in the countryside. The women of the Falcon Cycling Club ran one in an abandoned streetcar near Ocean Beach.

Through the League of American Wheelmen (L.A.W.), founded in 1880 in Rhode Island, cyclists across the country joined the movement. Bicycle organizing was already in full swing by 1887 when the *New York Times* editorialized ". . . since bicycles have been declared vehicles by the courts, they should be declared by statute entitled to the privileges and subject to the duties of wheeled traffic." As local agitation grew into a national clamor, the L.A.W. became the umbrella organization for the wider good roads movement. Bicycle agitation spread globally and locally. Candidates for local office found that unless they supported good roads, they stood little chance against well-organized L.A.W. chapters.

The San Francisco Movement

The 1896 protest was tied to the campaign to pass a City Charter that nullified unused street rail franchises. The charter was a core project of the Southside Merchants Association and the cyclery owners of the Cycle Board of Trade were unanimous in support. The protest offered a chance to rally San Francisco to the cause.

Cyclists risked crashing upon the raised steel slot in the roadbed through which cable cars gripped the cable, or slipping on the unpaved trackways. Most cyclists hated "the slot" and the street railways that ran upon it. Companies were killing old franchises to maintain their monopolies but leaving the tracks in place while more and more Mission District bicyclists needed access to downtown. They wanted abandoned rail tracks removed, pavement between the rails and reduction of the height of the slot, Market Street sidewalks reduced and overhead wires put underground when streets were rebuilt—common practices in eastern cities. They also wanted a road from their neighborhood to Golden Gate Park, and because thousands were riding there at night, they wanted illumination with electric lights like Central Park.

Meeting at the Indiana Bicycle Company Thursday before the parade, cyclists discussed their greatest opponent, the Market Street Railway, whom they blamed for the sorry condition of their main thoroughfare. "A person takes his life into his own hands when he rides on that street" someone said, accusing the streetcar company of sprinkling the street when many wheelmen and women were heading home from work. Another predicted that "with good roads, urban workers would ride to their places of business ...a good thing because it would cut into the income of the tyrannical street railroad." They had a friend in the Street Department, a wheelman himself, who promised that all obstacles would be

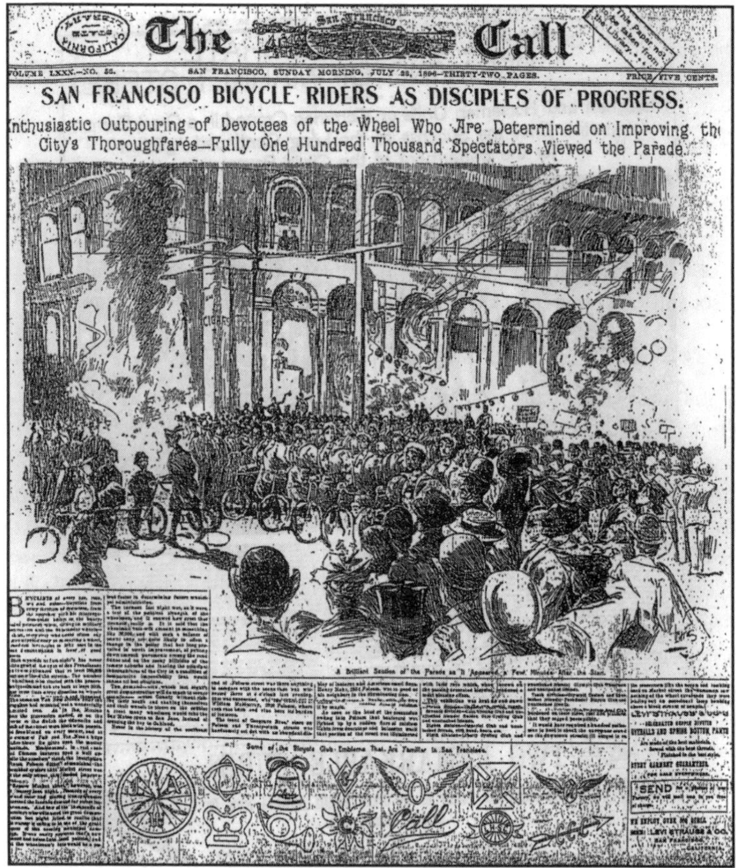

The San Francisco Call

VOLUME LXXX.—NO. 56. SAN FRANCISCO, SUNDAY MORNING, JULY 26, 1896—THIRTY-TWO PAGES. PRICE FIVE CENTS.

SAN FRANCISCO BICYCLE RIDERS AS DISCIPLES OF PROGRESS.

Enthusiastic Outpouring of Devotees of the Wheel Who Are Determined on Improving the City's Thoroughfares—Fully One Hundred Thousand Spectators Viewed the Parade.

removed from the route Saturday and streets would not be sprinkled.

Folsom Street was the main boulevard through the Mission and cyclists worked diligently for pavement from 29th to Rincon Hill. The July 25th rally would celebrate the opening of a new portion. The *Call* interviewed owners and managers of some of the numerous cyclerys in town, who spoke as one. Each was a sponsor of "the agitation" and each would close early on Saturday. In San Francisco that July, their demand was "Repave Market Street," their motto, "Where There Is a Wheel, There Is a Way."

A five-year wheelman named McGuire, speaking for the South Side Improvement Club stated: "The purpose for the march is three-fold; to show our strength, to celebrate the paving of Folsom Street and to protest against the conditions of San Francisco pavement in general and of Market Street in particular. If the Press of this city decides that Market Street must be repaved, it will be done in a year." Asked if southsiders were offended that the grandstand would be north of Market, McGuire exclaimed, "Offended! No! We want the north side to be waked up. We south of Market folks are lively enough, but you people over the line are deader than Pharaoh!"

The Emporium Department Store paved Market Street at 5th at its own expense, using tarred wooden blocks laid over the old basalt as an example of what Market Street should look like. Unfortunately, much of the Emporium's efforts would be undone during the commotion later on Saturday evening.

Several politicians had been invited and most sent letters assuring their friendly disposition toward the wheelmen. With the appointment of so many vice-presidents to the parade committee including the Mayor, two Congressmen, both Senators and the City Supervisors, political notice seemed assured. From the Cycle Board of Trade and the Southside Improvement Association, the call went out to bicyclists and "all progressive and public-spirited citizens to participate."

The Great Bicycle Demonstration July 25, 1896

Thousands of spectators from "the less progressive sections of the city" were expected. The decorations committee had distributed 8,000 Chinese lanterns. Citizens along the route were invited to decorate their properties, cyclists encouraged to decorate their wheels, with prizes offered for the finest displays.

By early evening, homes and businesses along Folsom Street were ablaze with firelight as the committee made its rounds. Businesses decorated their storefronts; one with colorful bunting and flags surrounded by lanterns, while a homeowner used carriage lanterns to cast colored lights onto the street. The Folsom Street Stables were a mass of torchlight.

Promoters had wished to get electric lights strung the length of Folsom Street, but the mansions, businesses and walk-ups "were not content to burn a single hallway light as usual but were illuminated basement to garret, a full stream of gaslight in every room commending a view of the street, with an abundance of Chinese lanterns strung from eaves to buildings across the street." Calcium lights cast the brightest glow but many windows "were lit in the old fashioned style, rows of candles placed one above the other." Every window was full of cheering spectators.

The divisions gathered on Shotwell Street in their finest riding attire and street clothes or their most gruesome costumes. The largest (from the L.A.W.) dressed as street-laborers. The Bay City Wheelmen, YMCA Cyclers, the Pacific, Liberty, Olympia, Call and Pathfinders bike clubs were all represented. Members

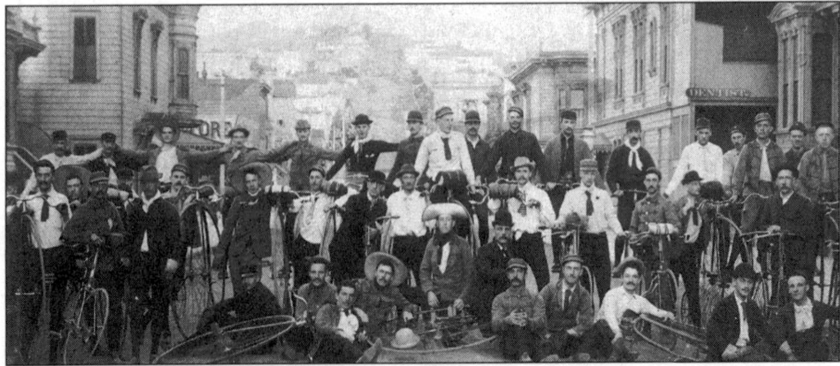

Bay City Wheelmen, c. 1890, San Francisco

wore insignias of their affiliations. "Unattached friends" were invited to join a favorite division.

Bicycles were adorned with ribbons and painted canvas with lanterns strung from the handlebars or from poles above—creating "a sea of Chinese lanterns as far as the eye could see." One was decorated with a stack of parasols, another intertwined with flowers and garlands, others "revolving discs of light guided by mystic men in garbs of flame." A few rode the old-fashioned "high-wheelers." Tandems were joined to create a pirate ship, another pair carried "a little chariot from which a child drove through the air two beautiful little bicycles." Many carried cowbells that "turned the night into pandemonium."

Clubs from as far away as Fremont, Vallejo, Santa Rosa and San Jose lined up alongside worker's divisions, letter carriers, soldiers from the Presidio and sailors from Angel Island. The SF *Call* stated cheerfully, "Though most of the column was composed of clubs, there was no restraining line to prevent the participation of individuals. Everyone was welcome to the merrymaking."

A few men rode in drag, one "in the togs of a Midway Plaisance maiden," another as an old maid beside a young woman as the "Tough Girl." Uncle Sam rode in bloomers next to a downhome hayseed. There were meaner stereotypes: Sitting Bull and Pocahontas, a man in bloomers mocking "the new women," one in blackface, one "imitating a Chinese in silks."

One riding club did not attend. For three years, the Colored Cycle Club of Oakland had sought membership in the League. Three days earlier they were again denied. But the Sunday *Call* would exclaim, "Bicyclists of every age, race, sex and color—bicyclists from every stratum of cycledom, the scorcher to the hoary-headed patriarch . . . turned out for the great demonstration in favor of good streets."

The parade president had invited liverymen and teamsters to join the march, and though many southsiders had to rent horses, they planned to "pay a silent tribute" later at the reviewing stand near City Hall, "to that noble and patient animal, for he is still with us."

The Parade Begins

Late in starting, the Grand Marshall "hid his blushes in the folds of a huge sash of yellow silk" and called the march. Orders had been passed down that candles not be lighted until commanded, but the streets were ablaze as the horsemen began. As the order to march came down the line, the glowing lanterns began to bob and weave above the crowds. Fireworks filled the air and the new pavement hummed beneath the wheels.

The children's division proceeded with the Alpha Ladies' Cycling Club in their first public ride. It had taken some effort to induce the Alphas to attend, yet the women's clubs were greeted with heavy enthusiasm. The procession quickly stretched ten blocks in "literally a sea of humanity." The children and a few others dropped out at 8th Street, but the majority of cyclists pressed on, all the while "good-naturedly" bombarded by Roman candles.

By 8th Street, the cyclists were forced to dismount and push their wheels

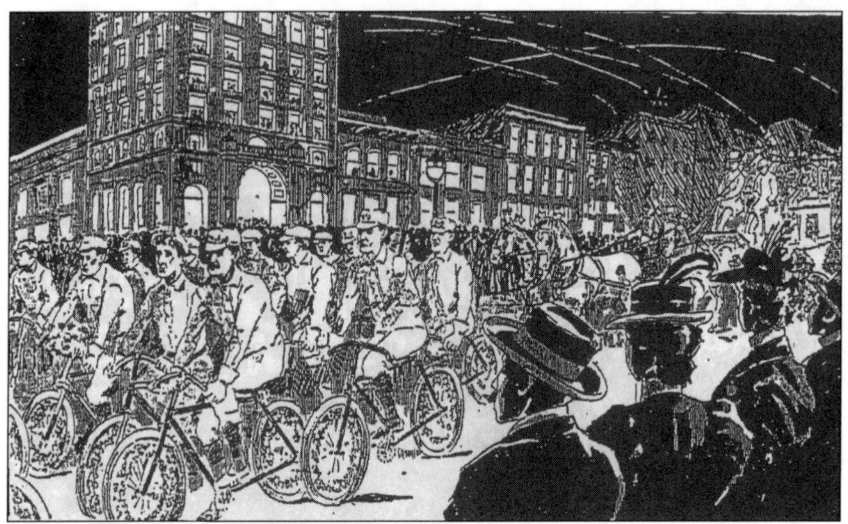

through a narrow strip above the rail tracks as the police began to worry about the "over-enthusiastic crowds." Upwards of 100,000 San Franciscans "watched the energetic wheelmen speed upon their whirling way." The disturbance caused by the streetcars and the narrowness of the space available in the center of the street began to separate the bicycle divisions.

At Market, streetcars were "so burdened, their sides, roof and platform sagged perceptively." The crowd filled the street and only a few lanterns appeared above the spectators. Riders had planned to dismount and push for three blocks to show "the pavement is too bad for any self-respecting wheel to use," but ended up pushing much of the way. Approaching Powell and Market, "the cyclists encountered a surging mass." Bells of a dozen trapped streetcars added to the chaos. When a number 21 car got too close to one division, some in the crowd began rocking it, attempting to overturn it.

Not surprisingly, some in the crowd had destructive intent, including, "an army of small boys from the Mission who ruthlessly smashed and stole the lanterns." The *Chronicle* decried, "They stole them by the score and those they couldn't pluck they smashed with sticks . . . others filled respectable spectators with dismay by their language." Before the last cyclists had passed up Market Street a larger disturbance broke out among the spectators. "The hoodlums began a warfare upon the streetcars," gasped the *Chronicle*. People were pulling up the Emporium's tarred blocks and throwing them beneath the streetcar wheels and at the cars directly, breaking windows while passengers cowered inside. When a car stopped, they attempted to overturn it by rocking it and when one got away, they fell upon the next. Squads of police chased and clubbed the crowds back uptown.

At City Hall, both sides of Van Ness were "black with people," when the lead firewagon finally appeared, well after 9:30 p.m., greeted by a great roar. At the grandstand in the gathering fog, accompanied by bursting fireworks, the crowd cheered as each new division straggled in.

On the reviewing stand sat many important San Franciscans; a Senator, a Congressmen, several Supervisors and the fine ladies and gentlemen of San Francisco's southside community. A gigantic bonfire blazed in City Hall Square, another burned at Fell and Van Ness; fires glowed around the plaza. Behind the stage hung a huge banner lighted by the ubiquitous lanterns stating simply, "FINISH FOLSOM STREET." Under a festoon of lights, speeches of "varying qualities of oratory" received tremendous applause.

Julius Kahn, an enthusiastic wheelman, preached good roads and great civilizations. Senator Perkins promised pavement to the Park, and lighting too. The last speaker claimed the bicycle had solved the age-old question that perplexed both Plato and Mayor Sutro, who rarely left the Heights in the evening: "How to get around in the world!"

Aftermath

Although the disturbance at Kearny and Market was not completely out of character for San Franciscans, the cyclists, to say the least, were not amused. Meeting Sunday after the parade, argument raged. Someone shouted "Chief Crowley is dissembling when he declares he could not put enough men out for a bicycle parade," Mr.Wynne agreed. "They are perfectly able to be out in force around boxing night at the Pavilion when some 'plug-uglies' are engaged in battering each other."

The final resolution declaring victory was approved unanimously.

"The parade exceeded any similar events held west of Chicago and the objects of the demonstration have been fully accomplished and we have aroused the sympathy and secured the support of the well-wishers of San Francisco."

They decried the inefficiency of the Police Department and especially condemned the Market Street Railroad Company's "outrageous, high-handed actions in operating and insolently intruding their cars into the ride, thus breaking into the route and materially interfering with its success." A vote of thanks was extended to

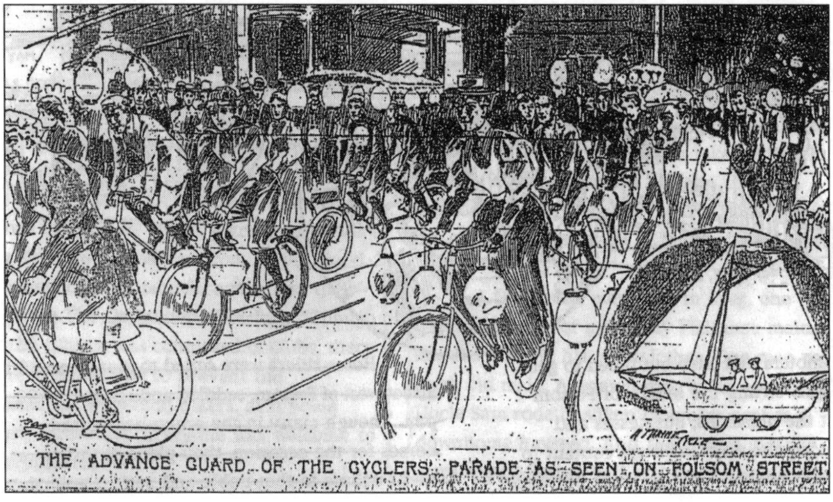
THE ADVANCE GUARD OF THE CYCLERS' PARADE AS SEEN ON FOLSOM STREET.

the Street Department for the fine manner in which it had prepared the road.

The Sunday papers estimated five thousand riders had taken part. The *Examiner* was effusive: "It was the greatest night the southsiders have have had since the first plank road was laid from the city gardens into the chaparral and sand dunes where 16th Street now stretches it's broad road." The *Call* heralded "An Enthusiastic Outpouring of Devotees of The Wheel."

That Sunday morning, the *Examiner* sent a reporter to Golden Gate Park to count cyclists, who had exclusive use of the drives. He recorded the number of women and men, types of wheels and clothing styles. "The men riding in the early morning, erect and never exceeding six miles per hour, wore knickerbockers, sack coats and scotch caps." These were "the best type of cyclist." Later, "the hard riding element appeared with a perceptible change in attire, their speed increased." The clubs followed and finally those on rented wheels, their garb "apparently hastily improvised." He observed numerous tandems. "Bloomer maids outnumbered their sisters in skirts 4 to 1." The paper published hourly figures totaling 2,951 cyclists between 7 a.m. and 5 p.m."

Great change took place, and swiftly. Cyclists rode in victory on a paved Market Street in 1898, but the victory was short lived. Roads were improved at about the time the bicycle lost public fascination to the automobile, and oil began to power transportation. Membership in the L.A.W. slipped heavily by the turn of the century. National bicycle sales dropped from 1.2 million in 1899 to 160,000 in 1909.

The bicycle remained an important option for workers and businesses for decades before being redefined as a child's toy following World War II. Its popularity rebounded in the 1930's and again strongly in the 1990's. In much of the world, it never left. Appearing between the horse and the automobile, the bicycle had helped define the Victorian era and aided the liberation of workers, women and children, as it changed concepts of personal freedom. On two wheels, individuals were free to move across distances at a greater speed than ever before, independent of horse or rail.

The Great Protest of 1896 remained unique for 101 years until, on another July 25th, in 1997, bicyclists again took over Market Street, this time as Critical Mass—in direct lineage from the wheelmen and wheelwomen of 1896!

When Market Street Reaches 'Critical Mass'

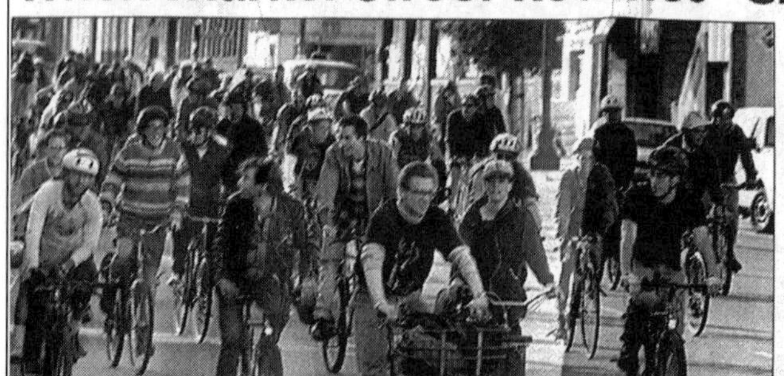

One Friday a month, bicycles become the dominant vehicle

BY SAM WHITING
Chronicle Staff Writer

Affecting a bike messenger's bravura, Paul Decker stands on his pedals, looks up Market Street and likes what he sees. Slowly migrating west are hundreds of bicyclists, clogging the Friday commute from the Financial District.

"When it gets going, it can span four or five blocks," says Decker proudly, "which is a pretty good piece of change."

From Decker's rear vantage, the pack resembles a cross between a contrary Tour de France and the Hell's Angels run to Bass Lake. Riders on all kinds of vin-

Critical Mass is a "happy coincidence" of two-wheelers who gather at Justin Herman Plaza, across from the Ferry Building, at 5:30 p.m. on the last Friday of each month. From there the bicyclists, numbering as many as a thousand, ride up Market, tying up the mad commute rush for as long as 20 minutes. The leisurely ride usually ends at Mission Dolores Park, or occasionally a more exotic destination, such as Ocean Beach, the Marin Headlands or on the last Friday of May, Candlestick Park, for a Giants night game and fireworks show.

For one hour of one Friday a month, the bicyclists own the road, and motorists must defer —

San Francisco Chronicle, June 16, 1994

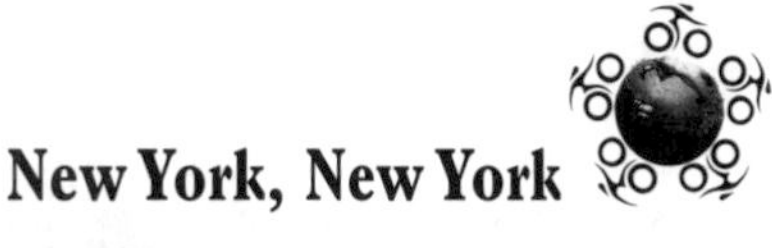

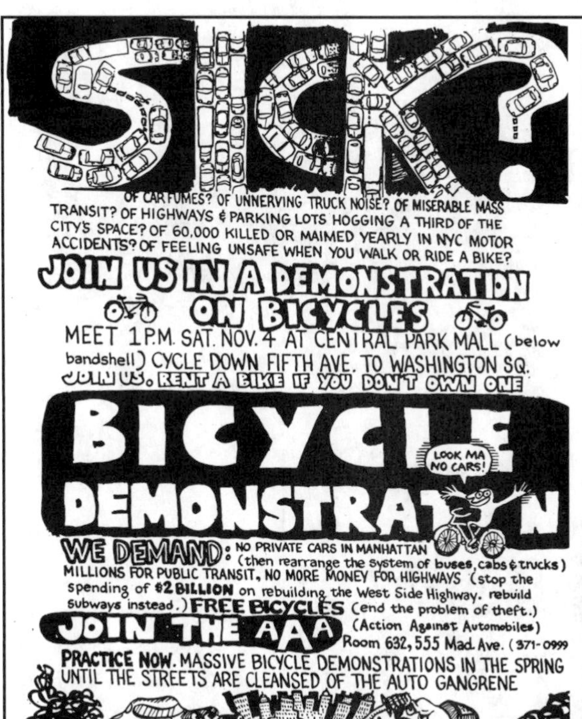

In New York in the early 1970s a movement of bicyclists arose against car traffic and highways. Mass bike rides were held demanding bike lanes amongst other things. Similar rallies erupted in Paris, France (10,000 cyclists clogged the streets on April 23, 1972) as bicyclists agitated for improved conditions in many places.

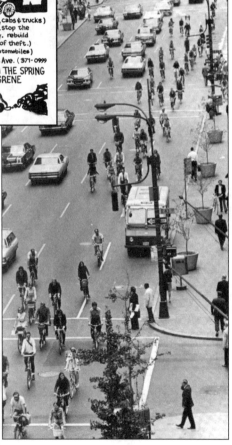

In the United States, the 1970s saw the widespread development of urban bike lanes in the wake of the energy crisis, though they were little used. But the mass rides of the time, especially in New York, were an important antecedent to today's Critical Mass rides. —*C.C.*

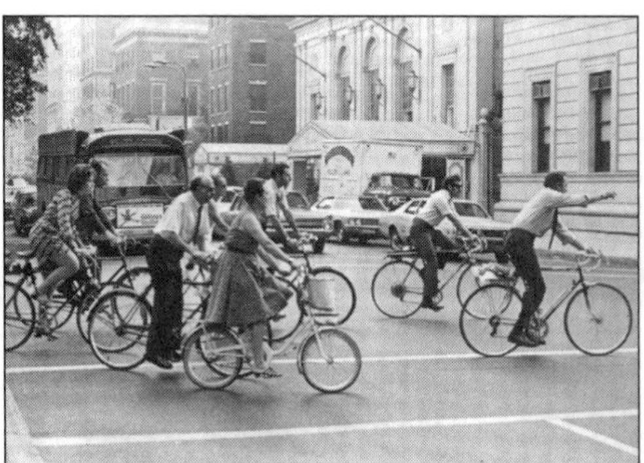

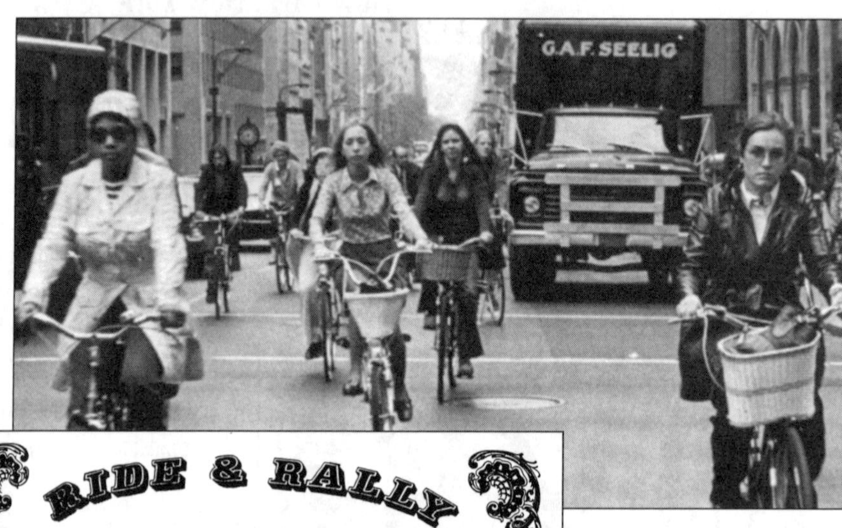

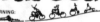

RIDE & RALLY

FOR A NEW YORK BICYCLE LANE NETWORK

TRANSPORTATION ALTERNATIVES

BIKE-IN

VIA THE AUTO SHOW

APRIL 7TH 1 PM

FROM CENTRAL PARK MALL at 72nd ST.

TO WASHINGTON SQUARE

Monte su bicicleta
venga con nosotros
Telefono: 220-3000

Music by Pete Seeger & other friends

Celebrate the SPRING!
Come RIDE with us!

Rain Date: Sunday April 8.

BOROUGH BRIGADES LEAVING IN MORNING:

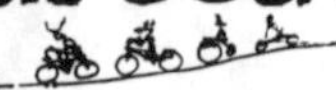

- Bronx: Poe Park (Concourse & Fordham Rd.) 11:00 am; call:220-3000
- Brooklyn: Grand Army Plaza, 11:00 am; base of Brooklyn Bridge, 11:45; call 287-6530
- Staten Island: S.I. Ferry at 11:15 am; call: 727-0697
- Queens: 63rd Road & Queens Blvd.; call: TW 7-2670 (eves) 939-7576 (days)

* For info or to volunteer to leaflet, call your borough no. In Manhattan, call: 865-9380

PLEASE POST

NYC Photos on previous page and above and below from *Bikes and Riders,* James Wagenvoord, 1972 (left) 1973 flyer

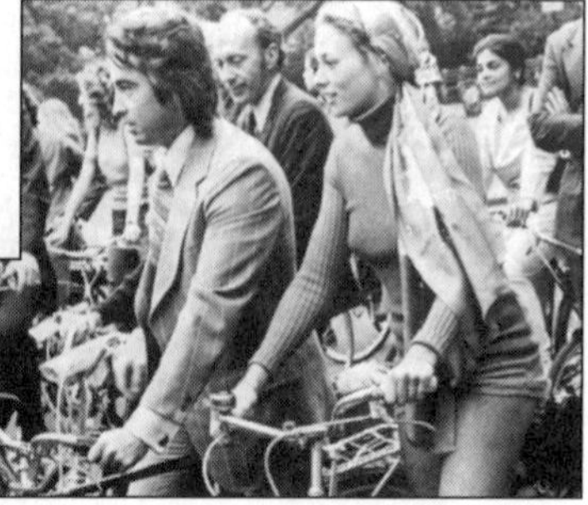

THE FIGHT FOR OUR STREETS

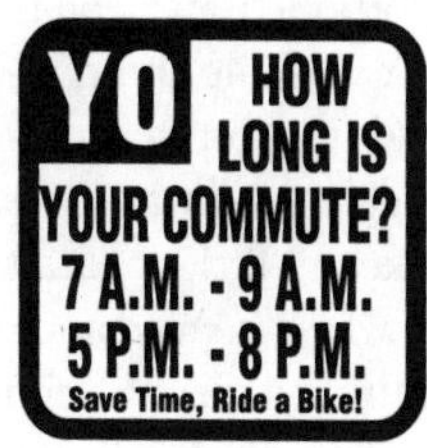

RIDING TO SEE

BY JOSHUA SWITZKY

Urban planners agree—Dense, compact, pedestrian-oriented cities structured around mass transit and bicycles with limited shared car services are the future. There can be no other future if we are to sustain the planet and our tenuous tenure on it. Depleted aquifers, choking haze, obliterated wilderness, loss of biodiversity, an obese populace, entanglement in foreign wars rooted in exploitation of natural resources, and a homogenous, cartoonish asphalt-covered cityscape not worth caring about are among the crises resulting from car travel and suburbanization. Critical Mass is most ostensibly a movement to assert and celebrate the bicycle's place in a modern eco-city, and the environmental arguments for greater bicycle accommodation are numerous and powerful. However what is often missing from discussions surrounding the motivation and effects of Critical Mass is the role of the bicycle in a humane city and the Mass' implicit critique of just how a humane city might look and feel.

The Bicycle and the City

The bicycle is ideally proportioned and engineered for navigating through a human-scaled urban landscape. A versatile and non-intrusive tool of transportation, the bicycle is swift and silent and graceful in motion. It can be held in your hand while walking on a sidewalk and chatting with a friend. Leaned against a lightpost outside a neighborhood cafe it takes up little space. It can squeeze through any opening or pathway, be out of the way when stopped and parked on a moment's notice for impromptu conversations or admiring a view. Cycling is an exercise in geography—natural, social, cultural, political. As cyclists, we become intimately familiar with our network of public spaces, and with a city's terrain and its inhabitants.

Though a solo act of transportation, riding a bicycle is a very social activity. Cycling not only exposes you to the natural elements, but to passing bits of conversation and chance encounters, to zigzagging down unknown alleys, to cruising through the farmers' market on your way to work. Cyclists are keenly aware of the sentiments of a neighborhood and the rhythms of a city. Intimate enough to engage with people on the streets and mobile enough to get a sense for the big picture, bicycles are vehicles of perception.

With sufficient numbers, bicycles can dictate the tempo and ambiance on a street, and this is exactly what Critical Mass accomplishes wherever it ventures. Critical Mass demands more than the mere apportionment of rightful space for cyclists in our road hierarchy. It demands a democratization and re-visualization of streets as vital public space, rightfully the domain of human civilization. CM acts out a re-occupation of streets under new ground rules regarding the balance between movement and destination, participant and spectator, serious dialogue and clowning levity. And above all, Critical Mass reintroduces the joyous spontaneity of living in contact with others into the regular course of city life.

Urban and Public

People gather in cities to make life rich, fulfilling, and enjoyable. Cities are meant to create mutually supportive communities and places for exchange. Ideas and experiences synthesize and fuse as they encounter one another in chaotic urban habitats.

No matter how much time I spend wandering around quiet mountain trails or loafing in numbingly-predictable-yet-comfortable suburbia, I am always drawn back to cities because of the great energy and diversity they provide—the untold mysteries harbored through every doorway and window shutter, new discoveries lurking just a step around each corner, exposure to new people strolling down the street, and odd juxtapositions of people adapting and transforming their environments.

City people are full of pent-up visions and ideas waiting to be expressed. Cities offer the physical space that gives life to this potential, these encounters of unknowns, this synthesis and debate of ideas. But what contemporary cities suffer from—especially American ones—is a lack of public space that is woven into everyday life. Instead, we are force-fed the familiar, the known, the one-sided gruel pumped through the ever-constricting mainstream channels of corporate communication.

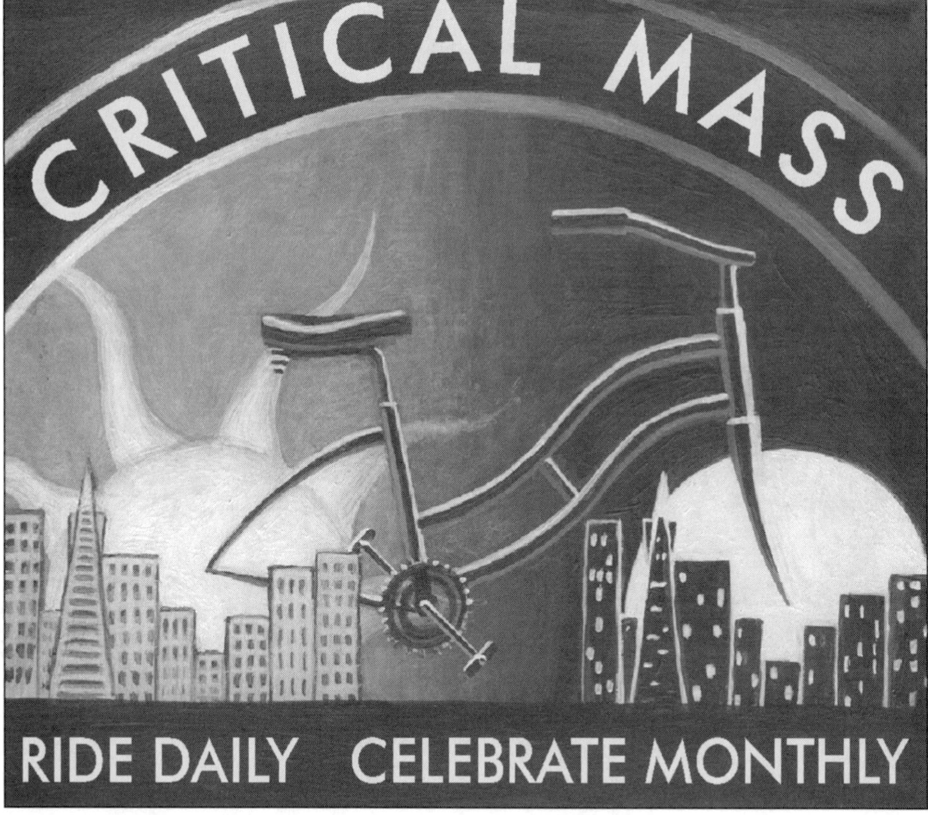
CRITICAL MASS
RIDE DAILY CELEBRATE MONTHLY

BETH VERDEKAL

In the age of private content-controlled, enclosed malls and sidewalk-less, single-use, subdivision pods, the only public space we know in common is that which we traverse by car. But in our cars we are usually alone, even if together on a "crowded" road. We peer at each other through tinted glass or stare at tail-lights, or sometimes we get out of the car to stand in line together to buy something. This is our only interaction. No conversations can be struck up in passing, no impromptu meetings or demonstrations or spontaneous theater materialize in this world (except the fascinating horror of the daily "accidents" which necessarily accompany automobilism). The only spaces designed for large numbers of people—stadiums and malls—are located on the fringe, isolated from daily life and populated only for special events, mostly sitting vacant. Drive-to or self-contained attractions are not functional public spaces. Good public spaces are integrally and seamlessly tied into the urban fabric and unavoidable parts of our daily routines. They are spaces that feel equally intimate when occupied by a single cyclist or a noontime concert. They are welcoming and accessible, not foreboding and monolithic.

Civil life and democracy themselves are withering. Freedom needs unprogrammed spaces to flourish; it needs space with equal and easy access to all people for it to function. Discussion, debate, exchange, openness—these are the things that cannot exist merely in the private enclaves of office buildings, houses, and malls. Ideas stagnate and die without fresh air. The Internet, while a welcome development, is a pale shadow of a real public commons.

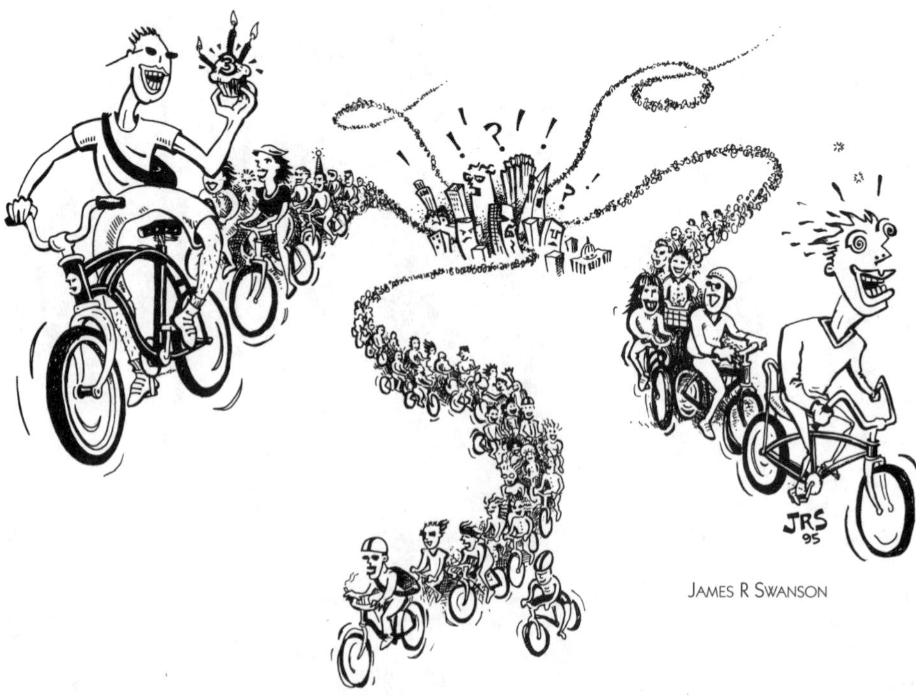

JAMES R SWANSON

In our technophilic and xenophobic society we are atomized more and more into segregated and isolating bubbles, whether in cars, chat rooms, office parks or living rooms glued to the tube. Increasingly tethered electronically to a tightening global web, we insulate ourselves from our immediate physical environment and shy away from physical interaction. This has led to more extremist, xenophobic, and myopic perspectives. We can relate to and tolerate "the other" less and less outside these bubbles. Especially in the security-paranoid wake of 9/11, the more we cordon ourselves off and shun contact, the more we fear unplanned mingling and interaction. This does not bode well for the future of cities or the prospects of cooperation and understanding in the global village.

In the age of the Internet and "cyber-communities," it's sometimes hard to think that we really need physical places to meet one another face-to-face. Yet we do more than ever. Democracy is not an institution that can survive or function properly while being inundated with mediated propaganda. Freedom cannot exist behind closed doors, nor can it be watched on TV. It must be acted out in the open, in plain view, on the stage of community life.

Critical Mass is uniquely skilled at plunging its participants into the messy, unpredictable public space of the streets. CM mixes spectacle with interaction, dialogue with movement. CM frees people from the conventional constraints of street behavior and liberates cyclists and pedestrians alike to utilize the full potential of public space.

Stepping off the Curb

Streets are our largest and most important piece of public open space in the city. They account for up to 30% of the total surface area of the city, yet we consider them only as afterthoughts. Streets are everyone's open space. We fret and tussle over every precious inch of our grassy parks, yet we overlook the massive wasted public spaces right outside each of our front doors, accessible to each and every resident. Streets could be our main stage. But somehow, around 1950, our growth and speed-intoxicated culture decided to sacrifice the *here* for the unending quest of getting to some amorphous *there*. Of course the there has equally been subjected to such values. Car culture is so obsessed with the grass that might be greener just a few miles' drive further out that *every place has become a no place*.

Our approach to the design and use of streets over the past 50 years has been to treat them as sewers—monofunctional conduits of ever-increasing volumes of effluent (motorized vehicles) at ever-increasing speeds, with all possible friction and volume-constraining elements (e.g. sidewalks, benches, trees, even buildings) stripped away to maximize flow. All humane elements, enriching texture, or quirks that create memorable places of interest have been subordinated to movement (and a very narrowly-constructed view of movement, at that). What we have been left with is no here or there.

Given how much they dominate our cityscape, streets should be more than means of getting from A to B, but should be places worth spending time in and of themselves. They should provide trees for shade, benches and stoops for rest, sculpture for amusement, and adjacent windows and doors that spill out with activity and intrigue. We have a right to expect streets to uplift our neighborhoods and provide space to move in a myriad of ways and tempos. Streets should be open to the possibilities for encounters and entropy.

We've created streets that enforce linearity—everything in its lane, moving forward as if we have blinders, and never back and forth or across and around or simply staying in place. Our world has been reduced to a network of interchangeable links with joints and endpoints of intersections, driveways, and parking lots. Critical Mass, with its amoeba-like swarming party that swirls and surges, turns streets into places that presuppose a different movement than perpetually forward. Riding in the Mass gives us a taste of a public street network with built in pauses and eddies, an organically linked series of events and spaces.

Critical Mass liberates cyclists to utilize the entirety of the street realm—breaking out of the linear confines of a lane mentality—and to not be afraid to weave exuberantly from side to side, pausing along the curb here, dashing forward there, looping when the time feels right. Pedestrians and other bystanders are also liberated by the example—seeing this free-form mass of cyclists taking liberties with the road space frees people to envision different movement possibilities and uses for streets—soccer matches, barbeques, dance performances, open markets, garden plots, hopscotch.

Space Crashes into Time

Changing the use of space as Critical Mass does also hints at changing the dominant *pace* of movement. A cross-section through a conventional American street would reveal two speeds—very fast and stopped. Streets are either raceways or parking lots. You're either at your destination or you're speeding there. Motorists habitually "jackrabbit" down streets between stoplights and stop signs—gunning the engine between intersections just to slam on the brakes, not understanding that moving at a moderate but steady pace will not only get them there at the same time, but will do so less stressfully and with less danger and annoyance to their surroundings.

Every new gadget, technological "advance," or improved streamlined design in our working and domestic lives is meant to speed up human labor to make us more efficient—either to produce more for the company or ostensibly to free our time for more leisure activities. But in practice, each new leap of productivity leads to further speeding up and rising expectations. Our lives start to resemble the mouse on the wheel. We spin our wheels faster and attempt to go farther but at the more hectic pace everything is blurred. The speedup taxes our concentration so much that we condition ourselves to tune out the noise. Unfortunately, the noise is what makes life interesting. This global speed-up has diminished our ability to appreciate, or even detect the existence of, the small details that give life richness, for these details—the shadows cast by a finely articulated cornice on an Italianate house or the wafting tunes emanating from a taqueria or the piece of poetry anonymously tacked to a telephone pole—are lost at 50 mph, or even 30 mph!

Critical Mass, and riding a bicycle in general, is a rebuttal to the relentless and enslaving speedup. We ride in CM at what is ironically called "rush hour," a term symbolic of the empty promises of the speedup. Movement, epitomized by "the commute," is one major aspect of people's lives that they hope to economize and zip through—movement viewed as wasted time. We treat streets as something to be rushed through, never savored or appreciated.

By slowing down—riding a bicycle, for example—the blurred background of streets and shops and parks and people becomes clearer. Critical Mass is a deliberate, communal act of decelerating the city to a humane and unstressful pace. Mass turns commuting on its head by converting it into a leisurely unhurried affair that encourages awareness and interaction with the tangible details of the city streets and its inhabitants. And by thus slowing down the pace, CM recaptures the street realm for a more intimate and local use. Motorists sitting through another gridlock on their crosstown race might not immediately appreciate the slowdown because Critical Mass playfully jabs at the futility of their "rush." Nevertheless, CM directly improves city life by establishing a human's pace, and manifesting it publicly.

In challenging these sacred cows head on—the type of "acceptable" movement and the pace of city streets—Critical Mass asserts streets as public space for celebration and dialogue, unsanctioned by the state and unsponsored by corporate benefactors. The Mass has a brilliant capacity to transform the cityscape through which it passes. Every time the mass of bicycles turns a corner and happens upon a routine street scene—cars rigidly queued and drivers idly seething in their lanes, pedestrians scurrying along a peripheral sliver of pavement, one-sided commercial billboards dictating to passersby passing as "dialogue"—the street metamorphosizes into a swirling, jingling festival of laughs and smiles on wheels.

To participate in Critical Mass is to catch a glimpse of the give and take among people that naturally belongs in public space. CM generates countless opportunities for exchange: cyclists chattering amongst themselves in the middle of pack, riders on the fringes of the mass engaging with pedestrians, cyclists engaging with motorists stopped in traffic, curious passersby questioning cyclists at the pre-ride gatherings. The ride itself creates a venue for distributing written literature—poetry and fiction, political action alerts and petitions, cultural screeds and artsy zines and party invitations—to other cyclists, to peds and motorists, and really anyone willing to stick out a hand. Critical Mass creatively appropriates urban geography with themed rides and route maps directing the ride to historical sites, natural features, or sites of current events, raising the space of the city itself from wallpaper to living stage.

But above all undertones of serious dialogue and social ruminations, the party atmosphere of Critical Mass is infectious. The sight of a roving carnival of smiles, cheers, tinkling bells, and good tidings taking over the otherwise mean streets lifts the spirits. The Mass regularly is greeted by hoots and hollers from third-story windows, honks from passing cars and buses, cheers from the sidewalks, waves from café tables. There is nothing so intoxicating as the exuberance of dancing in the streets.

My most rejuvenating and inspiring Critical Mass moment came in Boston, in an icy climate of reputedly icy motorists. On the Halloween 2000 ride, I took on the pleasure of "reverse trick-or-treating"—handing out sugary treats stapled to a CM flyer to drivers sitting in traffic while the Mass filtered by. At one particularly snarled intersection (which, mind you, was snarled long before we rode by), I approached a woman idling in a gargantuan SUV. I offered her a treat and she rolled down her window to accept my gifts. With a beaming smile she said, "I have something for you, too." She handed me a long-stemmed rose. I pedaled around with that rose affixed to my handlebars long after the petals fell off as a reminder of how enriching even a totally anonymous human encounter can be. The possibilities for such encounters are bleak these days, the spirits and hopes of human civilization wilting as these conditions worsen. Yet Critical Mass possesses a transformative power that shows these conditions are neither terminal nor inevitable.

Meet Me In the Street

Coloring within the lines and moving within the lanes—it's the act of automatons. Just like a canvas is meant to be filled with brush strokes and splashes of color, so too should a city be filled with people traversing its spaces, exploring and exploiting its nooks and crannies. Streets are the largest parcels of open space in any city and they belong to the people. The frenetic activity and entropy of city streets is exciting, it's infectious, it livens the pulse. The cacophony of ideas and mingling of cultures. . . the romance, the rock-n-roll, the revolution. . . It's in the streets. By injecting spontaneity and dialogue into city life, Critical Mass begins to define a humane city.

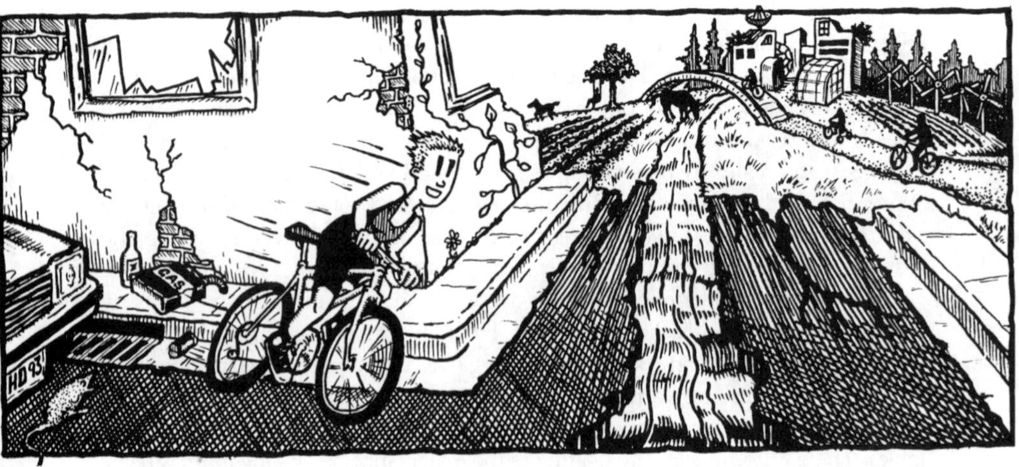

HUGH D'ANDRADE

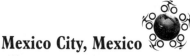

Mexico City, Mexico

BICITEKAS IN MEXICO CITY

BY AGUSTIN MTZ. MONTERRUBIO

Inside wheeled boxes, thousands of faces are the unsweetened reflection of the journey. The rush is the companion no one misses inside the car. It is increasingly difficult to navigate these slow tidal rivers that delay the arrival home. Meanwhile, in the Angel of Independence Plaza a group of human beings gather to create an urban conscience. Armed with bicycles, helmets, lights and informational flyers they sail into the sea of cars.

The uncontrollable chaos in the public avenues of the Valley of Mexico has brought forth again a sentiment against the public policies that favor the private car, disregard public transit and fail to appreciate alternatives.

In 1989 the Movement of Mexico City Bicyclists arose, demanding bicycle parking and bike lanes that would make possible and dignified bicycle riding through the city. The group grew fairly large, organized meetings that were heavily attended, but with all this they did not manage to gain influence, perhaps due to a lack of means to spread the message. As they didn't represent a general demand of the people, government functionaries limited themselves to giving tiny concessions. One of these was to reserve one lane for exclusive use of bicyclists on Avenida Insurgentes every Sunday. The Movement eventually vanished in the ebb and flow of social awareness.

Ten years later, *Bicitekas* began as an action group. It avoided complicated meetings that only served to vent frustration. Instead, a virtual community was established on the Internet where initiatives were planned that could be formulated in a horizontal structure.

Bicitekas made its first official "apparition" with an informational ride through the streets of the neighborhood called "Colonia Roma," to promote the creation of bikeways and bicycle parking facilities. A project to connect the most important Metro stations in the heavily traveled central zones was proposed and accomplished.

Bicitekas functioned politically, granting interviews, urging policies to "humanize the cities," affirming that our proposal was beneficial to the entire city.

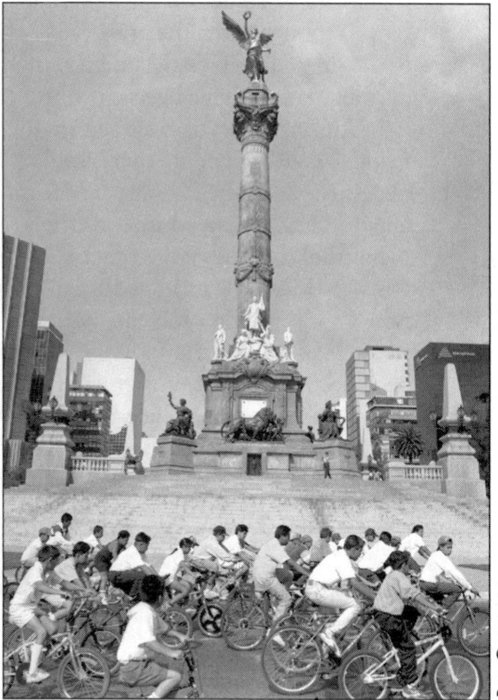

RICK GERHARTER

Movement of Mexico City Bicyclists, c. 1992

Bicitekas faced a bureaucratic labyrinth. The official apparatus slowed and rejected the *Bicitekas* agenda, offering a lot of talk and no action. Thanks to the fact that *Biciteka* adherents were journalists and graphic designers, they launched *Velo: The Magazine of Urban Bicycling*.

This began the editorial adventure that unleashed an urban action movement. Roberto Cruz is a lawyer that tries cases around the city, and like any other attorney, he went from court to court by car. By serendipity, he came across the first issue of *Velo* and it seemed to him a good idea. He decided to try his bicycle to get to work. Who would have thought that this professional would be converted into an administrator, spokesperson, and vital member of *Biciteka*? So, one by one, people joined the *Biciteka* movement and little by little are gaining ground and respect.

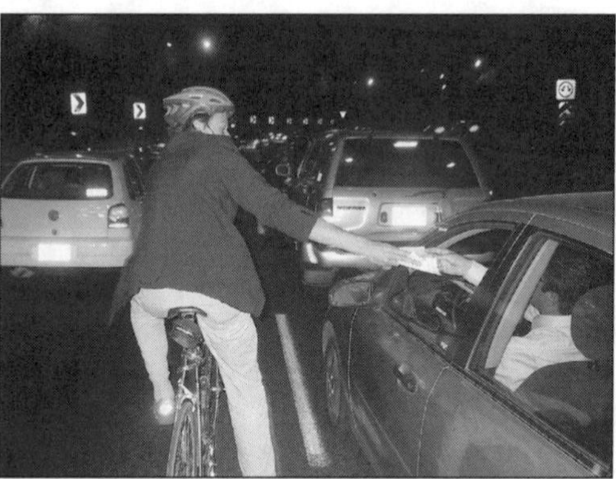

Agitating on the freeway in Mexico City against building a 2nd deck.

Every Wednesday night a ride of up to 50 bicyclists have taken the principal roads of the city. Since they started the Wednesday night rides, support and energy have been growing.

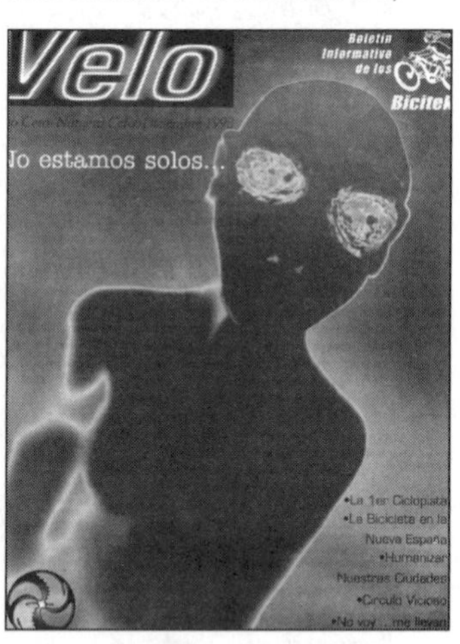

The presence of *Bicitekas* in the streets has made the authorities see that bicycling is a growing necessity, and already we are hearing promises about bikeways in various districts of the city. Nevertheless, the government of the Federal District (Mexico City) has chosen an absurd solution for the traffic problem. Bolstered by a questionable plebiscite, they are going to build a second deck on the main freeways that gird the city.

Work and perservence will bear fruit in the future; the pedals and wheels that have already begun to turn cannot be stopped.

Ciclistas Furiosas!

On the first Tuesday of every month, hundreds of "Ciclistas Furiosas," or enraged bicyclists, take to the streets of Santiago,Chile. Riding as slowly as possible, waving flags, and blowing whistles, they tangle up traffic to protest the city's dirty air, caused in large part by cars. The group, which began seven years ago and now boasts 5,000 members, emulates similar movements in the U.S. and Europe and aims to get people out of their cars, calling for bike lanes and car-free days.

—*Christian Science Monitor,* Aug. 16, 2000

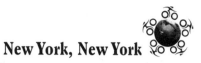

RECLAIMING THE STREETS OF NEW YORK
(for a world without cars)

BY BENJAMIN SHEPARD AND KELLY MOORE

In April 2000, 22 bicyclists, most of them regular participants in Critical Mass rode through Central Park in celebration of Earth Day. The police followed the group, stopped them, and ticketed them for obstructing traffic and for failing to have a permit for a "demonstration." This treatment was not unusual in New York that spring. A month earlier, twelve activists with black bandanas over their faces were targeted, profiled and arrested for wearing masks in public.

Yet, bicyclists and anarchists were not the only groups feeling the squeeze of growing informal and formal regulation of New York's public spaces. Squeegee guys, homeless people, cruisers, prostitutes, street vendors, and kids in baggy pants with their 40-ouncers were among the many on the long list of those thought to be emblematic of urban decay, threats to public order. They were targeted as part of a class cleansing of the city's public streets. A crowd control policy which had begun by cordoning off "participants" from "spectators" during the city's Halloween Parade/carnival had found its darkest expression in the racial profiling of those occupying public spaces. Unarmed immigrant Amadou Diallo and off duty security guard Patrick Dorismond had been shot by police for no other reason than being black in public. It was in this political context that Critical Mass and Reclaim the Streets-New York City decided to join forces to create a liberatory space beyond the socially sanctioned activities of shopping, driving and going to and from work which seemed to constitute the only safe way to use public space that Fall.

At their best, Critical Mass bike rides and Reclaim the Streets Actions create brief autonomous zones (see Bey, 1991). Born in London in 1995, Reclaim the Streets was part of a worldwide movement with local branches throwing road parties as both a protest against the corporatization of public space and as a living, dancing as example of what public space could be. Reclaim the Streets-NYC

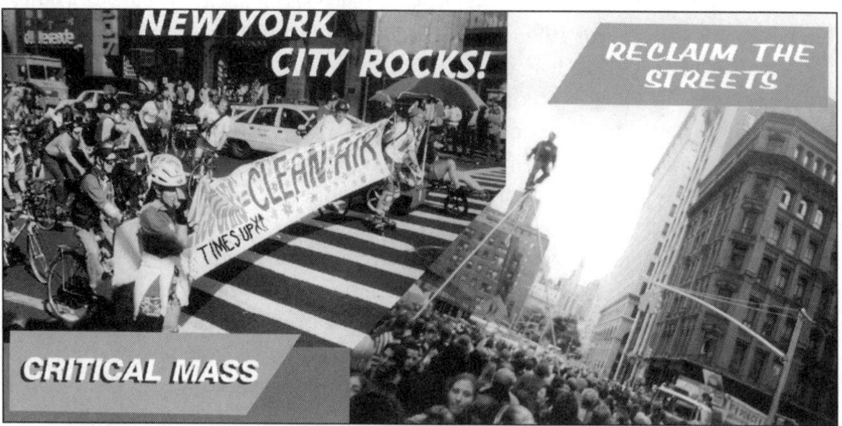

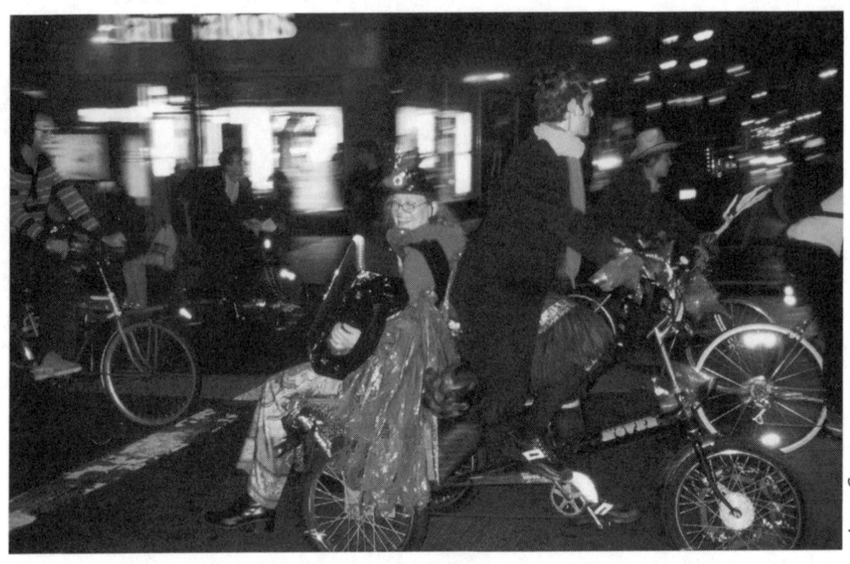

ALISA CLARK

Halloween Critical Mass, NYC 2001

was formed by members of the Lower East Side Collective, the Blackout Books Collective and Times UP! Its first action was an unsanctioned dance party on the corner of Broadway and Lafayette Streets in New York's East Village. Unlike its ambitious counterparts across the ocean who had recently torn a McDonalds restaurants from its roots, RTS NYC focused more on contested spaces such as community gardens or forming alliances with local labor groups (such as underpaid Green Grocers) than on hard core direct action. But this was not enough to prevent RTS from being featured on FBI Director Louis Freeh's list of domestic terrorist threats. While "Public Space for the Public!" had been the group's slogan, "God Bless Hysteria" became its mantra after its new notoriety. (For more information on RTS/NYC, go to www.rtsnyc.org and see Duncombe, 2002; for information on RTS international, visit www.gn.apc.org/rts).

Although Critical Mass rides had taken place sporadically in New York over ten years, it was not until 1999 that the ride became a regular feature of the rough and tumble urban political landscape. Time's Up, a local activist environmental group, revived the ride by linking it to a burgeoning Lower East Side activism of anti-gentrification, environmental, labor, queer and anti-police brutality movements. This mix of ingredients would become the basis for broader global justice movement which gained international recognition in 1999. In response to the new hyper-regulation of public space demanded by corporate globalization's hold on cities, a new generation of groups—from Sex Panic!, to Right of Way, to Surveillance Camera Players and More Gardens!—emerged to challenge the increasingly restricted parameters of public expression in the city. Public space was eroding, as were our rights to participate within these geographies of the public sphere (see Dunlap, 2000, Ferrell, 2001). Social spaces were filling with omnipresent technologies of surveillance and control (see Hardt, 2000). Concurrent with these changes, the impulse to respond became an imperative.

On any given last Friday of the month, New York Critical Mass rides are filled with a constituency of anarchists, village people, neighborhood wingnuts, vagabonds, commuters, kids, and art-and-revolution types, and the ubiquitous bike-messengers-with-attitude who made the ride famous in San Francisco. Every month the New York Critical Mass ride offers a different theme. One of the most popular and repeated rides is the Critical Mass for More Community Gardens, in which all the bikers decorate themselves and their bikes as the plants, whose very existence is under threat from zealous developers. This multi-focused ride publicized the city's campaign to destroy community gardens created on abandoned lots throughout the city. "Dress scary" flyers for Halloween brings out ghouls and goblins on wheels; each ride "theatricizing" possibilities for a more liberatory way of interacting in the city. A rejection of enforced monoculture, Critical Mass is about going from Q to E instead of A to Z, delightfully avoiding the linear functions of the every day. Critical Mass is a refusal to submit to "the magic" of the New York City Tourist Board's vision, preferring a plurality of urban storylines, multiple personalities, genders and hijinks in human interactions and public spaces. Substituting improvisation for hierarchies, rides have neither leaders, clear routes nor destinations.

In September 2000, Reclaim the Streets and Times Up!, two local public space groups, organized a Critical Mass action called "Reclaim the Streets for a World without Cars." We were there. It was blissful, utterly blissful.

The idea was born at a brainstorming session during the regular Reclaim the Streets meeting outside the Charas Community Center in August of 2000. More Gardens! and Times UP! helped drive the proposal, intersecting memberships between the groups contributing to create the movement which is Lower East Side activism. Ben and his comrades were thinking about what to do about the million people driving around Avenues A and B on Friday and Saturday nights, clogging up the Lower East Side. They were also trying to figure out how to localize the global justice movement after the A-16 protests against the IMF in D.C. and a major May Day Action in Union Square. The idea was to create a campaign for a Car Free Day in New York City.

What would make New York City a fantastic place for a day? A place were it would be easy for a plant to grow and for people to breathe, to have a conversation in public without feeling like you would be run over? Some skeptics thought that Critical Mass would be destroyed forever if riders showed up and were quickly engulfed by a RTS action and street party. Over the previous two years in NY, the police routinely intercepted protesters, street parties, and threatened to arrest Critical Mass riders. The message had been simple. If we were to stage an unpermitted party, we faced the scenario of mass arrests in which bicyclists would have their bikes taken away. In the end, a majority willing to challenge potential police repression was able to sway enough skeptics to find consensus, set a date and a theme for the action.

Ben: *I donned my leopard skin jacket ready for anything the evening was going to give me. I had wanted to look like Prince (but couldn't really pull it off). I recall going out in drag in San Francisco, trying to look like Donna Summer. My friends said I looked like Howard Stern. There were the usual "lord have mercy" pre-action jitters on the subway ride to the action. A friend said he'd felt the same way: Before he leaves for political actions, he sometimes looks at his bed in the morning, wistfully thinking about when he's going to see that space again. Arrests in New York City usually involve 24 hours or more.*

I couldn't have been more excited to see my comrades with green hair, pink jackets, crowns, hats, and the piñata. As more groups converged on Union Square, the site where generations earlier activists fought the battle for the minimum wage, the energy was growing. Our view was embodied in the drag anthem from Rocky Horror Picture Show, "Don't dream it, live it." We envisioned a public open to a vast new world of scenarios, dramas, and plot twists, most of which are rarely presented by just going to and from work. So, of course we had to dress up in the way we would want the city to be: A place where work dress codes and official uniforms of sameness were left behind for the possibility of a street where social categories disappear.

Kelly: *I have two notebooks at home, one called "I Love Bikes" and the other "I Hate Cars." In the bike notebook I write about all of the joyful moments on my bike, the ecstasy of seeing the world in a slower motion than most people ever see it, all of the different kinds of people and bikes I see, all the amazing things people can carry on their bikes, and the look of contentment on the faces of bicyclists. When I got back from the action, I wrote: "Could human experience get any better than this? Playful, festive, beautiful, expressive, and diverse." I dressed as a yellow and red sunflower, and so was my bike. No one would call me a "sunny" sort of person. It was great to ride eight miles down Broadway to Union Square feeling like I was lighting everything up. I was looking forward to a day when at least some people would stop abiding by rules that say be one kind of person, you are what you buy, disconnect from nature, art belongs in museums, faster is better, shut yourself off from strangers.*

Our legal info warned Critical Mass bike riders, "Reclaim the Streets actions pose an arrest risk. Our style of festival is their style of disorderly conduct." What emerged from our union on the streets, and continues to do so, was a series of competing urban narratives.

"What's going on here? You need to disperse, this is an illegal gathering," one cerebrally challenged police officer ordered when we met up at Union Square, recalling Foucault's paranoid sounding, yet quite on-the-mark point that, "the prison begins well before its doors. It begins as soon as you leave your house" (quoted in Hardt, 2000). Nine of us were strategizing about how to coordinate the event, which had planned and unplanned aspects to it. "Why is it illegal?" Hank asked (names are changed). "Because of Parks Department rules," she explained (see City Record, 1999). "But look at the numbers," Hank responded. "What do numbers have to do with anything? Disperse!" the officer responded. "Look," Hank pointed at everyone, counting, "one, two, three," up to nine. "There are nine of us here. That's not an illegal gathering," Hank replied, referring to the absurd "over 20" rule, whereby no more than 20 people may gather in a park without a permit. The cop walked off. The numbers of participants at the action served as both signifiers for a threat to order and a way to organize us into one interchangeable category. Yet the question remained, which reality is more real—our public theater, or their vision of racially, sexually, and economically segregated, increasingly sterile urban environment? Below that question lurks a further series of questions about who can or cannot walk in which areas without being profiled by police. Without access to public space or freedom of assembly, "any kind of talk about democracy basically goes out the window," one observer recently noted (see Ferrell, 2001). The point is clear: if you can't walk or ride a bike in the street, how can you be considered a citizen? (see Ribey, 1998)

A sermon by Reverend Billy, whose Church of Stop Shopping had been battling Starbucks, Disney, the sins of consumer narcosis and a suburban vision of urban life more appropriate for SUV's than bicycles, ushered us to the road. The Rev. exhorted his brothers and sisters to imagine a world where parking lots would be turned into gardens, where car payments, Armor-all, Turtle-wax, and automatic everything would no longer be an end point of labor. Adrenaline oozing everywhere, the crowd lurched forward, ritually sacrificing our *papier maché* model car and the hegemonic evils it represented. Cars had transformed the goings-on of urban transportation into a series of fits, starts, headaches and conflict-ridden, road-rage inspiring gridlocks. Where once urban dwellers had walked, bused, jogged, and actually dealt with each other's differences, the automobile functioned as part and parcel of an urban milieu of private privileges and secret panaceas, xanex, and prozac; its oil fueling yet another American addiction. Bent on consumption, our dependence on petroleum dictates the worst in American foreign policy: gulf wars and battles against terrorism. But we're getting ahead of ourselves. There was actually a bike ride aimed at detoxing us.

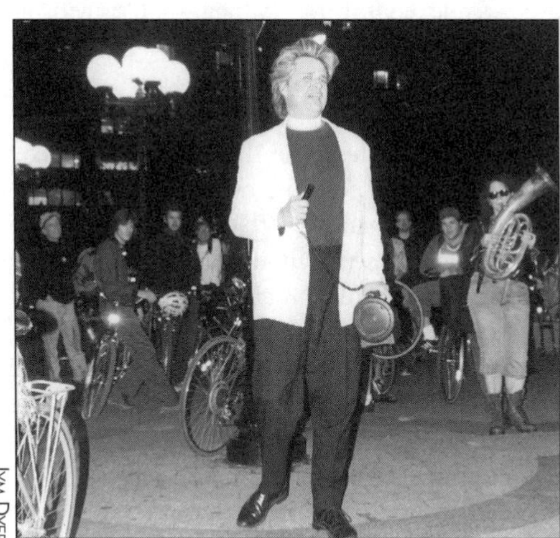

JYM DYER

Reverend Billy of the Church of Stop Shopping gives a rousing sermon at the beginnng.

We took off, five hundred bikers joyously intermingling, delighting and culture jamming one street after another of a city, which at least for one night, was not dominated by cars. There were the usual wacky bikes—some with small wheels, others with puppets—the tricycles, the skateboarders, the requisite jogger who runs with us, the choppers, the low riders, the disco bikes with boom boxes taped in front, dance music, the beats flying everywhere. Some chanted; others blew whistles feeling the air brush through their faces. One rider turned up his horn to produce the opening notes of *Thus Spoke Zarathustra*. "BAAAHHH, BAAAAHHHH, BBB BAAAAAAAAA!!!!" As we passed through Times Square a number of riders stopped, cars waiting at every corner of this intersection of the world, holding their bikes in mid-air in homage to the possibilities of a temporary autonomous zone, liberated for just a moment. 2001 was right around the corner. We zoomed out of the once-sterilized Times Square, reclogged with delights, possibilities, and spontaneity, our moving cavalcade zigging and zagging back to the East Village.

By the time we got to St. Mark's Church, where we were to meet to propel the RTS action, some ten paddy wagons and another 15 police cars were there to meet us. We felt that we were entering the lion's den. After getting word that the marshal on the bike ride had been pulled over for running a red light, the RTS organizers at the Church were temporarily out of touch with the Critical Mass ride. Things looked a little bleak; butterflies set in. But friends kept on coming to the Church, feeling the pulse of the early autumn night. Optimistic chit-chat contrasted with ominous forebodings in black and blue. We spread word of a quiet new destination for the action intersection point. We meandered through the East Village night, off to hit the "sale" at the Gap down the street on St. Marks where foot traffic is most pronounced. Instead of the usual RTS mass departure with horns accompanied by cops, two or three people left at a time. We looked for bargains, made conspiratorial winks, and the police—only prepared for conflict—hadn't noticed that most of us had left for a different meeting spot, without cops to crash the party.

Meanwhile, the larger Critical Mass ride did its thing, swinging and swaying up 6th Avenue, singing, meeting strangers, greeting tourists with "Join us, JOIN us!" "Less Cars!!! More Bikes!!!" echoed through the evening air. In answer to the usual "What's this?" queries from the sidewalks, we heard everything from "Living!" to "One kick ass bike ride!" to "The New World!" in response. The cops on minibikes laughed with, not at, the guy dressed as a huge pea pod and the woman dressed as a tree, but with a huge tree house perched at the top, filled with plants and miniature people. A cavalcade of bike riders and revelers careened though the streets, forming a Critical Mass, and led a crowd into our sound system and the dynamic process of spicing up bland, homogenous public space. Smack dab in the middle of 7th & A, our sound system, which had been sitting in the back of an old pickup, transformed the scene with sound. The crowd ditched their bikes, danced and boogied, people smiled, realizing their own power deep in the East Village night....

The real power of the Sept. 29 action was that we were not the things interfering with the movement of the automobiles that destroy the earth and keep people away from each other, we were not one bloc of "protesters," but people on foot, bikes, skates, and skateboards who moved together as a big amoeba of dazzling light, humor and joy.

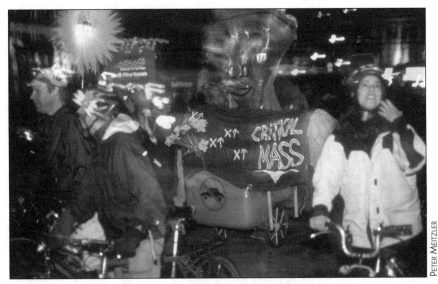

PETER MEITZLER

Time's Up and More Gardens Critical Mass, NYC 2000

Throughout the world, when people dance, significant bonds and important communities emerge and re-converge. Street parties and unsanctioned bike convergences result in a spectre of difference, profoundly threatening to the caretakers of the status quo. The police sat scratching their heads, not really knowing what to do at the threshold of another kind of city. And there were no arrests.

We learn early that the public sphere is not designed for drag queens, people of color, those who look different, or decide to form circles outside corporate structures. By the time the Rodney King verdict came along back in 1992, there was nothing else I could do but feel the sickness of betrayal and block traffic. Growing up, we are taught to believe in human rights, basic public morality, a system of checks and balances, accountability, democracy and government. While we have been taught to pledge allegiance to a system of laws, the power of this social contract ultimately resides with the people. When it fails us, we have no other recourse than to follow Rousseau's call to challenge the current social contract. Democracy in America is indebted to the enlightened notion that citizens are capable of revolution. The city of LA burned during that week after the five police were acquitted for brutalizing Rodney King, now some ten years ago. That was years before I got to NYC where police hostility toward otherness has warranted a report on human rights violations by Amnesty International. Currently, a federal investigation of misconduct by the NYPD has put the city on the verge of the same federal oversight the LAPD is facing, in part as result of the riots which brought LA to its knees (see www.web.amnesty.org/web/ar2000web.nsf/). Between the Rodney King beating and the Amadou Diallo murder, a generation of activists was born. Reclaim the Streets, Critical Mass, and a burgeoning global justice movement aimed at a do-it-yourself reclaiming of public space were part of this response.

There is another way of being in the city, in which people are not profiled by race or class. It's a space where difference intermingles within that broadway boogie woogie of bright colors, jazz, pastels, car horns, and the urban rhythms many would describe as part and parcel of the tradition of participatory democracy at its best. That's what Critical Mass is about isn't it, democracy. You can find it taking off from Union Square the last Friday of every month.

Join us.

References

Bey, Hakim. 1991. *T.A.Z. The Temporary Autonomous Zone, Ontological Anarchy, Poetic Terrorism*. Brooklyn, NY. Autonomedia.

City Record. 1999. Parks and Recreation: Amendment to Chapter 1 of Title 56 of the *Official Compilation of the Rules of the City of New York*. 16 August.

Duncombe, Stephen. 2002. "Stepping off the Sidewalk: Reclaim the Streets/NYC" in *From ACT UP to the WTO: Urban Protest And Community-Building in the Era of Globalization ed* by Shepard, Benjamin and Hayduk, Ron. Verso: New York.

Dunlap, W. 2000. In city canyons, slivers of public space erode. *New York Times*, 28 September.

Ferrell, Jeff. 2001. *Tearing Down the Streets: Adventures in Urban Anarchy*. Palgrave/St. Martin's Press.

Ribey, Francis. 1998. "Pas de pieton pas de citoyen: marcher en ville un manifeste de citoyennete" [If No Pedestrians, then No Citizens: City Walking, a Manifestation of Citizenship] *Revue des Sciences Sociales de la France de l'Est* 25: 35-41.

Hardt. Michel. 2000. "The Withering of Civil Society" in *Masses Classes and the Public Sphere* Edited by Mike Hill and Warren Montag. Verso Press, 2000

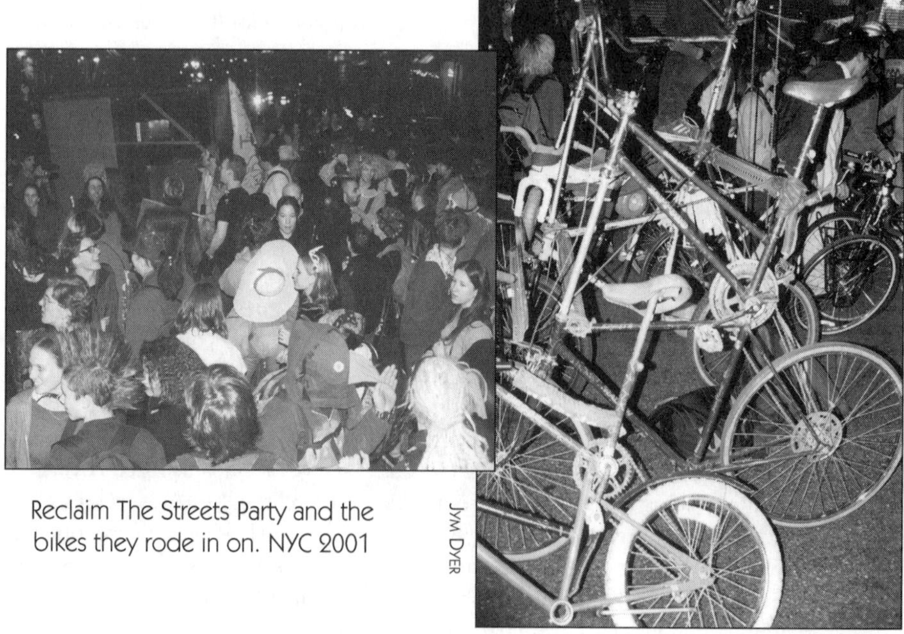

Reclaim The Streets Party and the bikes they rode in on. NYC 2001

Jym Dyer

CRITICAL MISSIVE JULY 2000

MARK REED, BROOKLYN, NY

"Just for a moment it feels as though we are creating a small rupture in the fabric of reality. Well, maybe that's a bit grandiose, but it does feel amazing to bring things to a halt for a second. The way I see it, we're doing everyone a real big favor."

RECAP: JUNE RIDE: The weather was perfect, the vibe was joyous, the food delicious, the band raucous— June critical mass was a spectacular success. We took off up Park Ave. South, took over the tunnel by 36th street (does it even have a name?), slalomed through the 42nd st. Viaduct, continued North for a while, then East to Broadway. We cruised through Times Square to the cheering of baffled, but enthused spectators, many of them unsure as to what we were up to but overjoyed to see all those bikes in the street, because BIKES ARE BEAUTIFUL!! From there we continued downtown to the East Villiage and to the beautiful Stannard Diggs community garden where we were greeted by a fantastic buffet and the pumped up musical collaboration of the Hungry March Band and Antibalas. Throughout the ride the vibe was kept wonderfully positive and informational (I have never seen so many cabbies asking for literature, as well as pedestrians and all kinds of drivers for that matter. People really do want to know what's up), and also really cooperative. I've never seen so many people help out with corking on a Mass ride in NYC! It was truly inspirational all the way around, and it didn't stop with the ride. After the riders arrived EN MASSE to the garden, and had danced for a while inside, the band decided to take their show into the street. Crowds followed and before you knew it we had reclaimed 6th street and were having an impromptu block party We held that street for two hours, until we were tired and people were ready to go home. Thanks and much respect to all those people who made the garden event such a blast, and thanks to all the riders for making the Mass a bigger and better event every month. Tell Your Friends!!

JULY RIDE: MUSICAL MASS: The theme of this months Mass is Music so grab anything that looks like it might have even the slightest potential for music playing and get to it! This is, after all, a celebration.

CRITICAL MISSIVE-JULY 2000

"Just for a moment it feels as though we are creating a small rupture in the fabric of reality. Well, maybe that's a bit grandiose, but it does feel amazing to bring things to a halt for a second. The way I see it, we're doing everyone a real big favor."

RECAP: JUNE RIDE: The weather was perfect, the vibe was joyous, the food delicious, the band raucous- June critical mass was a spectacular success. We took off up Park Ave. South, took over the tunnel by 36th street (does it even have a name?), slalomed through the 42nd st. Viaduct, continued North for a while, then East to Broadway. We cruised through Times Square to the cheering of baffled, but enthused spectators, many of them unsure as to what we were up to but overjoyed to see all those bikes in the street, because BIKES ARE BEAUTIFUL!! From there we continued downtown to the East Villiage and to the beautiful Stannard Diggs community garden where we were greeted by a fantastic buffet and the pumped up musical collaboration of the Hungry March Band and Antibalas. Throughout the ride the vibe was kept wonderfully positive and informational (I have never seen so many cabbies asking for literature, as well as pedestrians and all kinds of drivers for that matter. People really do want to know what's up), and also really cooperative. I've never seen so many people help out with corking on a Mass ride in NYC! It was truly inspirational all the way around, and it didn't stop with the ride. After the riders arrived EN MASSE to the garden, and had danced for a while inside, the band decided to take their show into the street. Crowds followed and before you knew it we had Reclaimed 6th street and were having an impromptu block party. We held that street for two hours, until we were tired and people were ready to go home. Thanks and much respect to all those people who made the garden event such a blast, and thanks to all the riders for making the Mass a bigger and better event every month. Tell Your Friends!!

JULY RIDE: MUSICAL MASS: The theme of this months Mass is Music, so grab anything that looks like it might have even the slightest potential for music playing and get to it! This is , after all, a celebration.

CORKING: To cork is to hold up traffic as the light turns from green to red in order to allow your fellow cyclists to ride safely through an intersection. It is a bold, exhilerating, and totally crucial act of support and cooperation. The people doing it are not "leaders" of the ride. THERE ARE NO LEADERS! It's up to us to ensure a safe ride, so if you see a car about to dash into an intersection where there are riders flowing, CORK IT!!!

We're not blocking traffic, We ARE traffic

A PERSONAL HISTORY OF PORTLAND CRITICAL MASS

BY FRED NEMO

Sometime in August of '93 Sara spots dozens of flyers around town that go something like "Tired of being run off the road by cars? Of riding alone, afraid, intimidated? Come to a Critical Mass planning meeting..." She's been especially frustrated with car behavior recently, so the invitation strikes a chord. On the appointed day, I accompany her down to the Howling Frog Cafe, but don't pay much attention to the proceedings, only noting the 20 or so cyclists of widely varying aspect, mostly listening to some folks from San Francisco rant about cars.

The afternoon of the last Friday in September finds over a hundred cyclists congregating in the South Park Blocks by Portland State. There are quite a few familiar faces, several of them from Citybikes, where Sara is one of the owner/mechanics. It's a gloriously balmy day, and once we get going I begin to experience an unfamiliar sensation. It is joy.

The combination of camaraderie and the feeling of utter safety is a potent mixture, and seems to inspire a cosmic unity of movement among our diverse crowd of bikers. It seems even the couple of bicycle cops escorting us feel it. And when John Benenate up ahead, in his scarily low-to-the-ground paraplegic's recumbent, goes sailing through a red light with a whoop and a holler and the cops blithely ignore it, it seems a revolutionary moment.

Well, it was great fun, but in the ensuing months I'm otherwise occupied on the last Fridays, though Sara religiously attends. She reports back that someone's superiors apparently weren't too happy about how things went on that maiden ride, for now there is rapidly escalating and progressively more irrational police attention. On a cold and blustery November ride there are 15 riders and over 20 police—on bikes and motorcycles and in squad-cars. On the clear and crisp January ride, someone has a flat, so the Mass turns into a residential side-street to wait, and almost half the riders are given tickets for impeding non-existent traffic. But the rides persist—they're not the huge amount of fun the first one was, but they're nevertheless exhilarating, a definite social event, and even incrementally educational for the cops.

The July ride has been especially large, raucous, and rude. For the August ride, Sara asks me to come help rein in some of the anarcho-cowboys of my acquaintance, who are attracting so much extra police attention that it's threatening to spoil the ride. This day, I am cited three times for nonsensical or non-existent violations, each ticket for $290. When I contest the tickets, two of my cops fail to appear, and the third one is caught in perjury, so the judge feels compelled to bump the ticket down to $30. In the process, this innocent bystander (by-rider?) has been turned into a flaming radical. Henceforward, someone better call their friend to come down

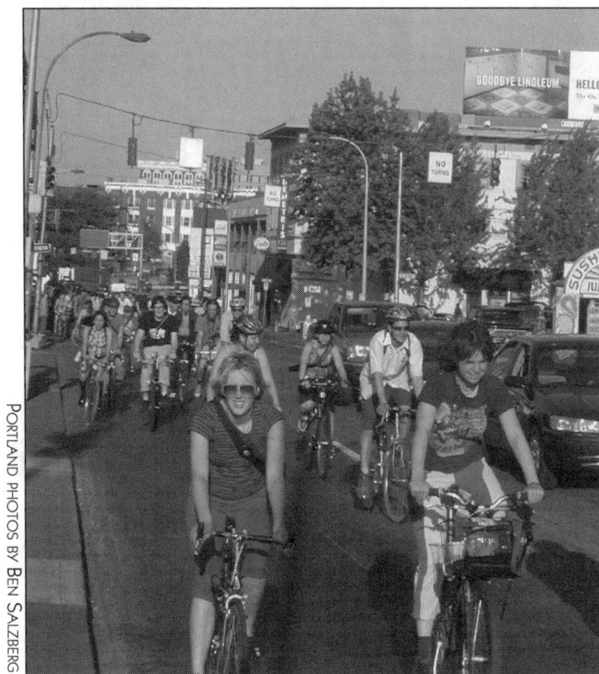

Portland, May 2001

PORTLAND PHOTOS BY BEN SALZBERG

and rein *me* in.

Two rides later, people are so tired of the police's unrelenting rudeness and inexplicable anger ("Why?" we keep asking ourselves—most Portland cops, in my limited experience, tend to be funny, smart, and interesting—but not these guys), that we decide to inaugurate a fresh meeting spot and not give them the route map as we always have. Heretofore the map had been proffered cheerfully, and always accepted with a snatch and a grudging look.

Our cops are so annoyed at the disinvitation to their monthly opportunity for misconduct and unprofessional behavior, that when they finally catch up with us just short of the ride's end, the only punishment they can come up with is to surround us and proclaim that we have disobeyed an (imaginary) order to disperse. Twenty-three of us are issued 30-day exclusion orders from the public square downtown for violating an obscure ordinance (which requires a permit for four or more people "demonstrating").

At the subsequent hearing challenging the exclusion orders, the first two cases are quickly dismissed. Douglas Squirrel's adept cross-examination makes his cop look especially foolish. When my case looks about to be dismissed as well, my cop jumps up and blatantly perjures himself (his sergeant, by the way, the one who supposedly gave the order to disperse, is also in attendance, making him complicit in this felony). This earns me a tongue-lashing.

Fortunately, there's someone to turn to: Ed Jones, the very funny—and very smart—lawyer who has been tirelessly representing Critical Massers with exhorbitant tickets for the past year (*pro bono*—and with an unprecedented 65% acquittal rate). Ed steers us to another lawyer, the celebrated Filipino-American pit-bull cop-litigator Spencer Neal.

So in December of '94, seventeen of us sue the city of Portland in federal court. Within a year, we've won, the City has to pay us over $50,000 and all police harassment, as if by magic, comes to a complete halt. The police documents uncovered by the suit nevertheless give no clue as to why we were being

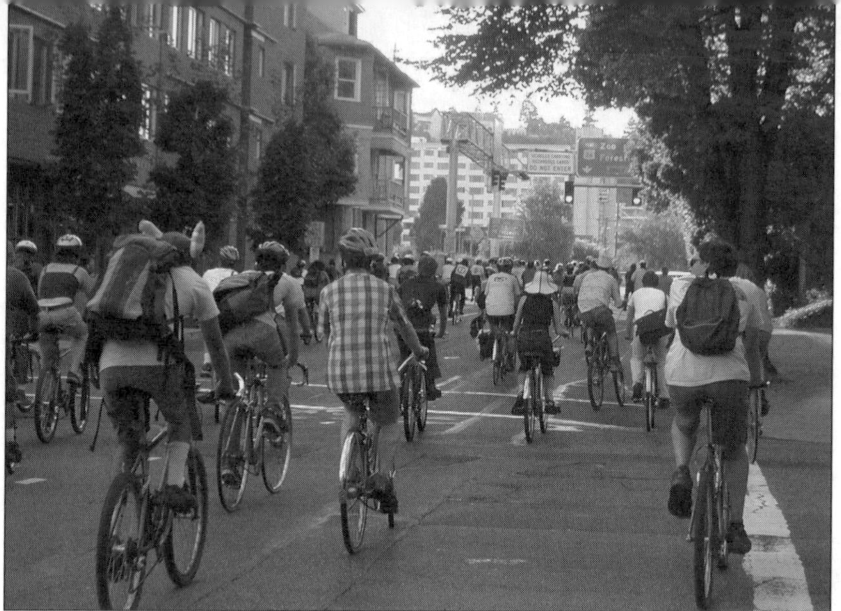

Portland, August 2001

harassed to begin with, except, perhaps, for the curious fact that not one of them ever refers to "Critical Mass," always designating us the "Anarchist Bike-Rally."

By this point, Portland Critical Mass is small but hardy: about 30-40 riders in the worst of the winter, 60-80 the rest of the year. It's takes us a long time to shake off the habits acquired during two years of intense and hostile police escorts, but our rides are always fun now. The '96 Halloween ride is outstanding—70 riders, 25 in costume, eight outrageous choppers, numerous recumbents and trailers, Slim's fine penny farthing, and the *pièce de la résistance*: Karl towing a trailer with a *full drum kit* being played by a seriously kick-ass drummer-dude. All the costumes really help inspire motorists to be content to wait through their green lights.

Two years later, word has spread that the Halloween ride is the one not to miss, and indeed it is huge—a couple hundred of us, scores of ultra-outrageous costumes—and it is a blast. One small thing, though: as we come off the Burnside Bridge, the police are waiting for us—probably, seeing as we're occupying all available lanes, some impatient citizen on a cell phone is responsible—and they pull over a couple of riders, possibly for straying over the center-line in the absence of oncoming traffic. The entire Mass stops dead in one of the busiest intersections in the city and very quickly a chant goes up: "Let them go! Let them go!" And they let them go! And the ride continues.

The next ride happens to fall on the day after Thanksgiving. The police department has assembled an elaborate arrest station with armored buses for Buy Nothing Day protesters, but the latter are so law-abiding that the police seize the opportunity to remind us of our unacceptable behavior the previous month. Out of the blue, and in response to no discernable law-breaking save one safely and courteously executed illegal left turn, they arrest 18 riders for "disorderly conduct," impound their bicycles (which, incidently, take weeks of pressure to get returned), and take the perpetrators to jail. Then tell the newspapers that we'd obstructed the path of a fire truck. But since there are about two thousand wit-

There has been a growing trend in our rides that has me very concerned. I am seeing too much anger in the Critical Mass riders. Nothing is accomplished when an angry motorist or cop and an equally culpable, angry bike rider are yelling at each other. If our hearts are full of anger, all we will reap is angry reactions from the people we disagree with. It is possible to change some peoples minds, but this is never possible with anger. Critical Mass rides should be fun. They should not create more hatred of bike riders. There should be no reasons for cops to handle a rider abusively, and if we break laws, we should know being ticketed or arrested is part of the playing field. On the matter of arrests: everyone should have a partner to look out after her bike and to keep track of his progress through the arrest labyrinth. Someone being arrested has --usually-- made the choice to be disobedient and a few riders should stop and follow through to support her, but its no cause to call the whole Mass to riot. Cops are out there, don't be surprised if they enforce the law.

There is a lot in our society that needs fixing and maintenance. The bad problems that Critical Mass is trying to address should not be represented in the attitude (and method) of the riders. Be nice, be reasonable, break some laws, obey the laws that make sense, respect your enemy (or else he will never be your ally), be zany, have fun, and spread fun to other people!

nesses—it was at Pioneer Courthouse Square on the busiest shopping day of the year—they back-track on that one and the next day drop the charges, causing the press to do a sudden back-flip and, for the first time ever, give us a good round of favorable coverage.

The arrests and their subsequent publicity have wide and unexpected repercussions in two areas, one in cyberspace and one on the rides themselves:

Sara is one of those arrested, and writes a stirring article in protest, highlighting, among other things, local cases of law-breaking car drivers causing grievous injury or death, and receiving more lenient treatment than the 18 arrestees. She writes it for the Portland daily—which is a little too dependent on auto ad revenue to run such an article—but it's published in *Oregon Cycling*, our excellent monthly. I e-mail copies of the piece to a few friends, one of whom, legendary gadfly Jason Meggs of Berkeley Critical Mass forwards it to a string of California bike lists (and the entire Berkeley city government), where it ignites an insane flame war (accessible at the pdx cm website or www.monkeychicken.com) between Critical Massers and devotees of John Forester's *Effective Cycling* over the correct strategies to advance bicycling. Several bike lists have to shut down due to the overwhelming traffic and cross-postings—one man receives 250 posts in 5 minutes. This skirmish takes a surprising trajectory—with many near-victories for the vehicularists, and featuring staunch champions and murderous knaves (on both sides) at every turn. It's a debate between two old and sophisticated cyclist communities, both of which have given much thought—and much life-and-death clinical practice, to their respective styles of civil disobedience. It's a violent, hilarious, and scandalous true-crime soap opera and a neatly-sketched profile of the future landscape of bicycle culture.

The other unexpected repercussion of the arrests results from the thoroughgoing media coverage of the Police Bureau's blatant dishonesty and patently unconstitutional harassment of clearly non-violent and essentially law-abiding cyclists. How does it impact our actual rides?

It brings out the aggro boys, on both sides. Starting in January of '99, we are visited by a semi-organized self-appointed "leadership" contingent that institutes several rigid new "rules": a) always take up all lanes—and if a car tries to sneak through, surround it and harass the driver. b) if the oncoming lane of traffic clears, try to have someone occupy it and play chicken with approaching cars. c) always cork (set a cyclist to dismount and block the cross street's green light for bikes to pass), even when the head of the ride has a red light or the rear of the ride is strung way behind. To most of the long-time riders, these young men (when we pow-wow with them, they have women spokespersons, but we never see any women engaging in the above behaviors), in their courting of the worst police elements, are deliberately seeking a decline in our numbers. Within a year, starting with the as-always outrageous Halloween ride (on which all 200 riders cross the Hawthorne Bridge the wrong way), battles with the police have escalated into routinely brutal arrests—never once of an aggro boy, by every account. All the children, parents with children, and young people, most of the old-timers, and anyone who cannot afford a ticket or an arrest, stops coming. The grumbling is ongoing, and increasingly thunderous.

This is not to suggest that on another level we are not having some fabulous rides. For one thing, we have several large and venerable factions who, when they come out in force, tend to relegate the anarcho-troublemakers to the sidelines. The Union Chorus, for instance, with their sea-chanteys, bike-songs, and trick riding, or the Chunk 666 krew and its deranged off-shoots —you've seen them —bikes that have 9-foot-long forks and are built to come apart after 3 1/2 miles, or are 9 feet tall, or lean back so far that it doesn't look sane—forget safe—to ride.

Back when the problem started, veteran masser Moses proposed splitting the ride into a confrontational group and a celebratory group—a good cop/bad cop Critical Mass. In November of 2000, anticipating official retaliation for the excesses of Halloween, not to mention the dreary prospect of both aggro-boys and police (our standard escort now consists of a half dozen paddy wagons, ten squad cars, and 15 motorcycles—to restrain maybe 55 riders) has brought Moses' dream to fruition and the Wuss Ride splits off. For 3 months we have two rides, maybe 40-60 bikes on the "original recipe" ride, no more than 25 on the Wuss Ride, although, I must say, when nine of the 25 are boys in dresses, riding synchronized, such a contingent draws a trifle more attention than the numbers might suggest.

The necessity—the very existence—of the Wuss Ride so enrages a devoted faction whose sympathies straddle the aggro/wuss divide, that they take aggressive action on two fronts. They start discussions with the city and, like some kind of cycling Borgs, assimilate the anarcho-cowboys. In March of 2001, City Councilman (and Transportation Commissioner) Charlie Hales agrees to ride and observes the police misbehavior first hand. It's indicative of the compulsive nature of the cops' harassment of us that the open presence of a City Councilman doesn't constrain it. Now Ayleen, Ben, Patrick, and Alex have the political edge to negotiate a history-making compromise. In it's most simplistic form, the deal boils down to this—Let us cork (responsibly), and we'll keep a lane free for passing cars.

Since the Spring of 2001, Critical Mass has been peaceful and joyous, with a very small bike-cop escort (and these are officers—in dramatic contrast to our cops of 8 years ago—who are clearly enthusiastic cyclists), no more arrests, and warnings instead of tickets.

In the course of this brief account, I've omitted many essential people and events (like our several great and solemn memorial rides in honor of beloved cyclists killed, like Peter Siracusa's unrelenting peace-making efforts) and largely neglected to convey the sheer color and exhilaration that has infused even the most difficult and weather-impacted rides and made even the bummer confrontational ones pretty damn fun.

As for the lessons learned by the great holistic organism (like a school of fish, as Ed Jones once tried telling the judge) that is Portland Critical Mass, off the top of my head:

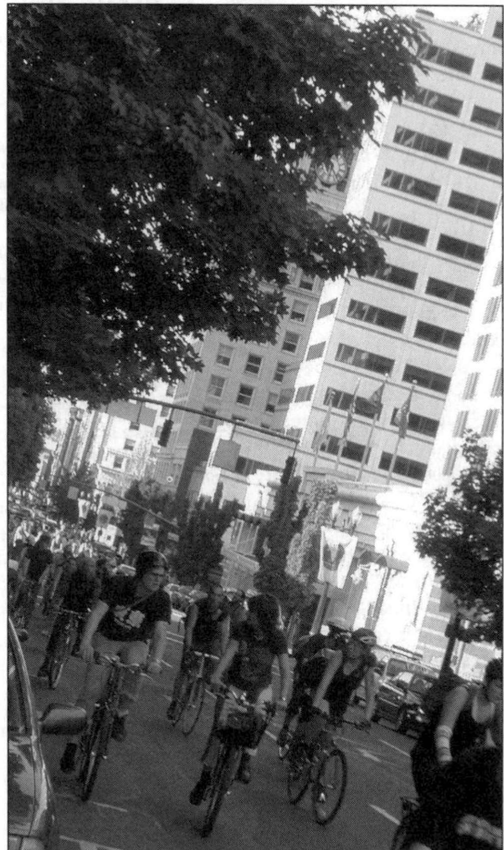
Portland, May 2001

1. As when riding alone, anticipate what's ahead, carefully track all threats.

2. Witness! If the police are breaking the law—videotape them. If they're committing perjury—document it. Remember: the knee-jerk police response to non-violent civil disobedience is perfectly tailored to advance the cause of its practitioners.

3. Negotiate! Talk to other riders, cops, the media, city officials.

4. When something's not working, change tactics. Be as versatile in negotiating your city's political landscape as your bike is in negotiating its physical landscape.

5. Costumes! Music! Funny bikes! Celebrate!

From the PDX list-serve:

From: rail hed
Sent: May 26, 2001 3:10 AM
CRITICal MASS,

i think the ride lass nite was great, i didn't see one rider thrown to the sidewalk. it was the first time i brought any one my kids and she was like WHAT?? where is all the action? She sed she smiled the whole ride. I lost the group at one point but found them when i was ready to cross the bridge then it semed to peter out at the pedestrian walkway on the eastside.

the cops were corking for us???!!!! i saw it! it is like 8 less cop cars! whoo whoo.

also it does seem to me enyway that keeping one lane for cars does get us spread out more but it gives us more visibility IF WE CAN CORK and keep together. we are going by a particular area for a long time. we hold up cross traffic longer but allow traffic to move with us more.

best, r

From: fred / Sent: November 1, 2001

Perfectly awesome ride. 522 riders—that would come to one out of every thousand Portlanders. 450 costumes. 15 polite and helpful bike cops—they allowed corking and only once took any action at all, and that was to herd a few riders out of the oncoming lane on Burnside. Zero anger, zero tickets, but some challenging riding, what with sudden bottlenecks and the sheer number of riders.

At one point on S.W. Broadway I heard some onlookers exclaim, "look! there's cops riding with them!" so I yelled back at them, as a Halloween joke, "They're not really cops!" Then one of the cops remarked to his buddy, "that's really sort of true." I don't know exactly what he meant, but they were unlike the cops we've come to expect on these rides. It was so excellent not to have all the squad cars and motorcycles. When she left the ride to go home, Sara approached the nearest cop contingent and thanked them for coming on the ride, and received friendly acknowledgement of her appreciation.

We included: 2 side-by-side tandem contraptions, one of which was dressed as a jellyfish, and steered by ghostly mariners, A bottle of ketchup that performed karaoke. Several scary Clintons and Reagans—one nude Reagan clasping the, er, rear of its rider. Many magnificent noisemakers—Sara's cymbal, Michael's elephant horn, etc., etc. Anthrax, Frida Kahlo, many many magnificent women—of both genders A stunning array of chunks (choppers) and recumbents. A man with a giant tampon affixed to his helmet. The Holy Father Wigs, kimonos, and fishnet stockings galore. Hideous giant skulls, an E.T. dummy, and A myriad of children—of all ages

I could go on and on.

In fact—we do.

What's with all the bikes?!?

This is **Critical Mass**, an unofficial, unorganized group ride to celebrate **bicycling** here in Portland!

Why are you blocking the road?

We try to stick together for our own **safety**. For that reason we may ask motorists to **wait** for our ride to pass.

Who's in charge?

Everyone you see here. We all can and do control the ride. There are no "leaders" and few "rules".

This isn't a **protest**, it's just a **ride**. Each person rides for their own reason, agenda, mission, drive, whatever. Our common ground is a **bike** that propels us through the city. Imagine for a moment if we were each in our own car. Then how tied up would traffic be? **Critical Mass** was begun in San Francisco by cyclists who were tired of riding in **fear of cars**. Riding together, *en masse*, the group becomes **impervious to auto traffic**. For a moment one can imagine a **city free of cars** and the problems they create. It's also a lot of fun. If you have a bike, please, come ride with us. **Critcal Mass** occurs on the last Friday of every month. Riders congregate under the west side of the Burnside Bridge at 5:30 pm. Some of us might look a little surly, but all are welcome, honestly.

Thank you participating in Critical Mass!!

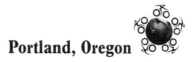

TO THE MASS

BY MEGULON-FIVE, PORTLAND, OREGON

It is the last Friday of the month. I spend some time contemplatively drinking a beer and repairing last night's damage to my ride in preparation for the mighty Critical Mass. The efforts complete, I mount my steed and ride towards the gathering point, only to be reminded that I forgot to fix that rusty brake that won't release its death grip on my rim. No matter, I anticipated a setback such as this, and have alloted the time necessary to smack the offending component around and lube the shit out of it. Once again I am awheel, and as the gathering point draws near I encounter my comrades on their own choppers, tallbikes, and battlewagons. We hail and are well met, becoming one clot among the many converging from all directions towards the shelter of the Burnside bridge, traditional meeting place for massing cyclists since the days of yore. Pedestrians and motorists mistake us for the Critical Mass ride itself, and we wave to them cheerfully, for it does not matter; whenever two or more cyclists are gathered in its name, there Critical Mass will be among them. In fact, nuts to the ride, perhaps we should ditch it and derby in the park tonight? The idea is debated back and forth with volleys of shouts as we ply the streets, but no, our destination does not change—we wish to be with our people, the people of the wheel. And as we come within sight of the milling throng, we are glad that we stuck with the plan, because there they are: the crusties on their barely functioning found bicycles, the technogeeks on their expensive yuppie rides, the nerdy guy with the basket bike, the clever mechanic, that one messenger, the shy kid, the loudmouth old dude, the ordinary people who just like to ride the Mass. They're all there, and we love them all, even if we don't like a lot of them. The socializing ends and the ride begins as we take to the streets once more, and wherever we go, we own. Better yet, we give it freely back, minutes later. Is it our fault that the drivers following us can't think of anything better to do with it than what they've been doing every day? We've made our mark. People around us have seen it, and that's swell, but it isn't really important, after all. What is important is that we can feel the mark within ourselves. Critical Mass is a part of us. When the ride is done, we will still own the streets every other day of the month, and we are still a part of the community of Massers, until the month rolls around and it is time to ride together again.

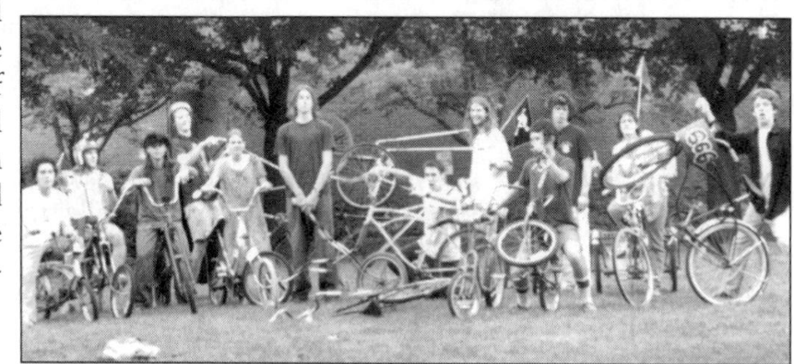

The Chunk 666 scene

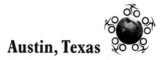

AUSTIN CRITICAL MASS: THEN AND NOW

BY MICHAEL BLUEJAY

Critical Mass in Austin has changed a lot over the years, and is very different today from the Critical Mass of old—so much so that I rarely ride any more. I think I know a bit about Critical Mass, since I've probably ridden on more local CM rides than anyone: I started in the early days, and was just about the only one who kept riding, even though there was nearly complete turnover every two years or so. Twice when it slowed down in the summer, I was one of only two riders to show up for the ride! (The others were John Dolley one time, and Tommy Eden another.)

After the first Critical Mass, the police turned out in full force for each ride for the next year or so, waiting for the group before it even got started. Dozens of motorcycles, squad cars, and bike cops lined Guadalupe in front of the University Co-op, not to mention the paddy-wagons and unmarked cars, which would videotape us as we rode. Police looked for any infraction, no matter how slight, and made numerous false arrests (not just tickets, but arrests) for things like riding on the sidewalk or asking why another cyclist was being arrested. Of course they handed out plenty of bogus tickets, too.

Critical Massers filed a Freedom of Information request to get copies of the police video. Naturally, the police tried to keep us from getting the tapes, but they were unsuccessful. The police edited out some scenes that were especially embarrassing to them, but they did a sloppy job of it. (At the end of one tape, the last few minutes of the tape repeats itself, indicating that they'd re-copied it and left something out of the middle. Duh!) Even so, there was plenty on the tapes that was damning. CM'ers took the tapes, along with some video that riders took, showed it to the City Council, and then amazingly, the police stopped showing up before the rides.

But probably the best way to demonstrate what CM used to be like is to contrast it with what it's become.

CONFRONTATION: Early Critical Mass was certainly wild, but it wasn't typical for cyclists to go out of their way to piss off motorists. Now, however, it's more common for cyclists to yell at motorists, and seem to look for any excuse to start an argument. I stopped riding CM in October 2001 after what happened on that ride. Before the ride I had addressed the crowd and encouraged them not to be confrontational and not to do things that would openly invite the police, such as taking up every single lane on every single roadway. After I spoke, someone else stood up and invited everyone to ignore what I had said. The crowd seemed more receptive to his message. On the ride, cyclists actually stopped in the middle of the street and faced traffic while straddling their bikes, just because they could. One motorist, frustrated by the delay, ran over my bike and knocked me to the pavement. (Sound familiar?)

One of the silliest things some CM'ers do is to ride as slowly as they can in front of a vehicle, practically begging to get hit, and then to act all surprised, shocked, and

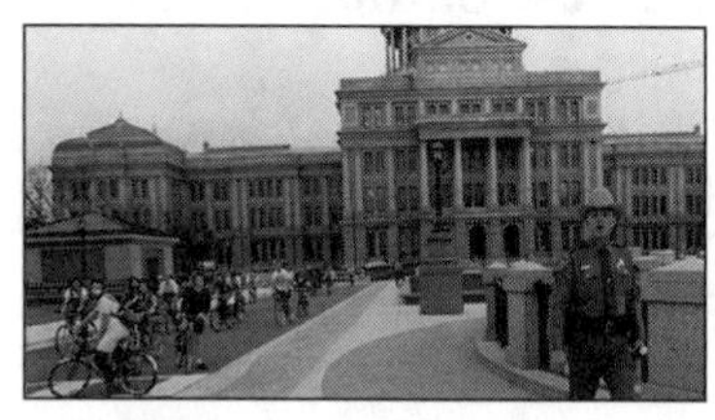

Austin, Texas, Capitol (left) and West Mall (right)

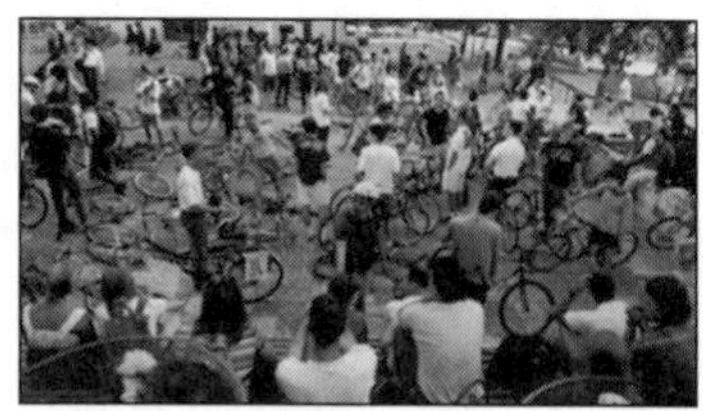

indignant when a motorist accidentally bumps them. Now, nobody harps on injustice to cyclists louder than I do, but it has to be real injustice. Trying to get hit and then having it happen just barely isn't injustice. It's just stupid.

SOLIDARITY: There used to be a feeling of unity among the group. Not so much so any more. Now when the mass gets split at a red light, those in front are more likely to keep going rather than slowing down or pulling over to wait for those behind. When I was hit on last October's ride, none of the CM'ers stuck around to be witnesses for me when the police arrived. (Thanks a lot, guys.) I was lucky to run into witnesses around town after that.

CELEBRATION: Early rides were an event. People came with high-bikes and other crazy homemade bikes, many mounted various musical instruments to their bikes, and people showed up in costumes, even when it wasn't Halloween. Several rode around half-naked. Cyclists had flags, banners, and trailers. We made cool fliers, handouts, and t-shirts. We had potluck dinners afterwards. Perhaps all these things helped us focus on ourselves, as a celebration of biking. Maybe it's the absence of this kind of fun that lets the attitude drift more towards anti-car instead of pro-bike.

CM AROUND THE WORLD: I run CriticalMassHub.com, an international site serving as a directory of all the CM rides all over the world. And yes, it's kind of ironic that I still maintain the CM Hub though I hadn't ridden in my own local CM in a year until this month.

I get email weekly from CM'ers all over the world. And as far as I can tell, Austin may have the distinction of having one of the more confrontational rides. Australian CM'ers have been known to hold signs saying "Sorry for the delay" and to hand out flowers to motorists. And it was from the Athens, GA folks that I got the idea for the Courteous Mass....

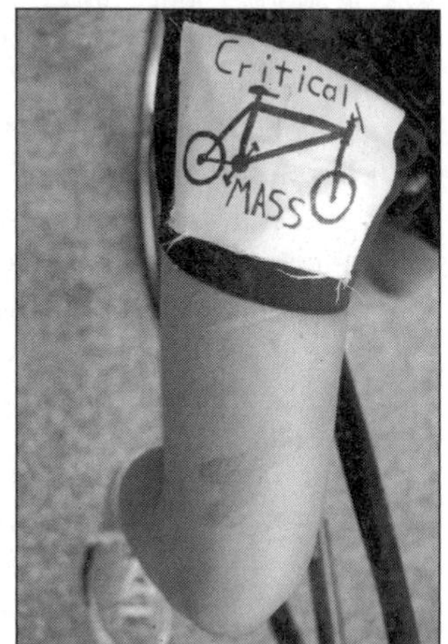

Whither CM?

Around 1996 we started a "CM-Lite" ride that would follow traffic laws, in response to all the people who said they wouldn't ride Critical Mass because not all riders obeyed all the laws. The result was a phenomenal failure: We only got a tiny handful of riders, and the ride lasted only a few months.

Now there's talk of resurrecting the second ride, and calling it Courteous Mass. Details are still being worked out, but it looks like it's going to happen. Stay tuned for more details.

Los Angeles, California

RIDE A BIKE, GO TO JAIL! CRITICAL MASS DNC 2000

By Scott Svatos

Riding a bicycle in Los Angeles is a dangerous proposition. Cars, trucks, and other motorized vehicles dominate the urban landscape. Air quality is lousy. The freeways are off limits. Bike lanes are few and far between. Even when bike lanes are available they are intermittent and usually shared with buses and parked cars.

These factors are certainly not unique to Los Angeles. But what is unique to this city is the degree to which these conditions are actually enforced by the city.

This was the lesson learned by a group of bicyclists at the August 2000 Democratic National Convention when 71 riders found themselves behind bars for challenging Los Angeles car culture.

THE RIDE

The Los Angeles Police Department was determined to make a strong show of force at the Democratic National Convention in downtown Los Angeles. Earlier in the year they had failed to stop crazed sports fans in the same area from burning cars and breaking windows following the Lakers basketball championship victory. And still smoldering in LAPD memory were the Rodney King 1992 riots where police found themselves trying to stop angry mobs from burning and looting a large section of the city.

The police strategy for the DNC was a military one—line the streets with police, fill the air with choppers, and confine protesters to limited areas surrounded by chain link fence and concrete. On Monday, August 14, the day before Critical Mass DNC got underway, a street concert and rally outside of the Staples Center was cut short as police dispersed protesters with rubber bullets and batons, and continued with the arrests that by the end of the week would number in the hundreds.

Meanwhile, inside the Staples Center, the country's elite was kept safe from messages of fair labor practice and environmental justice. Politicians went about their business smooching babies and accepting large checks from their industry sponsors. And what better place than the Staples Center to make these transactions—a building whose name alone is a symbol of corporate power.

The Critical Mass Ride the next day, Tuesday, August 15, started well enough. A diverse group of approximately 250 riders gathered outside of the public library at 5 p.m. on a warm summer afternoon. Among the numbers were overseas nomads on touring bikes, college undergrads on Barbie cruisers, masked anarchist types on garage sale giveaways, hippies on mountain bikes, couriers on expensive street racers, and everything in between.

News of the ride was spread by word of mouth and on various websites. "Bikes not cars" was the dominant theme of the ride. It was but one of many protest actions

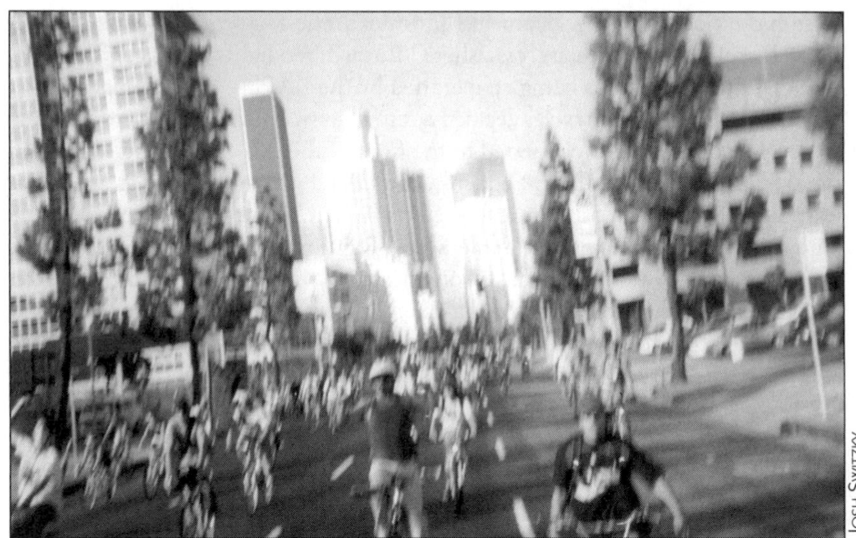

Los Angeles Critical Mass riding to the Democratic National Convention

taking place in the streets that week and many of the participants on the ride were first time Massers drawn from other events.

The core of the crowd was from Los Angeles, but there were plenty of riders from San Francisco and other locations that made the trek to L.A. (most of them by pedaling) to participate in this monumental ride. Not only was this a chance to bring awareness of bicycles and larger issues of air pollution and non-motorized travel to a major political function, it was a chance to do so in a city known for it's poor air quality and unapologetic love of internal combustion.

Critical Mass took to the streets, making a couple of laps around Pershing Square, the staging point for DNC week protests, before sidetracking briefly into residential neighborhoods. The *Los Angeles Times* would later report that Critical Mass "snarled" traffic in the downtown area, but most of the riders were surprised at how few cars were actually on the streets. The late afternoon ride started well after most of the business elite had left their skyscraper offices, boarded their SUVs, and driven home for dinner in the suburbs.

The colorful chain of bicycle riders eventually wound its way past the Staples Center. They were kept from getting too close to this mighty symbol of democracy by a standing army of police, tall fences, and cement barricades. There was constant noise from the Mass—dinging bells, squeaky horns and chants ranging from "Whose streets, our streets!" to "More bikes, less cars!"

It is an understatement to say that the police were a constant presence on the ride. Not only were groups of officers posted on most of the corners the ride passed, but the ride was followed by police cars and motorcycles, and surveilled from above by helicopter. Carefully unshaven undercover cops betrayed their identities by gabbing on police radios while riding side by side with Massers. The police actually appeared before the ride began, but they seemed unclear whether to stop the ride, join the ride, or just intimidate the Massers. At some intersections, bicyclists found themselves ushered through red lights by officers directing traffic. Critical Mass was being chaperoned by the LAPD—or so it appeared.

Eventually the motorcycles decided not to follow Critical Mass, but to surround it. Several police motorcycles jetted to the front of the ride, while others walled in the sides and sealed the flank. Suddenly, the LAPD was leading the group—or at least a sizeable chunk of it. Critical Mass was ushered down a one way street and onto a narrow walkway next to some Metro Rail lines. The police then split the group into two sections and turned on the sirens. One group found themselves pinned between the Metro Lines and a chain link fence. Another group was simply surrounded in the street by police. Any riders not surrounded by police hit the road at top speed. One rider posted news of his escape on the web later that night:

> *The motorcycle cops turned into the cyclists and were tagging, running into and running over bikes. At this point total chaos broke lose. Bicyclists were screaming, dropping their bikes and trying to get away. Also at this point a metrolink train boxed the cyclists in. As the motorcycle cops charged us, more police also came from the rear. It appeared there was no way out. People practically had to ride into the train. POLICE GAVE NO WARNING. THEY JUST CHARGED US WITH NO THOUGHT FOR THE SAFETY OF THE CYCLISTS. I was stopped momentarily by a cop on a motorcycle but was able to jump the curb onto the sidewalk and take off, zigzaging down alleyways and streets. When I was leaving I saw cyclists knocked off their bikes and pinned down by cops who were cuffing the Massers with plastic handcuffs. I'm lucky to not be in jail right now.*
>
> —Dale "Hayduke" 11:55 p.m. Tuesday, August 15, 2000.

Officers howled at Massers to get off their bikes and face the fence or lie in the street. Those riders that were confused or too slow were pulled off their bikes by force, shoved against the fence or thrown to the ground. Bikes were grabbed from cyclists and tossed on the road or Metro rails where ostensibly riders could not grab them and escape. Over the next several hours, Massers were cuffed, fingerprinted and photographed in the street before being loaded onto police buses and hauled off to jail.

CRITICAL MASS IN JAIL

Despite police presence throughout the ride, cyclists were never told of breaking any laws or given a chance to disperse before being arrested. After much ambiguity, riders were eventually presented with misdemeanor charges of "obstructing a public way" and infractions of "failure to stop at a traffic light" and "failure to stop at a stop sign." Riders' bicycles were impounded by the LAPD, slapped with a bar code, and held as "evidence." The message was clear: Los Angeles takes any threat to its car culture very seriously.

Most of the riders spent two or more days in jail. The exceptions were the two reporters the LAPD accidentally roped in with the rest of the Massers and who were released later that evening. One of them wrote later in the *Chicago Tribune*:

What could be more fitting than getting arrested and cited for "reckless driving" of a bike in a city with three major problems: clogged traffic, the resulting pollution and a police department with one nasty reputation for dealing with the public?...

Cmdr. David Kalish of the LAPD alleged in a Wednesday morning news conference that I "had committed all the same violations that the other people did." This is true, if he was referring to stopping at red lights, going through intersections as police or crossing guards stopped side-street traffic, and being escorted by two dozen L.A. bike cops.

The arrested group of cyclists included college students, activists, teachers, couriers, technogeeks and reporters. There were several seminary students, multiple law students, and a few bike riding adventurers from overseas. While many of the men in the group found themselves bored and frustrated at spending two or more nights in jail—including times exceeding 12 hours after release had been secured in court—the women were treated much worse. Under suspicion of riding bicycles down streets intended for cars, they found themselves strip searched and body cavity searched multiple times, including after release was secured in court. The men were not strip searched at all and were mostly just forced to endure verbal abuse from jailers who learned their lingo from lockup movies and high school gym coaches ("this is my hall, and you better learn to shut the fuck up in my hall.") Some members of the group were denied medication or immediate treatment for injuries sustained from rough cuffing by the police. One female rider suffered permanent nerve damage from abusive handling by officers.

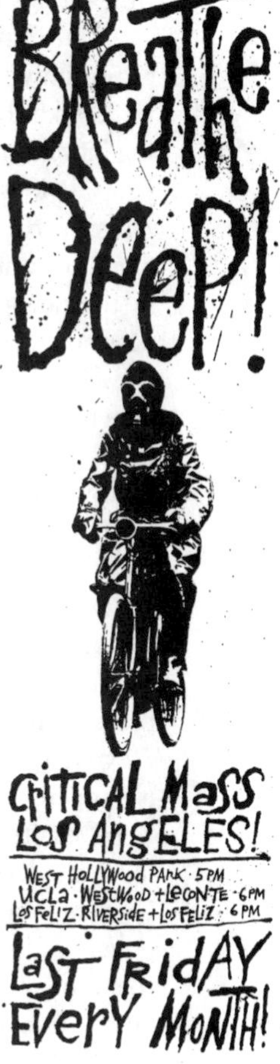
Breathe Deep!
Critical Mass Los Angeles!
West Hollywood Park · 5PM
UCLA · Westwood + Leconte · 6PM
Los Feliz · Riverside + Los Feliz · 6 PM
Last Friday Every Month!

THE AFTERMATH

A month after the initial arrests, charges were dismissed for all 71 Critical Mass cyclists snared during the demonstration. The riders were represented by lawyers with the National Lawyers Guild, Midnight Special Law Collective, and public defenders office. According to the *L.A. Times*, "veteran attorneys who normally handle felonies—including death penalty cases—were assigned by the public defenders office to represent the cyclists because the lawyers were angered by the nature of the arrests and reports that female cyclists had each been subjected to at least two strip searches in the County Jail."

Soon after charges were dropped against them, Critical Mass DNC filed suit against the LAPD and L.A. County Sheriff's Department challenging their arrests and seeking redress for the injustice that occurred in the streets and in jail. At the time of this publication, Critical Mass DNC is still in court-ordered mediation with the police.

To say Los Angeles is a car town might be a cliché, but it is not an exaggeration. This city is a tangle of streets and freeways

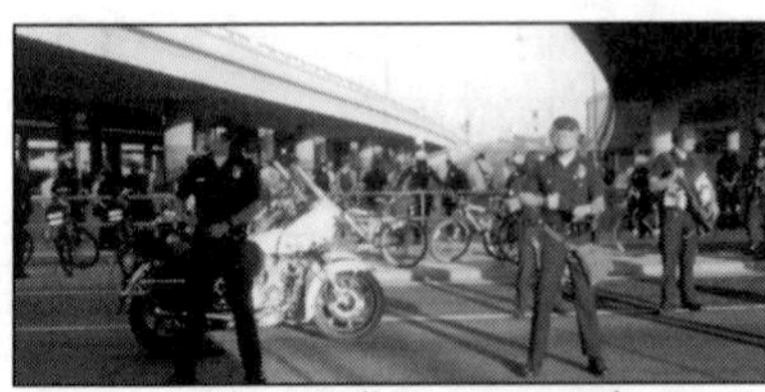
JOSH SWITZKY

Los Angeles police trap and arrest Critical Mass riders.

encased in a blanket of fuel-injected haze. Alternatives to the automobile are few and far between. This makes Critical Mass in Los Angeles all the more urgent.

Critical Mass in Los Angeles is a decidedly political event. Since the number of riders are fewer than in some other cities, the dangers are higher, and the population is often less than sympathetic if not entirely confused at why people even bother to ride a bicycle here. In the traffic lanes, bikes compete with SUVs, while in the bike lanes, bikes compete with busses—and not the clean burning kind.

Los Angeles is also a city of many geographical centers. Major sections of the city are long distances from one another and separated by many miles of difficult, dangerous roads whether one is travelling by car, foot, or bicycle. For many, biking in Los Angeles first involves a car ride to get to the location to be biked. Because of these conditions, Los Angeles Critical Mass actually consists of multiple groups that sometimes coordinate and other times go their own way.

The Critical Mass DNC ride was unique in that it brought many riders together not only within the city but within the state and country and from overseas as well. Additionally, many first-time Massers joined the event, some actually borrowing bicycles to ride in support of more bikes and fewer cars.

Obviously, the DNC ride was not well received by the city. The mayor of Los Angeles, Richard Riordan, himself an outspoken bicycle rider, did not have a kind word to say about the bicycle protesters after the arrests. His defense of law and order in the newspapers that week completely ignored the positive message of Critical Mass and of the other actions taking place.

Today, Critical Mass Los Angeles is a small but spirited pocket of resistance. The riders that mass in Los Angeles are not numerous, but they are dedicated, well educated on local laws affecting bicycles and alternative transportation, and involved with other environmental and progressive agendas. Many of the regular riders participate in Critical Mass as only one component of a wider program of bicycle and environmental advocacy.

Although the DNC arrests did not shut down Critical Mass Los Angeles, CMLA certainly did not grow in size because of them. The police action the day of the arrests cast a chilling cloud over Critical Mass in this city, as well as street protest and freedom of expression in general here. Simply put, protest in Los Angeles carries with it the threat of jail or police violence, and riding a bike here is dangerous no matter what your reason for doing so.

Despite this condition, the arrests and their accompanying coverage in the local media challenged Los Angeles car culture with a voice of resistance. Critical Mass plaintiffs are hopeful that their continued mediation with the police and sheriff's departments will result in positive reforms of some kind in this city and that biking in L.A. will someday be as common as fender benders on the freeway.

San Francisco, California

VICTORIOUS CRITICAL MASS LAWSUIT

Howard Besser was the only person who pursued to completion a lawsuit against the City of San Francisco for its illegal mass arrests in the wake of the July 25, 1997 police attack on Critical Mass. In the end Besser collected $1,000, double the amount he was initially awarded in Small Claims Court, after the City appealed to Superior Court and lost a second time. Following is a greatly abbreviated excerpt from his Trial Brief, useful to all who face similarly trumped up charges resulting from participating in Critical Mass.

HOWARD BESSER, Plaintiff vs. City of San Francisco, Defendant

For about two hours the evening of July 25, 1997 about 5,000 bicyclists rode through San Francisco as part of the monthly Critical Mass bike ride. Plaintiff was among a group of 100 bicyclists surrounded without warning by the San Francisco police, arrested, handcuffed, and taken to jail. Everyone in this group was charged with failure to disperse, unlawful assembly, disobeying a peace officer, and blocking traffic. All 100 mass-arrestees had their bicycles confiscated, and the Mayor threatened to keep them permanently. Plaintiff was finally able to recover his bike a week later. Plaintiff filed a claim against the City of San Francisco, then successfully sued the City in Small Claims Court. The City then appealed to Superior Court.

Though there were clearly crowd control problems and vehicle code violations committed the evening of the arrest, police should have acted against people who violated the law, rather than arbitrarily arresting a group of people in order to set an example. The evidence will show that the arrest was illegal. Furthermore, it will show that throughout this case the Police Department and the City has exhibited a pattern of obstification and reckless disregard for individual rights, from the punitive measure of confiscating and holding the bicycles to legal maneuvering to make it difficult for arrestees to challenge the false arrest.

Critical Mass Background

Monthly Critical Mass bicycle rides have taken place in San Francisco for almost a decade. For over a year prior to the July 25, 1997 ride, police had provided an escort for the riders. Riders believe that these police escorts waved them through while blocking cross-traffic at intersections, knowing that a mass group of bicyclists would be less disruptive to cross-traffic if the officers blocked that traffic long enough for the crowd of bicycles to pass. (The alternative of making bicyclists stop at red lights might be advantageous for cross-traffic at the lead light, but those stopped bicyclists would cause a gridlock of bicyclists behind them having nowhere to go, blocking cross-traffic for many blocks behind the lead light. Mayor Brown was even quoted as saying "The cyclists make a good point by saying the situation may be made worse by saying you can't run any red lights. I don't want to get hung up on this business of running a red light." ["Mayor Brown Backs Down on Bike Event; U-turn on Critical Mass catches police off-guard," *San Francisco Chronicle*, July 22, 1997, page A1])

Several weeks before the July 25 1997 ride, Mayor Brown was quoted in the newspapers saying that the Critical Mass event should be stopped. Over the next few weeks his position vacillated, and he actually showed up at the start of the ride to give a speech and joke with the bicyclists.

Plaintiff, along with most bicyclists in the crowd had no reason to believe that this ride would be any different in terms of police escorts and having the crowd of bicyclists pass through red lights to keep the large group from forming gridlock. Not until after the arrests did plaintiff discover that he was on an unsanctioned ride and was not being waved through intersections. If police did warn that the ride was unsanctioned, warning was at an isolated location, and did not reach most of the bicyclists.

The Arrest and Incarceration

About 8:30 PM (sun beginning to set) on Friday evening, plaintiff joined a group of bicyclists riding west on Sacramento from Davis, planning to meet friends at the Powell Street BART station and go back to his home in Berkeley. This group was stopping at each stoplight. The group passed a disturbance just before Sansome, but most (including plaintiff) continued on. Just past Sansome plaintiff stopped beside a police wagon and asked an officer a question, then continued west on Sacramento. There was a crowd of bicyclists stopped at the Montgomery Street stoplight, and it took some time for plaintiff to notice that the congestion was not because of the light, but rather because the police had formed a line across Sacramento and were not letting anyone pass. After a while the plaintiff noticed that there was also a line of police at the other end of the block, and that everyone on that block (about 100 bicyclists) had been hemmed in. Plaintiff approached an officer and asked what was going to happen, and the officer said the plaintiff would find out in due time. Plaintiff waited between 15 minutes and half an hour before an officer came out with a bullhorn to announce that all those encircled would be arrested.

No audible order to disperse was given while plaintiff was present, and no opportunity to disperse was given. One by one, each of the 100 encircled people had their bicycles tagged and taken away, were handcuffed, and were put into the back of a police van. Arrestees offered no resistance, no shouts, no chants. Plaintiff was placed in a van without any windows or interior light, and was unable to even see the other arrestees in the van. About an hour later plaintiff was transported to county jail and placed in a holding cell that eventually filled up with about 60 males.

After several hours in the holding cell, plaintiff was processed for release around 1 AM. At the processing, plaintiff told sheriff's deputies that he had missed the final BART train home, and requested to spend the night in the holding cell. Sheriffs told him that if he wanted to spend the night there, he would have to spend not just Friday night, but the entire weekend in jail and would have to go before a judge on Monday. Plaintiff decided that release was preferable than an entire weekend in jail, and tried to hitchhike home to Berkeley. After trying for over two hours (at two separate freeway onramps), plaintiff gave up and tried sleeping in some bushes near the freeway. In the morning plaintiff took BART home. Plaintiff spent the weekend highly agitated over the arrest and loss of his bicycle.

The Bicycle Confiscation

Sheriffs deputies handling the release processing had told plaintiff that he could retrieve his bicycle Monday morning at the Hall of Justice. Plaintiff crossed the bay and went to the Hall of Justice Monday morning, only to be told that the bicycle was not ready for release. Plaintiff was told to call back on Tuesday.

When plaintiff returned home to Berkeley, he heard news radio reports indicating that the City was considering permanently confiscating the bicycles. He then picked up newspapers and read quotes from Mayor Brown saying "I think we ought to confiscate their bicycles." ["Brown: Take bikes of busted cyclists", *San Francisco Examiner*, July 27, 1997, page A1]. He also read an article where the "San Francisco Police Chief will ask the district attorney's office to hold on to the bikes seized in Friday's Critical Mass, at least until those arrested show up in court... Lau's recommendation comes a day after Mayor Willie Brown first raised the possibility of seizing the bikes and either auctioning them off or donating them to charity." [S.F. Police Chief To Ask DA to Keep Confiscated Bikes", *San Francisco Chronicle*, July 28, 1997, page 1]

Plaintiff became very upset and agitated that his only means of transportation was going to be auctioned off. Plaintiff made repeated calls to lawyers and City officials, as well as trips to San Francisco to try to get his bicycle back. Plaintiff was unable to sleep and was inattentive at work for the next week. And plaintiff had to take taxis and busses to get to meetings and appointments that week.

Legal Arguments

The mass arrest of 100 bicyclists was illegal and contrary to proper policies and procedures. The arrestees were not part of an unlawful assembly, and even if one could conceive of their conduct as illegal, they were not given proper warning to disperse and a chance to disperse, as required by the penal code... Both the penal code and Federal Appellate Courts say that individuals must be given a chance to disperse, but no such chance was given by the SFPD that evening. If the police did indeed read a dispersal order somewhere in the vicinity of the arrests, they made no attempt to avoid rounding up and arresting bicyclists who had bicycled into the area after an announcement was made. It is quite telling that no one in the vicinity (except perhaps police officers) appears to have heard a declaration of unlawful assembly or an order to disperse.

There was no cause to declare plaintiff a member of an unlawful assembly. Unlawful assemblies require violent or illegal acts (PC 407), and plaintiff and witnesses were not engaging in violent or illegal acts. Illegal acts most certainly occurred that evening (and violent acts probably did as well), but police do not have the legal right to round up a random group of bicyclists in the City just because a few isolated illegal acts occurred somewhere. There must be a direct tie between the illegal act and the individuals who are declared the unlawful assembly. There were 5,000 bicyclists participating in Critical Mass that evening, and very few illegal acts. Police should have addressed the individual illegal acts.

A close reading of the law indicates that, unless one is given proper warning, one cannot be a participant in an unlawful assembly. According to the California Criminal Jury Instructions (CALJIC 16.241), both "an unlawful assembly [must have] occurred" and the defendant must have "willfully and knowingly participated in the unlawful assembly". Yet on July 25 1997 no one in the arrested crowd appears to have heard it declared an unlawful assembly, so they could not have been willful and knowing participants.

The charge of "Refusal to Disperse" was also blatantly illegal. The penal code (PC 409) states the individuals must be "lawfully warned to disperse" (which they were not). Federal appellate courts have ruled (*Washington Mobilization Committee et al v. Maurice J. Cullinane, Chief of the Metropolitan Police Department et al*, No. 75-2010) that individuals must be provided with "fair notice and opportunity to comply" with a dispersal order for that order to be lawful. In this case, the arrestees were given no notice, and no one had an opportunity to comply.

The City Attorney may try to make the argument that just being a part of Critical Mass constituted an unlawful assembly. But this argument is contradicted by repeated SF Police statements to the press in the weeks before the July 25 ride. In these statements police spokespersons said that they thought that most Critical Mass-ers were well-intentioned and law-abiding, and that any crack-downs would only affect a few trouble-makers. "'It's a small proportion that wants to actually create traffic havoc, perhaps one percent,' said Captain Dennis Martell. 'The overwhelming majority are just there for another San Francisco happening.'" ["Brown Wants to Put Brakes on Mass Bike Ride", *San Francisco Chronicle*, July 2, 1997, page A1] In an article appearing in the Examiner several hours before the ride started, Police Chief Fred Lau indicated that police would deal only with the few trouble-makers, not try to condemn the entire set of riders: "Anybody who independently diverts away or commits some type of traffic violation or some other type of offense is going to be dealt with on an individual basis." ["Critical Mass' moment of truth", *S.F. Examiner*, July 25, 1997, page A1]

In their legal brief submitted to Small Claims Court, the City made the absurd claim that the bicycle confiscation was necessary for evidence as "instruments of the crime". First of all, the charges leading to arrest (failure to disperse, unlawful assembly) did not involve bicycles, and this stance on the part of the City lends credence to plaintiff's contentions that he was arrested for being a bicyclist, not for failure to disperse or unlawful assembly. Secondly, the City already had more than enough hard evidence to show that the plaintiff had been riding a bicycle that evening: bicycles were tagged and labeled at the arrest scene, and plaintiff was given a receipt.

The bicycles were not confiscated as evidence; they were confiscated to punish the arrestees and send a message to other bicycle riders. This was the message given by Mayor Brown when he advocated auctioning off the confiscated bikes, and by Police Chief Lau when he asked the DA to keep the bikes. According to an article appearing the *Chronicle* the following Monday, the bicycle confiscation was punitive in nature. "The tactic, which Lau announced to the *Chronicle* yesterday, is intended to send the message 'that we are not going to tolerate any more of this mob mentality'." [S.F. Police Chief To Ask DA to Keep Confiscated Bikes", *San Francisco Chronicle*, July 28, 1997, page 1]

Summary

The City's position, as articulated in their Small Claims Court Brief, strains credibility. They would have us believe that police audibly warned the crowd to disperse or be arrested, yet 100 adults chose to be arrested. They would have us believe that the arrestees were the same group of people who the City's Brief calls "an angry crowd" that chanted threats at officers when they tried to ticket bicyclists —yet this same crowd became docile and neither chanted nor acted hostile when they themselves were surrounded and arrested.

The City has come up with these unbelievable scenarios because they are unwilling to admit the truth —that they did not follow the law, and that they arrested and incarcerated 100 innocent individuals. Though officers may have warned of an unlawful assembly elsewhere, they made no attempt to follow the law and assure that the individuals they had arrested had heard the warning, nor did they give those individuals any chance to disperse. Police decided to make an example of innocent individuals to prove that they could be tough and crack down. And they continued to harass these individuals by illegally confiscating their bicycles.

The City Attorney's role throughout this whole affair has been shameful. Instead of making sure that the police followed the law, the City Attorney has stretched out the process of paying damages for almost two years—long enough that only one claimant has stuck with the process. The City Attorney even appealed plaintiff's $500 judgment against the City in the hopes that plaintiff would realize that the time and effort required for a Superior Court Appeal would be worth more than the $500 judgment.

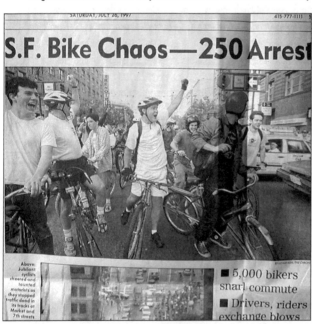

SATURDAY, JULY 26, 1997 415-777-1111

S.F. Bike Chaos—250 Arrest

Above: Jubilant cyclists cheered and taunted motorists as they stopped traffic dead in its tracks at Market and 7th streets

■ 5,000 bikers snarl commute

■ Drivers, riders exchange blows

San Francisco Chronicle, July 26, 1997

Minneapolis, Minnesota

NO SPACE IN THE FIRST PLACE

BY SAM TRACY

Minneapolis actually makes for some lively bike culture, cold winter nights or no. More people involve themselves through the warm seasons, for sure, but I'd swear there's more and more diehards every year. We support seventy-some bikeshops, tooling around on a nearly passable network of bikeways and dedicated street lanes. This likely owes something to a vaunted "progressive tradition" Governor Jesse Ventura is rapidly destroying, but the local "alt transportation" lipservice reduces bikes and busses to competition for the same scarce resources. Our downtown is a maze of contradictions. Transit has made some useful gains at the expense of bike lanes; the relentless drive to construct more parking dwarfs all of it. Well-seasoned transportation engineers try fitting the odd bike lane around purposeful increases in car capacity; the results suggest we're being modeled towards oblivion. Anyone without a car competes for table-scraps.

My friend Stephan, a New York courier, once told me the best place to ride is right down the yellow lines. 'Bike lanes' become 'cab parking.' This kind of blew me away at the time—I'm in Minneapolis—I've since been discovering he was absolutely right. Double-parking is not yet too big here, but doors are always opening for us, with no space in the first place. Minneapolis traffic approaches New York with record speed.

Riding the yellow lines does make it more difficult for someone to accidentally turn across your midsection, or snipe you from a driveway or something. Not always the thing to do; it's hardly a natural place to be. Might even require more attention—drivers are not expecting to see us there—so it goes. Only predictable thing is no space in the first place. I find myself riding the wrong way sometimes for the very same reason: we are already put in the position to "do things we're not supposed to do." There's nothing to prove; at this point it's just the nature of the beast.

Nicollet Mall, a federally-funded transitway, has been a particular bone of contention. It was once hugely popular with bikes. But to summarize a protracted political struggle, the bus company wanted to ban cyclists from the Mall, for reasons of insurance liability. When such a proposal was floated publicly in the summer of 1997, its reception was most unambiguous: Minneapolis saw the largest Critical Mass ride the city had ever seen. A thousand riders made all the networks, front-paged both our dailies the next day. This came together on three days' lead time, flyering all the bikes parked downtown. The ride itself was amazing, flat-out spectacular. We took every intersection we came across. Ended up back in the parking lot across from the downtown library, no arrests. But we lost in the end: the bus company made clear its choice of allegiances. A specific, liberatory solution had been proposed—re-routing the Mall's Southbound busses to the existing Southbound bus lanes one block to either side, converting Nic Mall's Southbound lane to a dedicated bikeway—and they choked it. The state's largest alternative transportation bureaucracy was not willing to confront the whims of car traffic on those two avenues; a supremely noble and principled position they could have adopted, for the sake of alternatives in transportation no less.

Cycling downtown has never been sketchier. And Minneapolis Critical Mass, lacking such an immediate, galvanizing issue, became somewhat less spectacular. An unfortunate dynamic emerges: those remaining true often seek to compensate for the (absent) natural mandate of a large ride by following more contentious routes, and the predictable antagonism that results discourages participation by inviting police harassment.

And so it came to the March, 2002 ride. I was not there, but descriptions were not uplifting: cops trailing the mass in ambush, sporting a flatbed truck for all the bikes they'd be impounding. They found their opportunity soon enough, when people ran a light to stay together, and they attacked. Maced at least one woman, put someone else in the hospital, arrested two others, ganked lots of bikes and flung arbitrary citations around like frisbees.

The episode runs smoothly tandem to the periodic Spring "crackdowns" on those confused, wayward cyclists who miss all the signs and challenge the Nic Mall bus sanctuary. It is a very old cycle—we want more people involved, reaction seeks to prevent this—in this we're only part of something larger. One big bridge to nowhere or the only thing left to do, depending who you talk to. Minneapolis has had its own taste of the new protest energy—the graceful and resilient Highway 55 occupation, a huge Mayday 2000 march, against-all-odds protests against an international animal genetics conference—police reaction to each has been absolutely surreal, beyond any scope or dimension. And so it goes: a friend told me about a Critical Mass meeting once. The cops had snooped out an email list and found out about it; they showed up that night to hassle people for not having lights on their bikes. (They also showed up at a meeting the other night, some hours after the doomed March ride, but this time just lurked outside. The aloof-watchfulness thing. Just creepy.)

It would be easy enough, considering circumstances, to simply cast cops as the "enemy" and be done with it: almost as if that's what is supposed to happen. The pressure applied is quite deliberate; we're supposed to get scared and fade away. The situation requires a certain political acumen—the cops are clearly desperate; it's probably best to act slightly scared and stupid once they pounce—but more than that, any attempts towards marginalization should be resisted proactively. They'd apparently like to force the whole thing underground; we should instead stride proudly towards the daylight. We have the right, it is cool, there is nothing going on at all. That's a tactical point, not a political one. Despite what anyone thinks of the police, we should know by now what to expect—it can appear they're only waiting for an excuse to flex on people—playing into that is pointless. Think about it. I've been busted for various things several times myself, but not everyone is up to risking arrest—for different reasons—equating this with "false commitment" is not the way to make friends. And we should be having

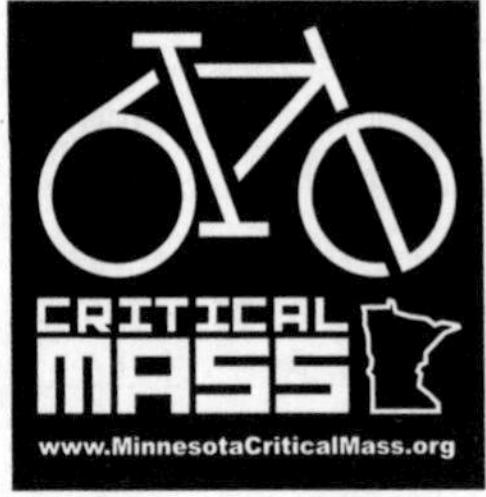

lots of friends with us if'n we're looking for bigger battles.

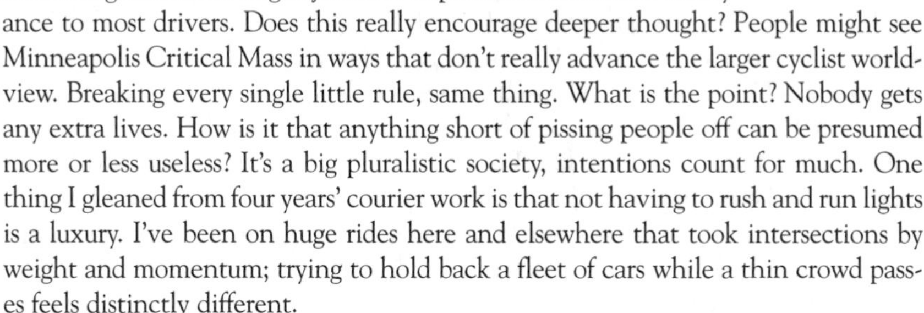

Matte Resist

It shouldn't be any question of roping people in to prop something up; we should at least be able to be forthright in our intentions. It's just nicer, it smells better. To the untrained eye, the aforementioned unfortunate dynamic reduces Critical Mass to a simple extreme-sports caper. Trying to hold Hennepin Avenue with 30 riders does not strike me as a good idea. It hands the cops an excuse; something that small might just be a disposable five-minute annoyance to most drivers. Does this really encourage deeper thought? People might see Minneapolis Critical Mass in ways that don't really advance the larger cyclist worldview. Breaking every single little rule, same thing. What is the point? Nobody gets any extra lives. How is it that anything short of pissing people off can be presumed more or less useless? It's a big pluralistic society, intentions count for much. One thing I gleaned from four years' courier work is that not having to rush and run lights is a luxury. I've been on huge rides here and elsewhere that took intersections by weight and momentum; trying to hold back a fleet of cars while a thin crowd passes feels distinctly different.

It brings to mind anti-globalization's intricate debate on the merits of violence and non-violence, which itself strikes me as an odd little contest. It's not like plans become magically waterproof; why not pass up the dualistic proclamations for an appreciation of flexibility? There might be a time and a place for everything, but in the meantime you probably should feel odd if you're the only one trashing things. The fluid approach is most definitely a good thing to have in mind on a bike, regardless of the circumstances. I took a really bad crash a few years back—I was knocked comatose, I almost died, the episode still colors everything I do—one particularly desperate result was an endless quest to deal effectively with traffic. For years I was in the habit of pointing my krypto lock at drivers' faces, when I had right of way and they challenged me, crossing Seventh on Marquette in particular. An odd bit of theater that actually worked somehow; at this point I am amazed it didn't get me run down. More recently I'm finding steady eye contact supremely useful; I don't take a lane unless I'm approximating traffic speed. This will be my thirteenth year without a driving license, assuming I live so long, and I'd really like to. Which is to say I don't rely on extreme sports for any special validation. When there is a choice to be had, trading up cycling's wholesome and subversive pleasures for a cheap, antagonistic shot in the dark comes out to some piss-poor compensation.

Flyers I've seen for Minneapolis Critical Mass present an odd inversion. The hand-lettered stick figure notices we see around are targeted for one slice of the activist demographic; those considered "truly down" or some such. Little badges-of-commitment. I'd flip that upside-down: a flyer's relative value might best be judged by the range of new faces it attracts. Yeah, stride proudly towards the daylight. Said flyer already competes with the show listings, the movies and all manner of commercial pabulum for anyone's attention. Take the time, do it right, get all fancy and shit. Flyers are proudly emblematic of their intentions—if there's no apparent interest to reach beyond an immediate circle, it should not surprise that the rest of the world busies itself elsewhere—let's play for keeps.

The first draft to this, done just after the March ride, ended with a suggestion for a Critical Mass walk. "They won't let us ride together, so we walk together." Right down Nic Mall, turn some heads. But things changed... The cop reaction to the March ride only added to our new mayor's frustration with the seated police chief, who has presided over some particularly brutal years. A confrontation ensued: the cops suddenly eased up in time for the April ride. April was very, very cool here. The crowd was huge, for Minneapolis Critical Mass, hundreds of people. Solidarity with the March riders. As with the August 1997 ride, a crucial and immediate concern got people out. And the ride itself was just a love boat, sailing all over the place, doing anything we wanted. I found myself again going down the yellow lines, up Lake Street and Hennepin no less. But this time I was busy hi-fiving maybe every fourth driver I came across, stalled-out in what would have been the oncoming traffic. "Hey, look at all the bikes!" People laughing, nodding, smiling outnumbered the grumpy ones. All kinds of folks reached a hand out to me. Cool.

Any point I might have made may have been lost beneath the moralist sweeping along somewhere behind me, whom I'd hear now and again, wailing some emotionally truncated syllogism or another. Yeah, that's right, people love being preached at, how could I forget? The cops, this whole time, brought up the rear. The proof once again that it can work. Big question is just how long the peace will last. Stephan tells me the NYPD has given up on Mass arrests in favor of a more benign escorting service. We can only hope for so much here. But who the hell knows!?

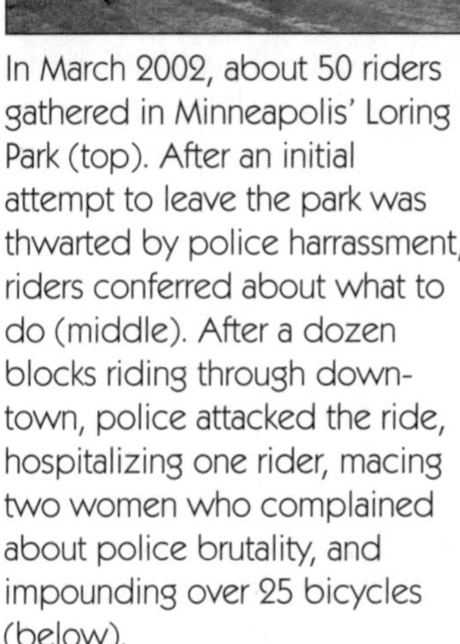

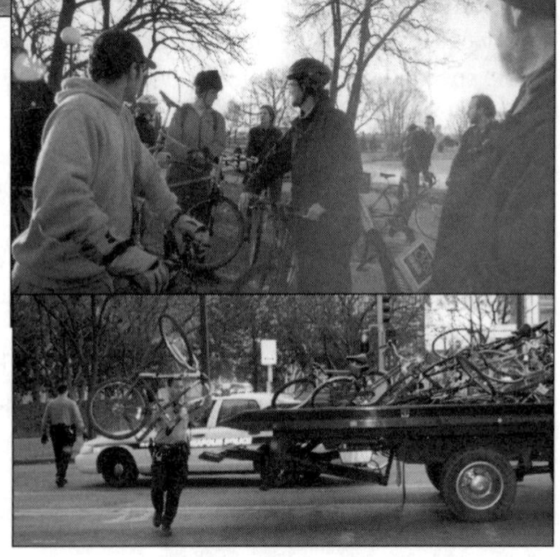

In March 2002, about 50 riders gathered in Minneapolis' Loring Park (top). After an initial attempt to leave the park was thwarted by police harrassment, riders conferred about what to do (middle). After a dozen blocks riding through downtown, police attacked the ride, hospitalizing one rider, macing two women who complained about police brutality, and impounding over 25 bicycles (below).

Francesca Manning

Vancouver, British Columbia, Canada

VANCOUVER CRITICAL MASS

BY MARK COATSWORTH

The city of Vancouver, with its wide network of bike routes and year-round friendly weather, is "bike accessible" at its finest. The city boasts a vibrant cycling community, with major groups such as Better Environmentally Sound Transport (BEST) and the The Bicycle People working to improve urban cycling conditions and promote alternative transportation options.

The Vancouver chapter of Critical Mass has been active since early 1997, when the first organized rides started taking place. Over the following years, it gained a strong following, with the monthly rides soon attracting crowds of up to 100 people. The founding of the Vancouver Indymedia center in November 2000 has helped attract media attention, as has *Momentum*, a cycling advocacy magazine which started in 2001. We meet on the last Friday of every month at the Vancouver Art Gallery, at the corner of Georgia and Hornby. The ride starts through the trendy Robson area, passing through the major fashion and corporate districts of the city. From there, it diverts to other heavy traffic zones in the downtown core. When there are larger numbers of cyclists, we often cross major city bridges. We have also been known to get adventurous and ride through shopping malls. Post-Mass festivities usually involve meals and drinks at the Brickhouse or the Buddhist Vegetarian Restaurant.

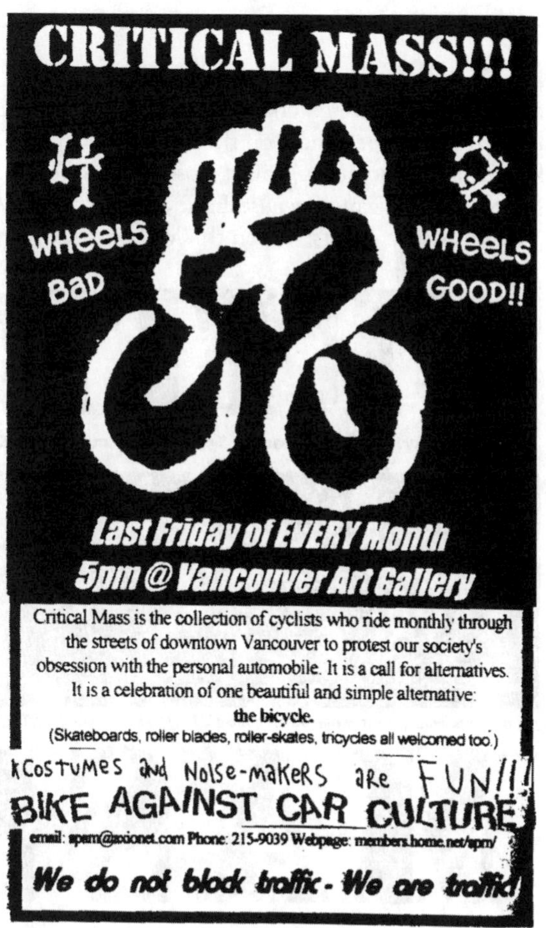
CRITICAL MASS!!!
4 WHEELS BAD
2 WHEELS GOOD!!
Last Friday of EVERY Month
5pm @ Vancouver Art Gallery
Critical Mass is the collection of cyclists who ride monthly through the streets of downtown Vancouver to protest our society's obsession with the personal automobile. It is a call for alternatives. It is a celebration of one beautiful and simple alternative:
the bicycle.
(Skateboards, roller blades, roller-skates, tricycles all welcomed too.)
*Costumes and Noise-makers are FUN!!
BIKE AGAINST CAR CULTURE
email: spam@axionet.com Phone: 215-9039 Webpage: members.home.net/spm/
We do not block traffic - We are traffic

Theme rides are popular among the Critical Mass crowd. Halloween

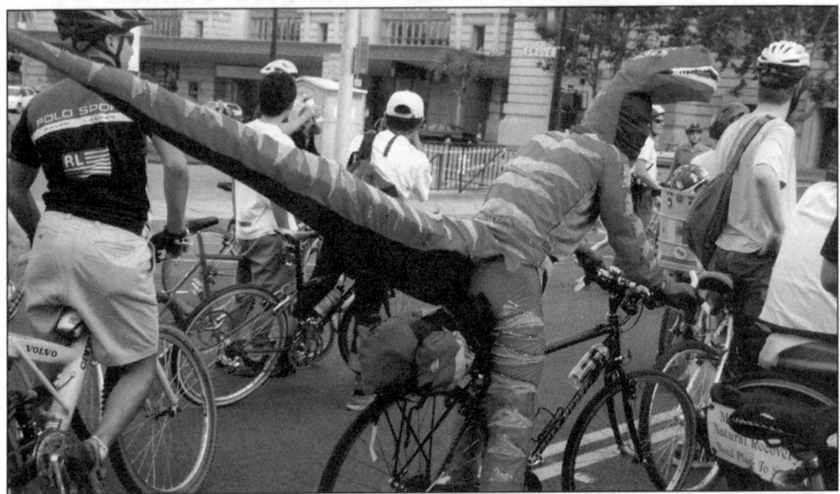

JANICE ROTHSTEIN

The infamous Vancouver dino "Because Extinction Stinks!"

and Christmas are big favorites, with riders taking to the road in full costume garb. A pedal-powered chariot, held together by inner tubes and duct tape, has made several appearances on the downtown streets. One cycling advocacy group known as "Dinosaurs Against Fossil Fuels" regularly ride in dinosaur outfits, sporting the slogan "Because Extinction Stinks!" Many rides are also centered around specific events. When the Molson Indy rears its ugly head each August,

CRITICAL

Last Friday of EVERY Month. 5pm @ Vancouver Art Gallery. bike against car culture!

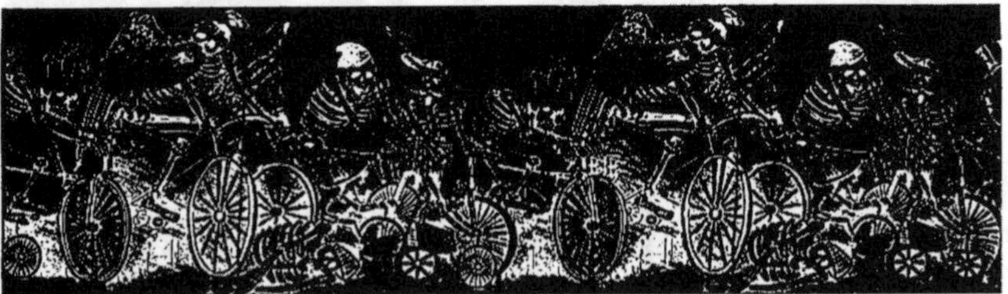

autosaurus@tao.ca ***We do not Block Traffic - We Are Traffic!!*** **http://members.home.net/cmass**

MASS

Critical Mass responds with the "Wholesome Undie" ride. Dressed in underwear and drag, cyclists storm the Indy track and race for the fabled ASSCAR Championship.

While Critical Mass is all about fun, there are also a lot of political issues that we try to address. Among Vancouver's major agonies in 2002 is the ongoing decline of Translink, the city's public transportation system. By combining increased fares with reduced service and fewer routes, they have made bus travel harder than ever. Moreover, with the B.C. Liberal party taking power in the 2001 provincial elections, government funding is getting cut for just about everything. Not just public transit, but social programs, health care and education funding have fallen under the strong arm of the powers-that-be. Critical Mass riders express their anti-appreciation of these evils in a variety of signs, stickers, pamphlets and songs. To show our support for bus drivers and transit users, we will open up a lane whenever possible to let busses pass through our bicycle crowds. Car drivers, in turn, show their support for us by honking repeatedly when they see the "HONK if you love bikes" sign.

WWW.MONKEYWRENCHCAFE.ORG/CM › LAST FRIDAY OF EVERY MONTH › AUTOSAURUS@TAO.CA ›
CRITICAL MASS
BIKES=
FREEDOM
SO RIDE TOGETHER

The Critical Mass scene in Vancouver has a great vibe, and is always lots of fun and adventure for those who attend. With any luck, it will continue strong for a long time, and convince more and more people to get on their bikes and ride.

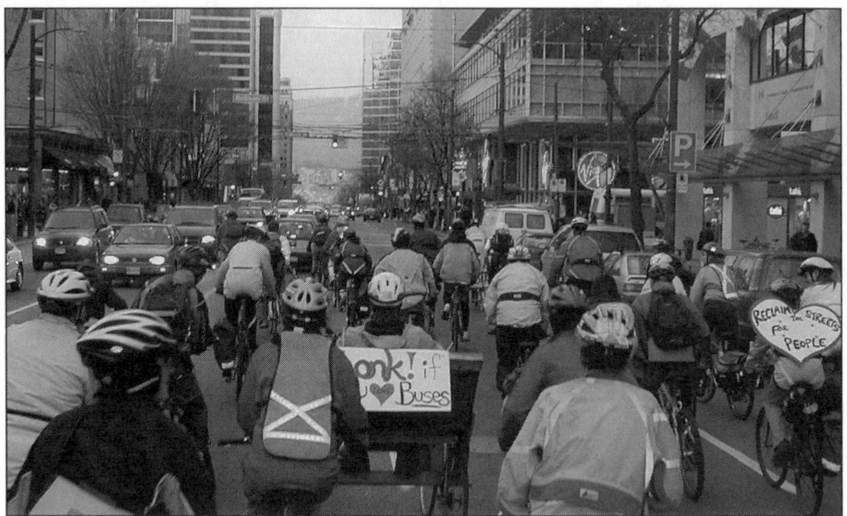
RECLAIM THE STREETS FOR PEOPLE
Buses

Rolling through downtown Vancouver, BC, March 2001

APPENDICITIS!

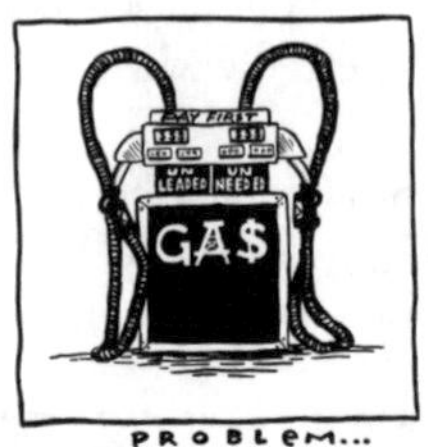

PROBLEM...

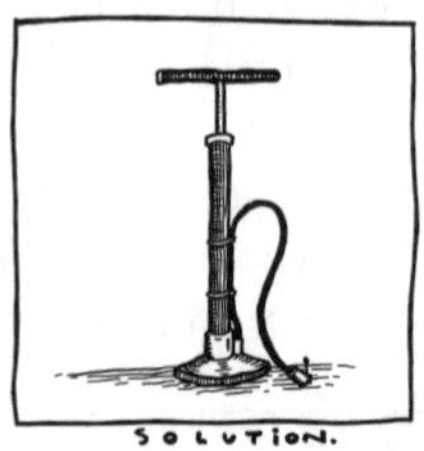

SOLUTION.

HUGH D'ANDRADE

A CRITICAL MASS CULTURAL GLOSSARY

BY JOEL POMERANTZ

In it's first decade, Critical Mass has developed its own culture and assumptions. Conversations about Mass are usually full of jargon. The event itself is full of arguments and celebratory shouts, even when it's calm and friendly. The whooping and yelling aren't just provocations or spirit-builders—they're part of the dynamic that makes the ride work. But what does all that banter mean?

Take the lane! Pedestrian alert! Ticket support! Thanks for corking!

Wait up—Let's regroup! Maniac driver—Escort needed! Hey, don't I know you!?

Here's a glossary to clue you in. Now, when you wish to pass the word on, or reinforce the idea, you can join in and yell too—it's rolling democracy! We who ride for the sense of community like it when there are the fewest confrontations, and when lots of people take personal responsibility for making the ride flow.

A careful reading of this four-page glossary will give you a good idea of what it takes to be an effective participant or instigator. Just don't say, "Go with the flow"!

agitprop 1. Old leftie term, shortened fr. 'agitation propaganda,' organizing materials, e.g. flyers, placards, booklets. 2. Invitations to join ***Critical Mass***, distributed in handfuls at the ***starting point*** to pass out to ***pedestrians*** and ***motorists*** along the ride route, reflecting many views of ***Mass*** (see ***xerocracy***).

bike Shortened fr. 'bicycle': Efficient machine to convert energy generated by bread and peanut butter into connectedness with fellow beings and the land; useful in transportation, art, meditation, celebration, recreation and cultural innovation.

build mass Wait to gather enough bicyclists to ride in a dense group, i.e. safely.

car Short for 'carriage' fr. *vb.* 'to be carried,' dates to a time when idleness was virtue.

cell phone contact Remote contact between ***minimasses***. For ***regrouping*** into one ***Mass*** or for ***route design*** on the fly. Arranged by exchange of numbers before riding.

clogging the streets 1. Usurpation and desecration of public space aggressively undertaken by short-sighted, profit-crazed corporate planners and their dupes, government officials, and *their* dupes, traffic engineers, and *their* dupes, motorists. 2. The occasionally rumored intentional main purpose of ***Critical Mass***. Such ill thoughts can be avoided somewhat by keeping a dense ride so that the group will be clear of any given intersection in a very short time.

Commute Clot ***Critical Mass***'s original name which...um...didn't catch on, used just for the first ride (Sept. 1992).

confrontation 1. The dynamic that automatically and inherently exists between ***Critical Mass*** and a society dependent on ***cars***. 2. The much publicized and unadmired tactic that pits individuals against individuals during a ride, distracting from the beauty of the ride and giving media sensationalists something to bite on.

cops Agents of a false sense of security or false sense of being controlled; sometimes perceive themselves to be in charge of safety, etc., sometimes treated by riders as ride leaders or as targets of abuse, either of which dilutes the ride's power. Best ignored or made irrelevant by ***keeping mass***, ***corking*** and other self-guidance techniques.

corking Leaving the flow of the ride for a while to plant your body and bike, in calm posture, a few feet from the front of stopped ***cars*** which would otherwise enter an intersection in use by ***Critical Mass***. Best accompanied by smiles and eye contact, or signs that say "Thanks for waiting!" and "Honk if you love bikes!" ***Corking*** a ***thinned out*** section of the ride undermines its own legitimacy and safety by tempting the aggression of the ***car drivers*** being corked, who no longer see a ***mass*** of bikes but are still blocked. *vb.* **to cork**, *n.* **corker**.

courtesy! Alert to other riders, meaning "Let 'em through!" e.g. ***Bus courtesy!*** or ***Pedestrian alert!*** Sometimes involves creative intervention to get cooperation.

Critical Mass **1.** Noncommercial, noncompetitive group biking event taking place, since the early 1990s, in a couple hundred cities around the world (often Fridays and monthly). Coined in San Francisco by Dave Snyder, October 1992, from comment by George Bliss, in the Ted White documentary film, ***Return of the Scorcher***. (Bliss observed, at an intersection in China, the method of accumulating enough cyclists to push past ***car*** traffic.) **2.** *not capitalized.* Threshold quantity of physical (or metaphorical) mass needed to reach a goal unreachable by small parts or quantities. **3.** Rider density, group coherence, tightness; the state of having enough bicycles in a given area to negotiate a given traffic situation as one entity. Sometimes shortened to '***mass***' as in, "Do we have ***mass***?"

cutting the red When front riders ignore a ***red light***. Dangerous and disruptive for riders near front and causes ***thinning out***, as opportunities to ***rebuild mass*** are fewer.

density The basis of ***Mass*** and of ***mass***. Created intentionally over time by use of ***agitprop*** describing techniques (see ***keeping mass***, ***rebuilding mass***, ***thinning out***.)

destination **1.** Secret that ***Massers*** are often rumored to keep even from ourselves. **2.** Park, viewpoint or other (preferably large) area which the rotating ***route designer*** picks to deposit the riders, ceasing responsibility for the ride's trajectory, after which point anyone who decides to continue their ride is encouraged to use ***dynamic street smarts*** to make route decisions.

distraction The bike equivalent of rubber-necking consisting of more people stopping than needed to solve a problem with a ***maniac.*** (see ***escort***, ***swarming***).

drive Push with moving force, as in "The profit motive will drive our society to the brink of disaster" or "You drive me to drink."

dynamic street smarts Group decision-making at the ride front concerning such things as "Where the hell do we go now that we've been separated from the group in front of us and we have no route map?!" or "These winter rides are pleasantly small enough to decide the route as we go, so are you too tired to ride to Glen Park?"

escort *vb.* Help a ***car*** out of a spot that obstructs the flow of riders. If you see intentional ***car***-trappers in a ***testosterone brigade***, ask them to ride on and then coax the ***car*** out of the ***Mass*** in the direction they wish to go so neither ***car*** nor swarm blocks our flow. You can yell, "*Keep going!*" to other riders and then yell, "*Homicidal Maniac Driver! Let 'em through!*" (You can wink at the ***car driver*** for added effect.)

hazardous obstacle! Yelled to indicate a ***car*** stuck in ***Mass*** created by ***swarming***.

high-five Opportunity on the ride to loop back toward other riders and become what motorists call "opposing traffic" (instead of opposing, we congratulate one another).

ignoring the red Middle and back of the ***Mass*** continuing through an intersection despite an unfavorable color emitted by traffic control devices. Keeps a ride safer, gets out of ***motorists'*** sights faster. Safest when accompanied by ***corking***. Dangerous if done where ride is ***thinning out***. Not to be confused with ***cutting the red***.

keeping mass Maintaining ride ***density***, our main safety mechanism, and our main P.R. mechanism too, since it gets us through and out of people's way faster. Accomplished by maintaining a very (sometimes frustratingly) slow, leisurely pace so as to ensure the safety of the many riders behind, as they struggle to ***keep Mass***.

leaders or **secret leaders** **1.** You! **2.** Anyone who participates—via email on various local discussion lists or in person at the start and end gatherings of rides—in the creation or distribution of ***agitprop***, ***route designs*** or strategy on ride particulars. Sometimes, but not often, found at front cajoling the crowd into following a route.

maniac driver or **homicidal maniac driver** A person in a ***car*** pushing through the group of cyclists (see ***escort***).

Mass **1.** *Critical Mass*. **2.** Any densely packed, mobile group of cyclists with bikes.

Massers Collected individual participants in ***Critical Mass***.

minimass **1.** *sometimes capitalized.* Smallish group bike ride occurring each week between monthly ***Critical Mass*** rides, usually shorter, mellow, social ride, possibly ending at a neighborhood watering hole. **2.** also ***splinter mass***; Group formed when a large ***Critical Mass*** splits up for safety reasons, creating multiple dense small groups rather than one spread-out large group. Often spontaneous reaction to ***thinning out***, carried out at an intersection where a light turns red under unfavorable conditions for ***corking***.

narrows A space which the ride passes through more slowly, such as an alley, narrow street, or pedestrian passage. To be avoided, except: Can be enjoyable late in the ride, or with only a couple hundred riders, or followed by a stop to ***rebuild mass***.

pedestrians **1.** Harried street-crossers whose rights-of-way you should always respect (see ***courtesy***). **2.** The wetware of every vehicle: ***car***, bus, truck or ***bike***.

racers **1.** People at front who don't stop and look behind them to see that they are getting far out ahead of the ***Mass***. **2.** *derisive.* (see ***testosterone brigade***.)

rails Well-meaning metal objects imbedded in pavement to facilitate streetcars, etc. Dangerous to bikes and (along with rough pavement) best avoided in ***route design***.

rebuild mass ***Build mass*** again during the ride by diligent use of slow riding, or by asking ***bikes*** instead of ***cars*** to wait a few light cycles at an intersection now and then so the ***thinned out*** (i.e. vulnerable) riders behind them can come together more densely. Best undertaken in a place where the crowd of bikes isn't antagonizing anyone unintended. (see ***density***, ***regrouping stop***).

red light **1.** Pretty decoration along the street which it is unsafe for mid-mass riders to heed when traveling as a dense group (see ***keeping mass***). **2.** Traffic control device for ***cars***. **3.** Convenient place for the front of the ride to stop, for many reasons: so already-moving ***cars*** don't have to screech to an angry halt; to ***keep Mass density***; to present a friendly face to the public; to give precedence to a crossing bus; or to hold discussion of route changes after ***cell phone contact***.

regrouping stop A way to express caring and love for the life and limb of those riders behind you (see ***rebuild mass***).

route design The cooperative process of trading off responsibility for thinking about ***Critical Mass***. Sometimes coordinated between interested parties (many of whom can be found on line or handing out ***agitprop***) with intent of minimizing ego and maximizing cooperation, democracy, safety and pleasure for participants (see ***secret leaders***, ***xerocracy***). When designing a route, avoid construction zones or ***narrows***, steep hills, ***rails***, and permanent traffic jam streets where stopped traffic inevitably brings impatience and ***swarming***. After a long downhill stretch or a ***narrows***, plan a location to stop and ***rebuild mass*** with a dozen preagreed loud helpers to halt the ride front a few blocks past the ***narrows*** spot. Competing route designs are voted on at the ride starting point.

splinter mass See ***minimass***.

splitting the Mass Getting the back of the group to stop at a ***red light*** in a large ***thinned out*** group of riders to create safer ***minimasses***.

swarming Surrounding and passing a ***car*** stopped at a light, rather than waiting behind it so that it won't obstruct ***Mass*** and create unneeded confrontations. Can be fun, but can create safety problems.

take the lane Expand the ride into a lane, dense with cyclists.

testosterone brigade Posturing, aggressive, confrontational riders who forget that the people stuck in ***cars*** are not all there by their own free choice. (see also ***racers***.)

thinning out Ride spreading out, usually due to speed of front riders. Opposite of ***Mass***, opposite of ***density***. Bad.

ticket support A "witnessing" activity conducted by a small, mellow and polite group when one of us (often a ***corker***) is singled out by law enforcement for a ticket or finger-wagging. If the face-saving atmosphere is friendly and not many ***cops*** are present, this activity can influence an officer not to give the intended ticket.

velorution **1.** 'Revolution' as spelled by a dyslexic. **2.** *quirky pun*. A swift change in society brought about by bicycling. Prefix comes from 'velocipede,' an old word for ***bicycle***, from Latin *velox*, meaning swift (as in 'velocity') and *ped*, 'foot.'

wait up! **1.** Commonly yelled if you want to let front riders know it's time to ***rebuild Mass*** by stopping and letting people catch up. **2.** A request to the group ahead to stop and pull over.

whoop start A simple, loud "WHOOP," meaning "*Let's go!*" used when the ride front is stopped at a ***red light*** and people are too busy socializing to notice the green.

xerocracy **1.** ***Critical Mass***'s form of self-government. You got an idea? Write it down and pass it out at the next ride. Include your ***route design*** suggestions. **2.** The method of ***route design*** in which the day's route is decided on the basis of who can convince the most people (preferably near the ride front) to follow their map, copied and passed out in the gathering before the ride.

BICYCLING OVER THE RAINBOW: REDESIGNING CITIES—AND BEYOND

BY CHRIS CARLSSON, SUMMER 1994

Critical Mass is nearly two years old. In terms of sheer numbers it is still growing, but the more profound goals associated with a developing political culture are substantially unmet. As a founder of CM and someone who has been on each and every ride in San Francisco I'd like to blurt a bit:

The growing pains we've experienced during the last six months, while not much fun, are in any case inevitable as an event takes on a life of its own. The July ride, nearing 3,000 riders, was an impressive display of statistical growth, but conversely it was what I've dubbed the "Stepford Wives" ride: it was characterized by an unusual zombie-like silence and lack of energy which underscored the basic anonymity in which even we regulars found ourselves engulfed.

Of course when we started out with 45 bicyclists in September 1992, I fantasized about Critical Mass becoming a big mass event, but it was never an important goal. Far more important to me was the lived experience of new communities, new friends, new social spaces, and most importantly, a new political space. Now that CM is so big, those of us who seek communitarian and utopian moments will have to make a greater effort to make them happen and can count less on the spontaneous combustion that has been a hallmark of the Critical Mass experience in the past.

I and a bunch of others informally planned routes and published most of the maps, Missives, and many other xerocratic documents, stickers, etc. during the first two years. A couple of dozen people found their way into the "process," which was amorphous and a bit clique-y but emphatically open. (We did jealously guard the secrecy of the process from those who might have shared it with the police, since it was and is our feeling that police involvement would inevitably destroy the free-spirited quality of the event.)

My guess is that the silent majority of riders for the most part would be happier if the police stayed home and don't want to deal with police one way or the other—they neither want to fight the cops nor submit to them. In general we've always sought to ignore the police, since we are merely using the city's roads to go where we're going, just like any other commuter or traveller. Our flaunting of traffic norms (essentially red lights and stop signs) was designed to ensure the safety of the mass of bicyclists AND that of the isolated motorist who unexpectedly and suddenly finds herself surrounded by hundreds of boisterous bicyclists in what can be an intimidating experience. We also run lights and stop signs to keep moving and bring the minor traffic delay to an end that much sooner, since individual motorists are not our enemy.

The tension provided by police attention has been an attraction to some Massers and a disincentive to others. In any case it, and our varied responses to it, have shaped our political culture. I, for one, hate it when the police cheerfully welcome us to our own event, as though they thought it up and were providing it to us as a service! Their presence insults me, but the police are not the issue. If I let my opposition to state authority tilt my CM participation towards engaging in antago-

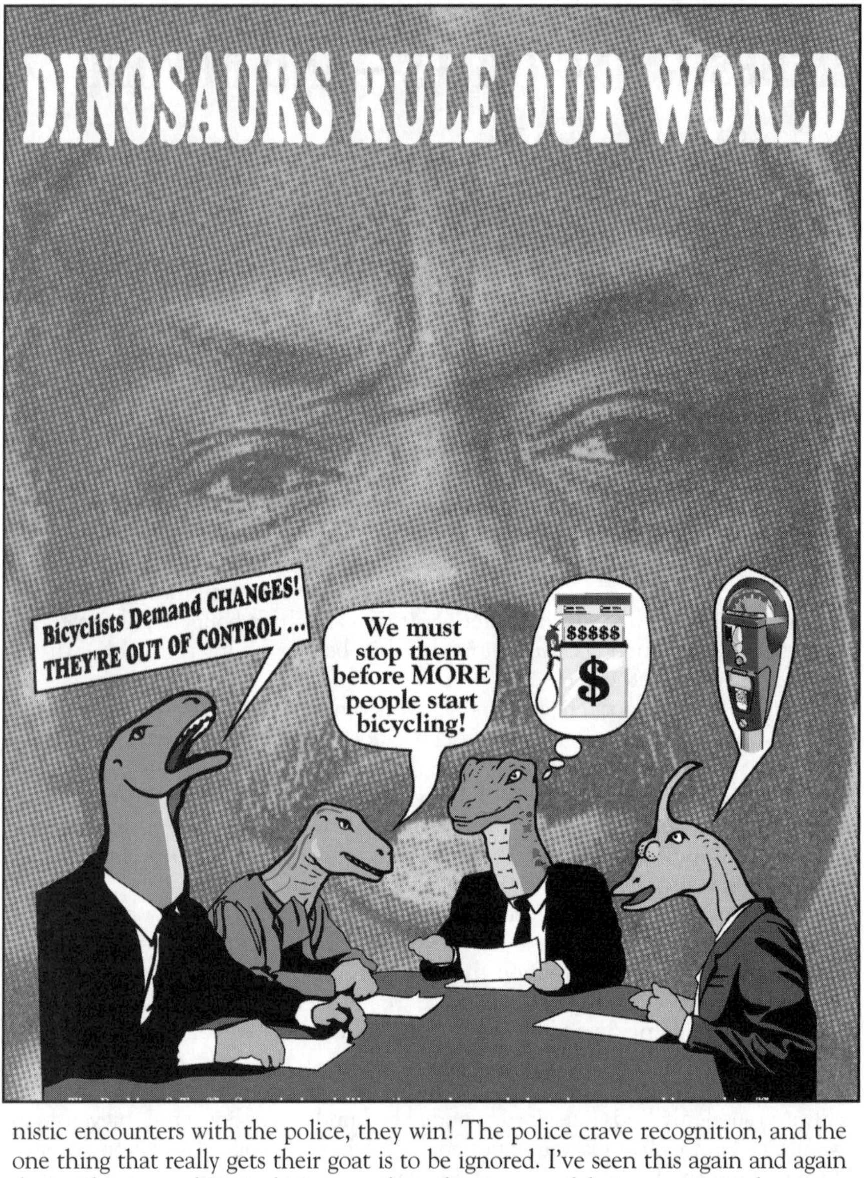

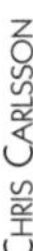
DINOSAURS RULE OUR WORLD
Bicyclists Demand CHANGES! THEY'RE OUT OF CONTROL ...
We must stop them before MORE people start bicycling!
$$$$$
$
CHRIS CARLSSON

nistic encounters with the police, they win! The police crave recognition, and the one thing that really gets their goat is to be ignored. I've seen this again and again during the years of Critical Masses—the police go out of their way to attack anyone who attempts to cork or establish dialogues with motorists or in various ways break out of the acceptable norm of a police-sanctioned and -controlled parade. (There is at least one individual who is seeking order, predictability and legal standing for Critical Mass, cooperation with the police, and a trajectory towards a bicycling Bay to Breakers, which may grow into a mega-event with refreshments, commercial sponsors, and entertainment at the end!)

To avoid the inevitable progression into an oversized, predictable and dull parade we might consider our original pretense: that we are merely *RIDING HOME TOGETHER* and break into 5 or 7 alternate groups heading for different neighborhoods at a designated midpoint, like the Civic Center or Market and Van Ness. I am already tired of the apparent attempt to visit every hilltop in town, and have never been interested in 17-mile endurance rides. This brings us to what must be a profound divergence among Critical Mass participants: are you participating to have a bike ride or a social experience? Most of us want both, I'm sure, but most of us can probably identify our primary motivation as one or the other. I want the social experience and I don't need the bike ride to be really long or necessarily go to obscure parts of the city. I actually liked the early days when we looped through downtown and ended up at a bar, Dolores Park or Golden Gate Park for hanging out. I think those who want to take really long rides should do so, but there's no particular reason to impose that on Critical Mass, certainly not every time.

We conceived Critical Mass to be a new kind of political space, not about PROTESTING but about CELEBRATING our vision of preferable alternatives, most obviously in this case bicycling over the car culture. Importantly we wanted to build on the strong roots of humor, disdain for authority, decentralization, and self-direction that characterize our local political cultural history. Critical Mass descends from the anti-nuke movement as much as it does from the bicycling initiatives of the past. It is as much street theatre as it is a (semi) functional commute, or at least it has been at its best. It is inherently anti-corporate even though there are more uncritical supporters of the American Empire and its monied interests riding along than there are blazing subversives, which is just another of the many pleasant ironies of Critical Mass.

The Bicycle itself embodies the counter-technological tradition that is the flipside of America's infatuation with technological fixes. Like the pro-solar movement in the 1970s, today's bike advocates tend to view the bicycle as something that is inherently superior, that brings about social changes all by itself, endowing it with causal qualities that ought to be reserved for human beings. I am a daily bike commuter, have been for most of the past 20 years, and am very fond of bicycling in cities. I greatly appreciate the bicycle for its functionality in short-circuiting dominant social relations, but let's not forget that it is merely another tool, and has no will of its own. When I bicycle around town I see things happening and can stop and explore them in depth with no hassles. I also see my friends and acquaintances and can stop and speak with them directly. This, combined with the absence of mass media pumping into my brain in the isolation of my car, sets up organic links and direct channels of human experience and communication. These links are potentially quite subversive to the dominant way of life in modern America, which is one of the reasons I like bicycling.

But bicycling is not an end in itself, just like Critical Mass is really about a lot more than just bicycling. Our embrace of bicycling doesn't eliminate an enormous social edifice dedicated to supporting the privately owned car and oil industries. Similarly, the infrastructural design of our cities and communities is slow to change in the face of our preferential choice of bicycling. Finally, we won't see any real change if we continue to act as isolated consumer/commuters, and in part Critical Mass allows us to begin coming together. But Critical Mass is far from enough, and until we begin challenging a whole range of technological choices at their roots, our lives and the planetary ecology are likely to continue worsening. Our capitalist society doesn't really care what we buy or which toys we like to play with, as long as we keep working within a system that systematically excludes us from decisions about the shape of our lives or the technologies we must choose.

The space we've opened up in Critical Mass is a good beginning. Out of it must grow the organic communities that can envision and then fight for a radically different organization of life itself! We will *never shop our way to a liberated society*. So questions of utopia lurk beneath the Critical Mass experience. What kind of life would you like to live, if you could choose? What of all the work that this society imposes on us, is *work worth doing*? What kind of technologies do we need? What direction do we want science to go (e.g. do we want to dedicate millions to military "defense" and a space program, or shall science address the basic research associated with redesigning cities, transit and energy systems, etc.)? Why do we live in a "democracy" in which serious questions such as these are never discussed, and if they are, only in remote academic journals and around the occasional kitchen table? Why is politics primarily a detached and meaningless ritual of popularity and money?

In general our culture is quite backwards when it comes to politics: genuine arguments are greeted with horror and discomfort because the antagonists aren't being "nice." Substantive disagreements regularly descend into personality squabbles wherein the real issues are quickly lost beneath the heated rhetoric of personal contempt. Most people seem to think politics is about elections and governments rather than the day-to-day compromises we have to make with each other to live. By that way of thinking, many Critical Massers on both sides of the question have concluded that Critical Mass is "apolitical" either because it eschews demands, lobbying, and policy declarations, or because it is celebratory and fun and not confrontational and angry.

Critical Mass is one of the MOST POLITICAL events of this depressing decade; its lack of formal leaders or agenda has opened it up for everyone to claim it for their own demands and desires. It has no further purpose than its continued existence, which in itself is an affirmation of communities that are otherwise invisible and easily ignored. How the newly self-discovered communities within Critical Mass evolve into more contestational political movements remains to be seen, and is a challenge that faces us all. Maybe some folks will begin direct action campaigns around open space, transit corridors, parks and wildlife corridors, etc.? Perhaps others will band together at work to demand that their employer dedicate 10% of their hours to work in the city helping build an ecologically sound urban alternative? Clearly, the daunting task of remaking city life on a humane and ecological basis is going to take a serious challenge to the status quo, one unlikely to emerge from existing entities that claim to be political. So take heart my friends, be patient but not lazy, wait but don't dawdle, act with intelligence, an open mind, and good will, and reject the easy ideological clichés. Life is very different these days, but not nearly as different as we would like it to be, and certainly not different in the ways that would make for an equitable, enjoyable, ecological and fulfilling human life for all of us.

HOW TO MAKE A CRITICAL MASS

Lessons and Ideas from the San Francisco Bay Area Experience

Originally published in 1993. Produced by Hugh D'Andrade, Beth Verdekal, Chris Carlsson, JR Swanson, Kathy Roberts and Nigel French, with help from many other friends.

"What's this all about?" ask amused and bemused pedestrians on Market Street as hundreds of noisy, high-spirited bicyclists ride past, yelling and ringing their bells. There are a wide variety of answers: "It's about banning cars." "It's about having fun in the street." "It's about a more social way of life." "It's about asserting our right to the road". "It's about solidarity." Critical Mass is many things to many people, and while many concepts expressed may evoke memories of past political protests, Critical Mass is foremost a celebration, not a protest.

Critical Mass got started in September 1992 in San Francisco as a way to bring these various populations together in a festive re-claiming of public space. San Francisco's prominent bicycle messenger community was enlisted primarily through word of mouth, while commuters were reached by someone standing in the middle of the financial district passing out fliers.

Beginning rather under a less catchy name—the Commute Clot—the ride drew an initial crowd of 48 cyclists, and these numbers doubled for several months following. Critical Mass has continued and grown in San Francisco, drawing about 700+ from month to month, with an October 1993 high of 1000+, but it has spread to other cities as well. With independent rides springing up all over the place, Critical Mass has begun to take on the character of a large scale, decentralized grassroots movement!

Ultimately, Critical Mass is just a bunch of cyclists riding around together, going from one point to another. (Someone coined the descriptive phrase "organized coincidence.") But the incredible thing is that, in attempting this simple task, so many important and interesting questions come up. Why is there so little open space in our cities where people can relax and interact, free from the incessant buying and selling of ordinary life? Why are people compelled to organize their lives around having a car? What would an alternative future look like?

In writing this, we have not set out to answer these questions. Instead, we are using our familiarity with only one of the many Critical Mass rides (San Francisco's) to help accelerate the spread of Critical Mass to other cities, and share ideas, tactics, solutions, etc.

It is important to emphasize, however, that no two rides will be identical, and while Critical Mass may be a common approach to a common problem, different contexts will produce different dynamics, pressures, etc. This text, then, is in no way intended as an "official blueprint" or strict set of guidelines set forth by some all-knowing committee. Rather, it is simply the brainchild of a small handful of Critical Mass enthusiasts in the Bay Area, and it will inevitably reflect our experiences, prejudices and beliefs.

Pre-ride planning

It should be relatively easy to set up a Critical Mass ride. Whether they are commuters, couriers, or ride just for the fun of it, every city has a population of bicyclists that are marginalized and threatened by the current transportation system. Perhaps more importantly, these groups are just the tip of the iceberg. Poor air quality, environmental degradation and the general decay of living conditions due to over-reliance on motorized traffic in urban areas are felt by everyone. There is a potential mass base for change in all these scattered, isolated groups, and a Critical Mass ride can serve as a rallying point to bring them together.

Xerocracy

In San Francisco the organization of the event has been as much a part of its success as anything else. Organizational politics, with its official leaders, demands, etc., has been eschewed in favor of a more decentralized system. There is no one in charge. Ideas are spread, routes shared, and consensus sought through the ubiquitous copy machines on every job or at copy shops in every neighborhood—a "Xerocracy," in which anyone is free to make copies of their ideas and pass them around. Leaflets, fliers, stickers and 'zines all circulate madly both before, during and after the ride, rendering leaders unnecessary by ensuring that strategies and tactics are understood by as many people as posssible.

Xerocracy promotes freedom and undercuts hierarchy because the mission is not set by a few in charge, but rather is broadly defined by its participants. The ride is not narrowly seen as an attempt to lobby for more bike lanes (although that goal exists) or to protest this or that aspect of the social order (although such sentiments are often expressed). Rather, each person is free to invent his or her own reasons for participating and is also free to share those ideas with others. Some people are there to promote human powered transportation as a viable alternative, others seek the respect of motorists and city planners and some take part simply because they like riding bikes and feeling a sense of community with all the other cyclists on the Critical Mass ride.

This "organic system" doesn't lead to chaos, but rather a festive, celebratory atmosphere. Great pains have been taken to avoid the common pitfalls of other movements, with much Xerocratic space being devoted to arguments against moralizing attacks on motorists and other unproductive tendencies. By presenting bicycling as a fun, positive alternative to the dreary destructiveness of car culture, Critical Mass has gained immeasurably.

Getting the Word Out

Getting the word out is the first step. Fliers are a quick, cheap way to reach a large number of people. With a few friends and a copy machine, you can have your area saturated with Critical Mass announcements within a few days. However, the public walls of most cities have already been plastered with so many announcements that alternative strategies are useful.

- Thin strips of xeroxed fliers can be attached to bicycles around town.
- Small stickers can be put on anything bicyclists lock their bikes to.
- Bicycle stores and bike-friendly businesses can put fliers in their windows.
- Word of mouth, announcements by friendly local radio DJs, etc.

Where and When to Start

The preliminary steps to setting up a ride are fairly straight forward: pick a time, place and route. Beginning the ride in some downtown area is obviously a good choice, since so many bicyclists and commuters are already there. A well-known public area, easily accesible to most bicyclists, where large numbers of people can congregate before the ride is perfect. (In San Francisco, Critical Mass leaves from a plaza adjacent to the financial district, which is conveniently located at the foot of the main traffic corridor.)

Choosing a time is even easier: you want to meet in the early evening, say 5:30, both in order to accommodate bicycle commuters who are on the streets anyway, and to gain visibility by making sure Critical Mass is part of the rush hour traffic. Having Critical Mass fall on a Friday marks it as the beginning of the weekend, and contributes to the celebratory feel of the ride. And what better Friday for the event to take place than the last Friday of the month? If Critical Mass continues to spread, the day may come when, on the last Friday of the month, the sun is always setting on a Critical Mass ride!

It is important that the meeting time and place remain constant, so that it is as easy for people to take part on a regular basis, and more people can join in as the ride becomes a regular event.

Planning a Route

Picking a safe, entertaining route is integral to keeping Critical Mass novel and fun. There are several things to consider when planning a route:

Safety

- Bicyclists of varying skills will be taking part; planning a ride with lots of difficult hills or a very long distance is not a good idea.
- The streets chosen should be large enough to accommodate large numbers of cyclists. (One way streets are especially good.)
- Keep it simple. A complicated route that veers all over the

Critical Mass isn't BLOCKING traffic—

We ARE Traffic!!

At the end of every workday, thousands of people pour into the streets, in what has become a central ritual of life in the late twentieth century —the daily commute. For most people, however, getting off work is not cause for celebration, or even relief. The ride home promises frustrating gridlock, disgusting air, and for us bicyclists, constant threats to our safety and well-being. But one day a month, the ritual is transformed. Hundreds of us get together and ride through the streets on bicycles, providing motorists, as well as ourselves, with a vision of how things could be different. We know that you aren't responsible for the organization of our cities around motorized traffic, and if we have contributed to your delay, **WE'RE SORRY!** But maybe you can take this opportunity to reflect on what a world without cars would be like.

Or better yet, join us next time!

CRITICAL MASS

San Francisco

Last Friday of each month:

meet at East end of Market Street (Justin Herman Plaza) at 5:30 p.m.

CRITICAL MASS IS MORE THAN JUST A BIKE RIDE.

It is a space where we come together to share a public life, to exchange ideas and swap stories, and to imagine together what a different life may be like... Critical Mass is an experiment in alternative political expression, an attempt to establish organic communities with the strength and vision to fight for a better way of life. Among other things, we want more places for pedestrians, children, bicyclists, public gardens, more parks and open spaces; but also a different social system: less rushing, less buying-and-selling frenzy, more enjoyment of social life, more community, more FUN!

place might look fun on paper, but will prove to be unworkable on the ride. People need to be able to read and easily memorize the route, so they know where they're going and what the ride is doing.

Pleasure

- Varying the route from month to month makes each ride a bit of an adventure, and reaches a wider spectrum of people.
- The mood of the ride is influenced by the area cycled through. A ride through a downtown area, where whoops and hollers can echo off tall buildings, and there is a population of motorists and bystanders to interact with, will create a more festive mood than a ride through an industrial or suburban area. The latter two tend to quiet down the ride, which could be used to vary the mood. It's up to you.
- Have an end point, such as a park or bar, where there's the possibility for cyclists to socialize after the ride.

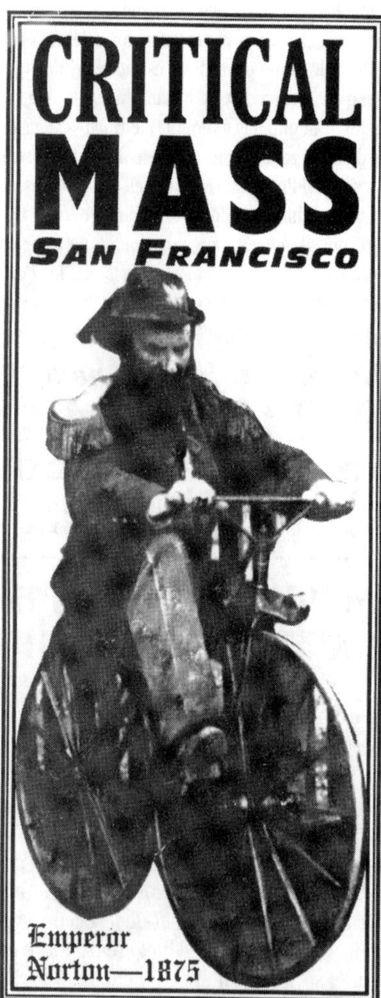

Xerocratic Aesthetics: If you want to communicate, make it easy to read!

Make sure the fliers passed out to participants are readable and tell people what they need to know about the ride. For instance, if there is a tricky intersection, or dangerous train tracks on the route, point it out on the map. Doing the route flier on a computer can make things easier (if you're computer literate, and has the advantage of being easy to read and reproduce). The route sheet can also double as an informational bulletin/newsletter, with troubleshooting ideas, news from the last ride, and ideas for future rides.

As the San Francisco Critical Mass grew beyond the point where a single bicyclist could see both front and tail of the ride (about 300+), a xerocratic publication, *Critical Mass Missives*, started to appear. It contains happenings on the previous ride, news of other Mass's around the world and discusses problems within or concerning the ride.

Traffic Tactics

When bicyclists take to the streets en masse, there will be a certain percentage of motorists who will not be amused. These motorists—a minority, to be sure—will have a hard time seeing a group of bicyclists as legitimate traffic, and may insist on forcing their way through the crowd. The interference of these frustrated individuals, trapped as they are in their cars, are a CONSTANT problem for Critical Mass. Tactics have to be developed, understood, and implemented by as many people as possible in order to ensure that this problem does not become too much of a drag on an otherwise fun and good-natured ride. Here are the ones we've found work.

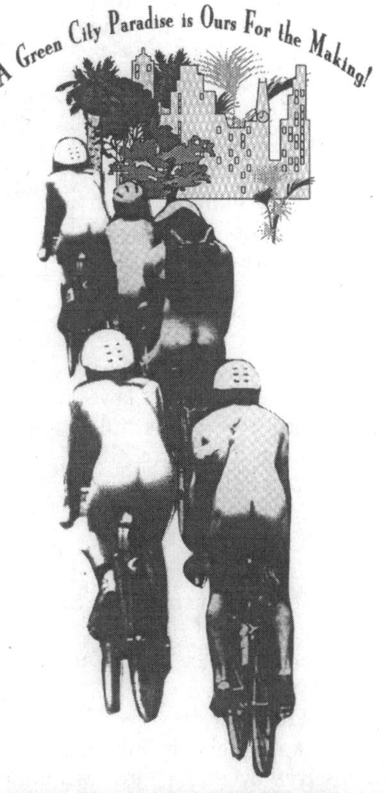

Density—Stay Together!

Think of Critical Mass as a density. It works by forming a mass of bicyclists so dense and tight that it simply displaces cars. Anytime the ride begins to spread too thin, with areas large enough for a car to drive into, you have a potential trouble spot developing.

The simplest and easiest way to deal with this problem is to encourage people to be aware of what's going on around them, and to act when they see things go awry. If a gap large enough for a car develops, someone needs to ride into it and call over a friend. If the head of the ride moves too fast and the Mass becomes too thin, someone in front needs to call out for people to slow down, and for the ride to regroup. The same goes for those at the tail of the ride, who may be riding so slow that the ride, again, spreads too thin. Diagrams on the route sheet pointing out trouble areas and regrouping points are a great way to bring all this across.

Density is vital in ensuring safety and a solid image of bicycling as practical, safe and fun for the ride's participants. When Critical Mass is still passing through an intersection after the light has turned red, in rush hour traffic, it is important to justify the long wait for cross traffic by maintaining a steady mass of bicyclists riding through the intersection.

Corks

Corks are the diplomats of the ride. Their title comes from their function. Here's how they work: one or two bicyclists block each lane of oncoming traffic as the ride goes through an intersection, making sure that even if a gap large enough for a car to drive through should develop, cars are stopped where they are. This tactic is especially effective if the cork takes a friendly, non-antagonistic stance with motorists, even holding up signs that say "thanks for waiting" and "honk if you like bikes!" Corks need to protect the rear of the ride, too, from cars turning into it. Of course, no one needs to be officially designated as a cork, and people will largely take on this role of their own initiative.

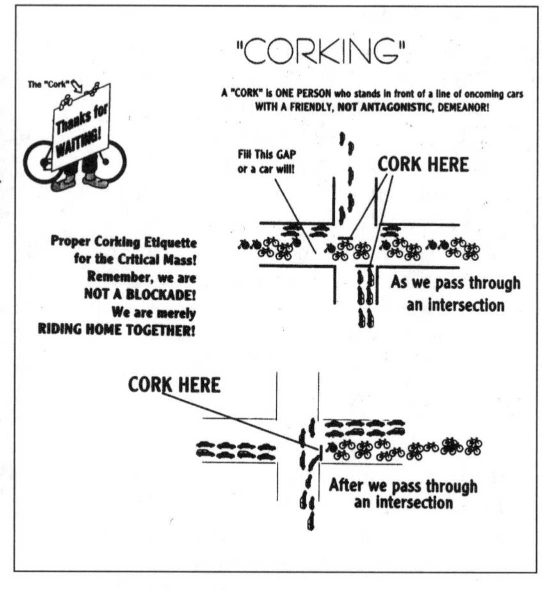

Red Lights

Should Critical Mass obey the same traffic laws that motorized traffic follows? Yes and no. For the most part, traffic laws were made for cars, as anyone who routinely bicycles through stop signs can attest, and they certainly weren't written with large groups of bicyclists in mind. So the answer to this question is obvious: Critical Mass should bend or ignore existing traffic laws where the group's safety and effectiveness will be served, and follow the law where it serves our interests and needs.

Red lights are a perfect example of this principle. When the head of the ride reaches a red light, it only makes sense to stop. This way, a) no one endangers themselves by riding into oncoming traffic, b) we allow motorists the simple courtesy of their right of way, and c) we give ourselves an opportunity to stop, regroup and form a solid Mass. But if, as Critical Mass passes through an intersection, the light changes, it does not make sense to break into two groups, and the ride should just continue through the intersection, shielded from the waiting cars by corks.

Breaking Mass

When the Mass thins out too much to justify holding an intersection through a red light, it can be useful for someone to yell out "BREAK MASS!" The first section of Critical Mass would continue through the intersection and the second part would wait for the light to turn green. If all goes well, the two groups will be reunited at the next light. This tactic is most often used when the Mass gets larger and less cohesive.

Fliers

As the ride goes along, people on the street, waiting at bus stops or sitting in their cars will want to know what's going on. You won't be able to stop and talk with all of them, and you'd be hard pressed to fit it all into one sentence even if you could. So for anyone that is curious, it really helps to have a small flier made out that lets people know what Critical Mass is, why we feel this action is necessary, and that invites them to the next ride.

These fliers can be made to fit three to an 8 1/2 sheet of paper so that they're inexpensive and can fit well in your back pocket. Pass them out at the beginning of the ride, make sure that anyone who is interested has a stack to give out, and watch as they get passed out to hundreds of people who otherwise would have never heard of Critical Mass!

Those who hand out fliers along the route are the real diplomats of the ride. Often the face-to-face contact by these cyclists and occasional rollerbladers have been especially helpful in diffusing tense situations arising from an angry car driver who has been made to wait. A cyclist will roll up to these frustrated commuters and explain the ride while handing them a flier. This shows people you've thought of them a bit, and it buys you some time as they digest the tract while the ride proceeds.

Like the corks, flier distributors lend an air of self-control to the ride for motorists and pedestrians. Corking and flier distribution is usually done on an ad-hoc basis, as needed, by cyclists who decide spontaneously to fill those gaps.

Know the Law

The above planning is the skeleton of what the Mass needs in order to be as enjoyable and carefree as it is. However, other issues arise as soon as bicyclists, hundreds of bicyclists, hit the streets. Traffic laws vary from state to state and city to city. Find out what the Vehicle Code says about bikes in your area. Know your rights; in California bicyclists "enjoy" all the rights and responsibilities of motor vehicles. Knowing the truth about what is in the book and being able to correct those who quote it wrongly empowers the riders on Critical Mass. You can obtain a traffic rules and regulations book at a Department of Motor Vehicles office.

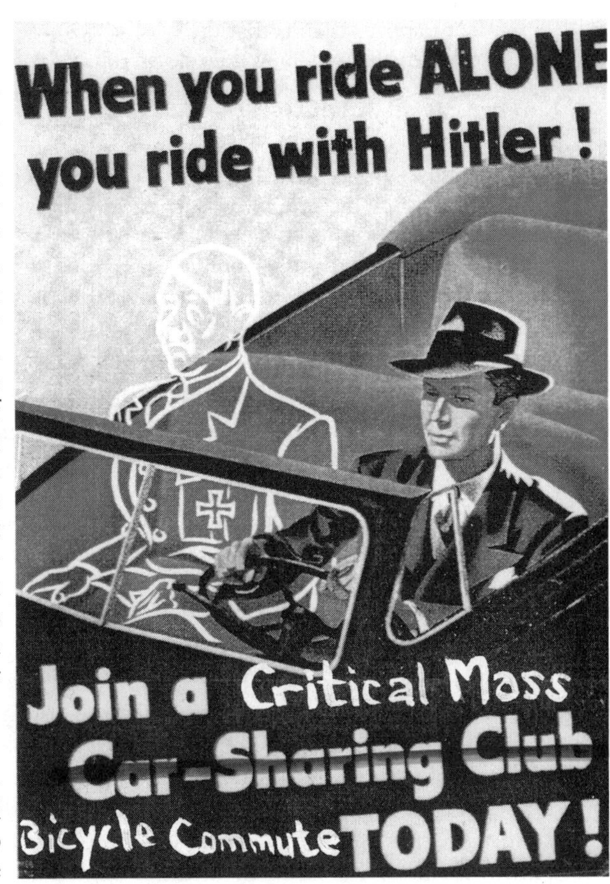
When you ride ALONE
you ride with Hitler!
Join a Critical Mass
Car-Sharing Club
Bicycle Commute TODAY!

Testosterone Brigade

What kind of approach do we take toward people who choose to drive, or who happen to be stuck in cars, maybe for business, when the ride passes? Just as important as devising strategies to deal with hostile motorists is the need to deal with those in the ride who may provoke them.

For some bicyclists, Critical Mass is an opportunity to berate motorists, now that WE own the road for once. Our society's over-reliance on motorized traffic is a massive and overwhelming social problem, and it won't be changed through the use of irritating, ineffective tactics by a small minority of pissed-off bicyclists. But a movement for change based on a reclaiming of public space and the building of human community, open to people from across the social and political spectrum, could contribute to a deeper and more fundamental change in the way our society operates.

Vanguards

One of the important things to realize is that the Mass will tend to follow whoever is iin front, whether they have a clear idea of where they're going or not. "Vanguard" types, frustrated that their self-destructive antics are not put up with in the middle of the ride, will generally sprint ahead of the ride, go through red lights when it isn't necessary, and try to block as much traffic as possible. Or, they may decide to lead the ride off the agreed route.

What happens then is that the head of the ride goes too fast, the ride spreads out, cars get in the middle of the ride, no one has any idea what is going on, dangerous situations occur pretty rapidly—your Critical Mass becomes a Critical Mess.

The way to counter this is to get two or three friends at the head of the ride who have some idea of what the route is and, more importantly, are committed to staying in a group. If you all stick together as a clump, you can influence the course of the ride by riding slowly, speaking out where neccessary, and trying to keep everyone together. If you do this, you have to be prepared to take a certain amount of shit from people who may see you as someone imposing your ideas on everyone else. But speaking your mind and actively asserting your initiative is not akin to being authoritarian—in fact, it's the essence of democracy.

Snails

Snails are a group of antagonistic bicyclists who poke slowly behind the rest of the mass. This dawdling causes the mass to thin out and angers car drivers who are waiting for the ride to progress through the intersection or who are behind the mass and impatient for the mass to get moving.

Again, make your opinion known and be comfortable with that type of interaction. Remember, these people are not out to have the best time for the greatest numbers. They are selfishly antagonizing motorists and destroying any positive association that the drivers might have had when the rest of the jovial mass passed them.

Cops

Public demonstrations tend to make the government look bad, since they vividly show that the government does not always represent or have the support of the people. Naturally, the police are concerned about popular demonstrations, and they generally take one of two approaches: either they attack the demonstration—exposing the force on which this society is based—or they attempt to portray themselves as the demonstration's sponsors and diligent protectors.

RADICAL PATIENCE

Many of us attracted to radical politics are very impatient—with the larger society, but also with ourselves and especially with people who don't see how much better life could be if our radical visions were pursued. This impatience with the slow development of organic human communities, communities that might really be able to construct a different logic to our daily lives, often leads to childish and simplistic confrontational stances. These postures are much more about reassuring ourselves that we are truly radical and willing to face danger than they are about contesting the organization of modern life.

If radical bicyclists are so hot to go on freeways, instead of blocking traffic lanes why not wait for rush hour gridlock and then overwhelm the already stopped cars with dozens or hundreds of bicycles streaming through the traffic, departing the freeway at the next exit after a convincing demonstration of the ease, superiority and pleasure of bicycling? Imagine the surprise and support one might generate if such an intervention was carried out with courtesy and friendliness?

It is a terribly rash assumption that someone stuck in their car is necessarily a big supporter of the status quo. Consider instead the complexities of human choices and constraints and try to create openings in people's minds, rather than assuming that someone who hasn't adopted your choices about what to buy, how to get around, and lifestyles in general is your conscious enemy and deserves your moral condemnation, rage, or self-righteous taunting. It's not easy to proceed politically when we take seriously how difficult, deep and personal are the changes we seek. But pleasure, passion, and patience can bring real progress. Remember, the Americans you scorn today must be your allies tomorrow if you are serious about changing life!

THINK GUILT'LL GET 'EM? THINK AGAIN!!

We are drowning in moralism! Worse still, it is a primitive consumer moralism! Many bicyclists and other social radicals fall back on the uncontroversial idea that people ought to do the right thing. But as soon as we start explaining what the "right thing" is, we run into trouble. A lot of people seem to think social change hinges on buying/using the correct products (bicycles, Birkenstocks™, used clothing, vegetarianism, etc.). This focus on good shopping leads people to ridiculous, philosophically retarded syllogisms like "Cars Are Bad, You're In A Car, You are Bad."

Motorists are not bad. They are not moral failures, nor thoughtless, greedy or rich, just because they are in a car! They might be triumphant proponents of the oil/car culture, but let's face it, not many people trust, believe in, admire or have any control over oil companies, car companies, government transit bureaucracies, or local transit systems. It's a stupid assumption that someone in a car necessarily embraces the values of this society at face value. We are probably right to assume that many, if not most, of the people we pass wish they could join us, and at least offer us good will.

Bicycling and other alternatives are self-evidently better than sitting in a traffic jam or waiting for an overcrowded bus. The more we can live up to that truth, the more people will jump in—not because they were made to feel guilty, but because they want the pleasure and increased health and convenience that comes from bicycling. People will get out of their cars and onto bicycles when they think it will make their life better, not because someone tried to make them feel ashamed for participating in an absurd, suicidal transportation system.

—Chris Carlsson, 1993

With the Bay Area Critical Mass rides, they have generally taken the second, paternalistic approach, allowing the ride to take place, blocking traffic for us and making sure their presence is felt as an "escort". On one occassion they even went so far as to announce over a bullhorn before the ride "Welcome to this event!"—an outsider might have surmised that the whole thing was planned and executed by the police themselves!

When police begin to arrest people or hassle riders, they are trying to provoke a confrontation which will justify a repressive crackdown—a confrontation

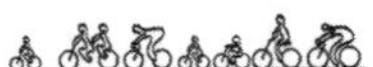

in which their victory is almost guaranteed. It is important not to take them up on the offer. When the police demand that the ride move into the right lane, do it. Then, when the coast is clear, go back. After a few more attempts to control the ride, the police usually give in and realize, short of arresting everyone, there's little they can do except ride along and actually act like the public servants they professed to be in the beginning.

The best strategy is to avoid breaking any laws you don't have to, try to reason with those individuals on the ride who display a tendency to get out of hand and don't give the police an excuse to stop your ride or bust anybody. Be up front and above board about the ride. After all, we're just riding home together in an organized coincidence, so give the cops the route sheet if they want one.

As much as they may try to own or control the ride, Critical Mass is a popular movement that operates independently of government regulations, and as such, we don't have any business with the police (although they may have business with us). Within the anti-authoritarian culture of the bicyclist milieu, refusing the arbitrary commands of the police might make sense. But the best approach to the police presence at Critical Mass is not to engage in some pathetic, losing confrontation, or embrace them as our saviors and protectors. Rather, we should ignore them and get on with the business of trying to build a Mass.

ALL TIED UP IN TRAFFIC?!?

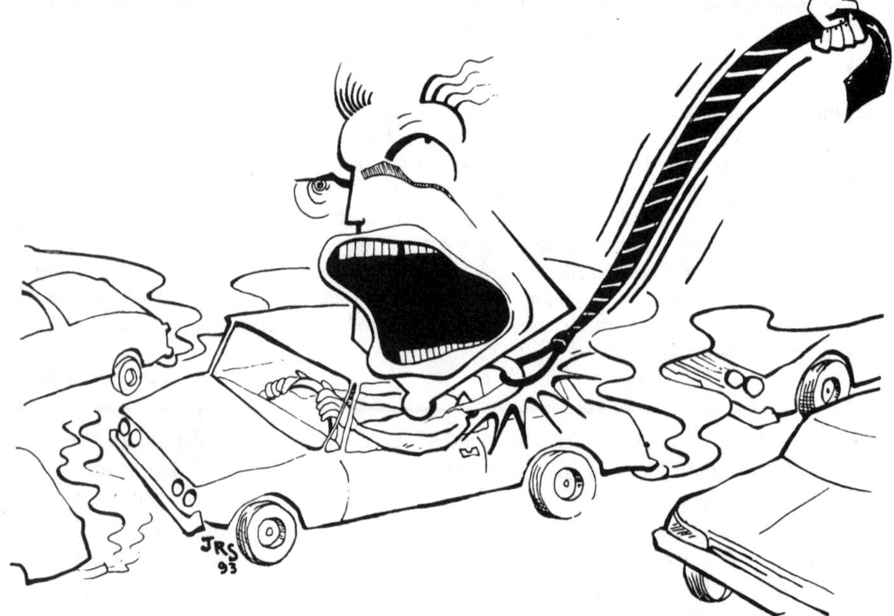

James R Swanson

Critical Mass Worldwide Directory as of May 2002

APOLOGIES FOR INFO THAT HAS ALREADY EXPIRED (COMPILED BY JYM DYER, www.critical-mass.org)

NORTH AMERICA

Albany, New York, USA
http://groups.yahoo.com/group/araalbany/
Albuquerque, New Mexico, USA
Amherst, Massachusetts, USA
http://www.massbike.org/mbpv/
Anchorage, Alaska, USA
http://www.alaskagreens.org/transportation.html
Ann Arbor, Michigan, USA
http://www.monkey.org/a2cm/
Atlanta, Georgia, USA
http://www.learnlink.emory.edu/~jmahr/
http://www.topica.com/lists/critical_mass_atlanta/
Arcata, California, USA
Asheville, North Carolina, USA
Athens, Georgia, US
http://www.bikeathens.com/activities/cmass/cmass.html
Auburn, Alabama, USA
http://www.blowupyourcar.com/
Austin, Texas, USA
http://CriticalMassHub.com/austin.html
http://www.topica.com/lists/austin-bike-news/
Baltimore, Maryland, USA
http://marathonexpress.com/criticalmass/index.html
Baton Rouge, Louisiana, USA
http://world.care2.com/brcriticalmass/
Bellingham, Washington, USA
http://www.epilogicconsulting.com/cmb.htm
Bend, Oregon, USA
Berkeley, California, USA
http://www.preservenet.com/CMEastBay.html
http://guest.xinet.com/bike/women/
Blacksburg, Virginia, USA
http://www.slac.com/tree/criticalmass/
Bloomington, Indiana, USA
http://silver.ucs.indiana.edu/~mreece/cm.html
Boise, Idaho, USA
http://members.tripod.com/~eckelberger/CriticalMassBoise.html
Boone, North Carolina, USA
http://www.boonenc.org/critiaclamass/
Boston, Massachusetts, USA
http://www.bostoncriticalmass.org/
http://www.topica.com/lists/bostoncriticalmass/
http://www.topica.com/lists/massbike/
http://www.cycling.org/lists/massbike/
Boulder, Colorado, USA:
http://bcn.boulder.co.us/transportation/bbc/bbcc-pictures.html
Buffalo, New York, USA
http://www.geocities.com/buffaloactivism/newcalendar.html
Burlington, Vermont, USA:
http://groups.yahoo.com/group/CriticalMass-BurlingtonVT/
Calgary, Alberta, Canada:
http://www.angelfire.com/ct/cmwd/calgcm.html
Article http://www.get.to/criticalmass/
Champaign-Urbana, Illinois, USA:
http://critical-mass.groogroo.com/
http://lists.cu.groogroo.com/mailman/archive/critical-mass/
Chapel Hill/Carrboro, N. Carolina
http://www.angelfire.com/ct/cmwd/articles.html
http://metalab.unc.edu/the_board/detours/recreation/critical_mass.html
Charleston, South Carlina, USA
http://www.charlestoncriticalmass.com/
Charlotte, North Carolina, USA
http://www.homestead.com/chaba/cmass.html
Charlottesville, Virginia, USA
Chattanooga, Tennessee, USA
http://www.chattanooga.net/cycleclub/btf_cmr.htm
http://groups.yahoo.com/group/criticalmasschatt/
Chicago, Illinois
http://www.chicagocriticalmass.org/
http://ness.uic.edu/archives/chi-crit-mass.html
http://www.bikesummer.org/2000/
http://www.bikewinter.org/
http://www.cyclingsisters.org/
Chico, California, USA
Cleveland, Ohio, USA
http://www.ecocleveland.org/g3w2b/archive.html
Columbia, Missouri, USA
http://www.deviant.org/~lamp/critmass/cm-main.cgi
Columbus, Ohio, USA
http://comacrew.homestead.com/criticalmass.htmla
Coeur d'Alene, Idaho, USA
Corvallis, Oregon, USA:
http://www.funkybikes.com/
http://groups.yahoo.com/group/CorvallisCM/
Courtenay, Vancouver Isl., Canada
Dallas, Texas, USA
http://www.uproarnow.org/critmass.html
Denton, Texas, USA
Denver, Colorado, USA
http://www.preservenet.com/CMDenver.html
http://groups.yahoo.com/group/CriticalMassDenver/
Detroit, Michigan, USA
http://www.criticalmassdetroit.org/
http://groups.yahoo.com/group/CriticalMassDetroit/
Edmonton, Alberta, Canada
http://www.cmedmonton.org/
Eugene, Oregon, USA
http://www.preservenet.com/CMEugene.html
Fairbanks, Alaska, USA
Fayetteville, Arkansas, USA
http://comp.uark.edu/~cdemcol/criticalmass.html
Flagstaff, Arizona, USA
http://www.sni.net/~bbaxter/cm.htm
Fort Collins, Colorado, USA
Fresno, California, USA
http://members.tripod.com/fresnomass/
Gainesville, Florida, USA
http://www.preservenet.com/CMGainesville.html
Garberville, California, USA
Goshen, Indiana, USA
Green Bay, Wisconsin, USA
Greensboro, North Carolina, USA
http://www.angelfire.com/nc3/criticalmass
Halifax, Nova Scotia, Canada
http://www.chebucto.ns.ca/CommunitySupport/Critical_Mass/
Hamilton, Ontario, Canada
Harrisonburg, Virginia, USA
http://harrisonburg_cm.tripod.com/
Hartford, Connecticut, USA
http://www.ctbike.org/cm.htm
Havana, Cuba
Headwaters Forest, California, USA
Honolulu, Hawaii, USA:
http://www.lorax.org/criticalmass/
http://www.topica.com/lists/cm-honolulu/
Houston, Texas, USA
Huntington Beach, California, USA
Huntsville, Alabama, USA
http://www.preservenet.com/CMHuntsville.html
Indianapolis, Indiana, USA
http://www.geocities.com/indycm/
http://groups.yahoo.com/group/IndyCritMass/
Irvine, California, USA
Isla Vista, California, USA
http://www.criticalmassmedia.org/islavista/
Ithaca, New York, USA
http://gee.netwater.com/mass/
http://groups.yahoo.com/group/ithaca-cm/
Kansas City, Kansas, USA
http://www.oldtowncyclery.com/CriticalMasskc.htm
http://groups.yahoo.com/group/criticalmasskc/
Kent, Ohio, USA
http://www.geocities.com/anthonyrhodes/
Kingston, Ontario, Canada
Knoxville Tennessee, USA
http://groups.yahoo.com/group/ilikebikes/
La Grange, Illinois, USA
Lincoln, Nebraska, USA
Los Angeles, California, USA
http://www.geocities.com/Yosemite/Gorge/7367/CM/
http://members.aol.com/lacritmass/
http://www.criticalmassmedia.org/
http://groups.yahoo.com/group/la-critical-mass/
Louisville, Ohio, USA
http://lorax.antioch-college.edu/louisville/mass.html
Lubbock, Texas, USA
http://www.angelfire.com/tx3/criticalmass/
Madison, Wisconsin, USA
http://www.mailbag.com/users/mattlogan/cmass/
http://www.kingresearch.com/jk/biking/pm.html
http://groups.yahoo.com/group/madisoncriticalmass/
Manchester, Connecticut, USA
http://www.crcog.org/bicycle.htm#CRITICAL%20MASS%20RIDE
Marin County, California, USA
http://www.preservenet.com/CMMarin.html
Memphis, Tennessee, USA
Mexico City, Mexico
http://www.laneta.apc.org/bicitekas/
Minneapolis and St. Paul, Minn., USA
http://www.angelfire.com/punk/mplscriticalmass/
http://www.minnesotacriticalmass.org/
http://groups.yahoo.com/group/bicyclelane/
Moab, Utah, USA
http://www.moabutah.org/critical/
http://concordia.pirg.ca/~rtm/
Montreal, Quebec, Canada

Newark, New Jersey, USA
http://groups.yahoo.com/group/NewarkCriticalMass/
Morgantown, West Virginia, USA
New Brunswick, New Jersey, USA
http://www.preservenet.com/CMNewBrunswick.html
New Haven, Connecticut, USA
http://www.preservenet.com/CMNewHaven.html
New Orleans, Louisiana, USA
http://studentweb.tulane.edu/~dsaad/mass.html
New York, New York, USA
http://www.times-up.org/
Norman, Oklahoma, USA
http://students.ou.edu/E/Grant.L.Elam-1/cm.html —
Oakland, California, USA
http://www.oakcal.com/
Oklahoma City, Oklahoma, USA
http://www.oktrails.com/okc_critical_mass.htm
Ottawa, Ontario, Canada
http://www.flora.org/afo/
Peoria, Illinois, USA
Philadelphia, Pennsylvania, USA
http://westphila.net/critmass/
Pittsburgh, Pennsylvania, USA
http://www.pghcriticalmass.org/
http://www.pitt.edu/~jucst7/cm/home.html
Portland, Maine, USA
Portland, Oregon, USA
http://www.subluna.com/CriticalMass/
http://mail.pdxbikes.org/lists/listinfo/cm
http://www.arborrhythms.com/~ben/cmass/
Portsmouth, New Hampshire, USA
http://www.geocities.com/nonmotorized
http://groups.yahoo.com/group/nonmotorized_revolution/
Prince George, BC, Canada
http://otaku.unbc.ca/cycling/criticalmass/
Princeton, New Jersey, USA
Providence, Rhode Island, USA
http://www.dutchmoney.com/criticalmass
Raleigh, North Carolina, USA
http://groups.yahoo.com/group/RaleighCM/
Reno, Nevada, USA
http://www.stickerguy.com/renocm/
http://www.topica.com/lists/renocm/
Rochester, New York, USA
http://www.geocities.com/CapitolHill/Congress/9892/green light/
Sacramento, California, USA
http://www.bclu.org/sactocm/
http://www.mutualaid.org/mailman/listinfo/sactocm
Saint Cloud, MN, USA
Saint Louis, Missouri, USA
http://www.stlcriticalmass.org/
http://www.topica.com/lists/STLCM/
Salt Lake City, Utah, USA
http://www.slccriticalmass.org/
http://www.topica.com/lists/slccriticalmass/
San Antonio, Texas, USA
San Diego, California, USA
http://www.subrosa.org/CM/
http://www.virtualswapmeet.com/CriticalMass/
San Francisco, California, USA
http://www.bikesummer.org/1999/
http://www.scorcher.org/cmhistory/
http://www.things.org/~jym/critical-mass/
http://members.aol.com/MitsuAvaco/critmas2.htm
http://www.ooto.com/cm/
http://guest.xinet.com/bike/peace/
http://users.lmi.net/mhoover/propaganda.html
http://www.notsosketchy.com/crm.html
http://www.icsi.berkeley.edu/~sean/critical-mass/
http://www.shapingsf.org/ezine/transit/critmass.html
http://www.sfgate.com/news/pages/1997/critmass.shtml
http://www.brasscheck.com/cm/
http://www.sausagefactory.com/dildoman/
http://guest.xinet.com/bike/superheroes/
http://www.topica.com/lists/sfbike/
http://www.topica.com/lists/sf-critical-mass/
San Mateo County, California, USA
http://home.earthlink.net/~daniweber/
San Jose, California, USA
San Marco, Texas, USA
San Salvador, El Salvador
Santa Cruz, California, USA
http://www.scruz.net/~paul/cm/
Santa Fe, New Mexico, USA
http://home.earthlink.net/~ttrowbridg/sfCmass/
Santa Rosa, California, USA
http://www.eudaemon.com/~ollie/ollie/sr_mass.html
Sarasota, Florida, USA
http://www.bicyclemessener.com/bicycleride.html
Saskatoon, Saskachewan, Canada
Seattle, Washington, USA
http://students.washington.edu/wino/
Silicon Valley, California, USA
http://www.topica.com/lists/sil-val-crit-mass/
http://www.cycling.org/lists/sil-val-crit-mass/
Smithers, British Columbia, Canada
Somerset, Massachusetts, USA
Spokane, Washington, USA
State College, Pennsylvania, USA
Toledo, Ohio, USA
Toronto, Ontario, Canada
http://www.semiotek.com/cm/
http://www.darrenstehr.com/biintro.html
Tucson, Arizona, USA
http://www.seac.org/seac-sw/critmass.html
Tulsa, Oklahoma, USA
Tuscaloosa, Alabama, USA
http://bama.ua.edu/~aec/cm.html
Vancouver, BC, Canada:
http://www.bikesummer.org/2001/
http://members.home.net/cmass/
http://members.home.net/spm/Critmass.htm
Verde Valley, Arizona, USA
http://users.sedona.net/~noillusions/criticalmass/
Victoria, British Columbia, Canada
Walnut Creek, California, USA
http://www.preservenet.com/CMWalnutCreek.html
Washington, DC, USA
http://www.dccourier.com/dcbca/solid.htm
http://www.2wrongs.net/dc-critmass/
http://lists.mutualaid.org/mailman/listinfo/dc-critmass-list
Waterloo, Ontario, Canada
http://imprint.uwaterloo.ca/issues/061695/News/n-04.html
West Lafayette, Indiana, USA
Worcester, Massachusetts, USA
http://www.topica.com/lists/wcm/

EUROPE

Denmark: http://www.props.dk/
Germany: phttp://www.critical-mass.de/index.htm
Italy: http://www.inventati.org/criticalmass/
Netherlands: http://www.dwars.org/
Spain: http://www.nousis.com/masacritica/
United Kingdom: http://www.zap20.ukgateway.net/ or http://www.critmass.org.uk/
Aachen, Germany
Antwerp, Belgium
Barcelona, Spain
Bergen, Norway
http://www.uib.no/People/sspeo/nvh/criticalm.htm
Berlin, Germany
http://www.critical-mass.de/
http://members.tripod.com/~ichwillkeinennamen/
http://www.fortunecity.de/olympia/adrenalin/195/
Biele/Bienne, Switzerland
http://www.propane-systems.ch/clients/cmbiel/english/index.htm
Bonn, Germany
Bratislava, Slovakia
Braunschweig, Germany
Brussells, Belgium
http://placeovelo.collectifs.net/
Budapest, Hungary
Copenhagen, Denmark
http://sunsite.auc.dk/sound_transport/enmass.htm
Cordoba, Spain
Cork, Ireland
http://indigo.ie/~woz/ccc/
Darmstadt, Germany
Dijon, France
http://www.chez.com/maloka/bikedemo.htm
Dresden, Germany
Dublin, Ireland:
http://rene.ma.utexas.edu/users/guilfoyl/Cmass/dub-flyer.html
http://members.tripod.com/~dublinbike/
http://www.connect.ie/dcc/
http://groups.yahoo.com/group/dublincriticalmasslist/
Duisburg, Germany
Dusseldorf, Germany
Edinburgh, Scotland
http://www.critmass.org.uk/cmed.html
Erfurt, Germany
Frankfurt/Main, Germany
http://www.frankfurt.critical-mass.de/
http://www.wiwi.uni-frankfurt.de/~rainerh/cmffm.html
http://www.vbr.com/adfc/cm/
Freiburg, Germany
Freising, Germany
http://www.freisinger-verkehrsseiten.de/allgverkehr/fahrrad/critmass-fs.html
Galway, Ireland
http://www.emc23.tp/panda/panda10.html
Geneva, Switzerland
http://www.criticalmass.ch/
Ghent, Belgium
Girona, Spain
Goteborg, Sweden
http://hem2.passagen.se/mancopac/

Hamburg, Germany
http://www.critical-mass-hamburg.purespace.de/cmhh.htm
Jena, Germany
Ljubljana, Slovenia
http://flag.blackened.net/agony/yugo.html
London, England
http://groups.yahoo.com/group/UKCM/
http://groups.yahoo.com/group/londonmasstalk/
Lyon, France:
http://antenna.nl/eyfa/trafrep.htm
http://sunsite.auc.dk/sound_transport/enlyon.htm
Madrid, Spain
Mainz, Germany
Marburg,Germany
http://members.xoom.com/cm_marburg/
Marseille, France
Milan, Italy
Munich, Germany
http://members.xoom.com/cmmuc/
Utrecht, Netherlands
http://huizen.dds.nl/~omtrap/
Nuernberg, Germany
http://www.geocities.com/Hollywood/3033/CM.html
http://groups.yahoo.com/group/cm-nuernberg/
Opole, Poland
Pamplona, Spain
Paris, France
http://www.souris-verte.net/
http://www.pacificnews.org/jinn/stories/4.01/980115-bike.html
http://www.pacificnews.org/yo/stories/98/980202-mass.html
Poznan, Poland
Prague, Czech
http://www.carbusters.ecn.cz/jizda/
Krakow, Poland
Stuttgart, Germany
http://www.geocities.com/RainForest/Jungle/7671/
http://www.geocities.com/Hollywood/3033/CM-Stuttgart.html
http://groups.yahoo.com/group/cmstuttgart/
Turku, Finland
http://members.nbci.com/cm_turku/
Warszawa (Warsaw), Poland
http://free.ngo.pl/rowery/
Wien (Vienna), Austria
http://akin.mediaweb.at/andere.gruppen/critical.htm
Winterhur, Switzerland
http://www.geocities.com/RainForest/8609/
Xixon, Spain
Zagreb, Croatia
http://flag.blackened.net/agony/yugo.html
Zurich, Switzerland
http://criticalmass.cjb.net/

AUSTRALIA/N.Z.

Critical Mass Australia
http://www.criticalmass.org.au/
http://groups.yahoo.com/group/cm-aus/
Adelaide
http://free.freespeech.org/activeadelaide/criticalmass/
http://www.adelaide.net.au/~jonivar/cm.html
http://groups.yahoo.com/group/cm-adel/
Auckland, New Zealand
Brisbane
http://www.dstc.edu.au/RDU/staff/aw/bike/cmass.html
http://groups.yahoo.com/group/cmass-bris-talk/
Cairns
http://www.altnews.com.au/cbug/
Canberra
http://www2.dynamite.com.au/rowead/cm.htm
Christchurch, New Zealand
Hobart, Tasmania
http://www.physics.usyd.edu.au/~eddie/cmass/cmOz/cmhobart.html
Lismore
Melbourne
http://www.ecr.mu.oz.au/~amorton/cmass.html
http://www.vmore.org.au/~damon/cm/
http://www2.one.net.au/~no_data/critmass.html
http://groups.yahoo.com/group/cm-melb/
http://groups.yahoo.com/group/cm-news/
http://www.mail-archive.com/cmass-melb%40vmore.org.au/
Mildura
Newcastle
http://www.physics.usyd.edu.au/~eddie/cmass/cmOz/cmnewcastle.html
Parramatta
http://nccnsw.org.au/member/cmass/parramatta/
Perth
http://storm.prohosting.com/pentar/
http://groups.yahoo.com/group/cm-perth/
St Kilda
http://groups.yahoo.com/group/cm-stkilda/
Sydney
http://www.nccnsw.org.au/member/cmass/
http://groups.yahoo.com/group/cmass-syd-news/
http://groups.yahoo.com/group/cmass-syd-talk/
Townsville
Wellington, New Zealand
http://www.preservenet.com/CMWellington.html
http://groups.yahoo.com/group/criticalmasswellington/
Wollongong
http://www.physics.usyd.edu.au/~eddie/cmass/cmOz/cmwollongong.html

SOUTH AMERICA

Bogota, Colombia
http://www.geocities.com/Yosemite/7584/
La Plata, Argentina
http://www.preservenet.com/CMLaPlata.html
Rio de Janeiro, Brazil
Santiago, Chile
Sao Paulo, Brazil
http://www.geocities.com/RainForest/Vines/7747/index-i.htm

ASIA

Chiang Mai, Thailand
Delhi, India
Hong Kong, China
Israel (Tel Aviv, Haifa, more)
http://bike.org.il/cm/
Kyoto, Japan
Mumbai, India
http://free.prohosting.com/~cgreens/critmass.htm
http://www.topica.com/lists/mumbaicm/
Pune, India
Quezon City, Philippines
http://www.fireflybrigade.org/rides.html
http://groups.yahoo.com/group/fireflybrigade/
Seoul, Korea
http://bike.jinbo.net/
Taichung, Taiwan
Taipei, Taiwan
http://www.geocities.com/Pipeline/Valley/4231/CMASSTAIWAN/
Tokyo, Japan
http://www.ecolink.sf21npo.gr.jp/criticalmass/
http://groups.yahoo.com/group/CriticalMassTokyo/
Yokohama, Japan

AFRICA

Johannesburg, South Africa
http://www.afribike.org/
http://www.saep.org/subject/transport/trnsprt4.html

About the Editor

Chris Carlsson was one of the founders, editors and frequent contributors to the San Francisco magazine ***Processed World (1981-93, 2001).*** He is a founding participant of Critical Mass and is one of the creators of the urban history CD-ROM *Shaping San Francisco*. He has also edited two books, *Bad Attitude: The Processed World Anthology* (Verso: 1990) and *Reclaiming San Francisco: History, Politics, Culture* (City Lights: 1998, co-edited with James Brook and Nancy J. Peters). He is currently working on a novel of a post-Economic San Francisco in the year 2157. A daily bicycle commuter since 1985, he survives in San Francisco as a graphic artist, editor, and typesetter. **ccarlsson@shapingsf.org**

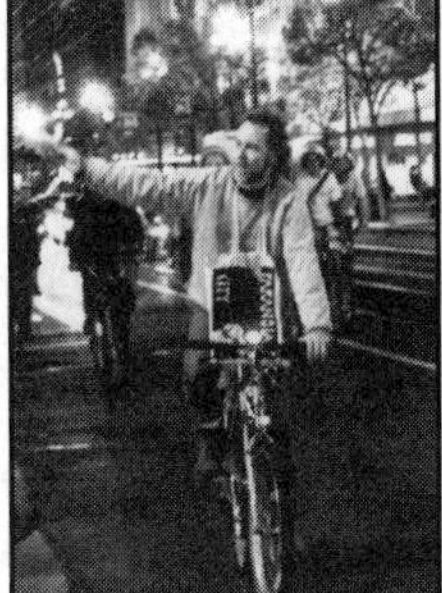
PETER MEITZLER

Chris Carlsson handing out flyers on Critical Mass in S.F., Oct. 1992.

Contributors' Notes

Matthew Arnison lives in Erskineville, Australia where he loves exploring science, media and activism.

Jessica Becker celebrates life in Madison, where she bikes, practices yoga, and works for the Wisc. Humanities Council.

Howard Besser is a Professor at UCLA's School of Education & Information Studies where he explores the social and cultural effects of new information technology.

Bernie Blaug is 38, from london, with almost 20 years stateside He's been dedicated to Critical Mass since it began 10 fast years ago. He commutes, races, tours, shops, exercises, relaxes, protests, and feels alive on a bike!

Michael Bluejay of Austin, TX has been advocating for bicycling since 1994. He was one of the original participants of Austin's Critical Mass. His main projects include Courteous Mass (an alternative to Critical Mass), BicycleAustin.com (winner of the Austin Chronicle's "Best of Austin Award"), BicycleSafe.com, and CriticalMassHub.com.

Iain A. Boal is a social historian of science and technics, who teaches in the Department of Geography at the University of California, Berkeley. An extended discussion of the political ecology of automobilism and cycling will appear in his forthcoming book on the history of enclosures old and new, *The Long Theft* (City Lights Press).

Steven Bodzin is communications director at the Congress for the New Urbanism, teaching and advocating for real estate development that creates real neighborhoods, rather than sprawl. He is a journalist and activist with a particular interest in bicycle transportation and enhancing traditional cities.

Sarah Boothroyd is an activist and artivist with two arms and two wheels. This spawn of Raincouver (on the Wetcoast of Canada) is currently dwelling in Montréal, where she relishes sculpting oddities out of words, out of fabric, and out of sound.

Guido Bruidoclarke is a former bike messenger and current bike advocate. He is the editor of the longest running cycling zine in the world. www.hideousewhitenoise.com.

Michael Burton is a founder of Chicago Bike Winter, the Campaign for a Free and Clear Lakefront and the Chicago Critical Mass Legal Defense Fund. He resides in Chicago, Illinois.

Mona Caron rides her bicycle between gigs as a muralist, illustrator and teacher of illustration. She designed the world famous Duboce Bikeway Mural in San Francisco. www.monacaron.com.

Hank Chapot is a San Francisco native, Mission High graduate, green activist, natural politician and master gardener blessed with a compulsive interest in earth science, history, art, sex, politics, bicycles and rock music.

Mark Coatsworth is a twenty-year old university student currently residing in Toronto, Canada. His involvement with Critical Mass started in November, 2000, when he attended his first ride in Vancouver.

Travis Hugh Culley, a former bike messenger and author, lives and rides in Chicago. He wrote *The Immortal Class*.

Hugh D'Andrade is an illustrator, designer, and agitator based in San Francisco, who can't remember things.

Jym Dyer works on software by day, freelance environmental writing by night, and spends too much time in front of a computer. He handles code and transportation issues for Faultline.org, a project of the Earth Island Institute.

R. Wiley Evans lives and works in San Francisco as a freelance audio developer, composer, and tuba player, and has been known to appear publicly as Dildo Man.

Jeff Ferrell is the author of *Crimes of Style: Urban Graffiti and the Politics of Criminality* and *Tearing Down the Streets: Adventures in Urban Anarchy*, and co-editor of three books: *Cultural Criminology*, *Ethnography at the Edge*, and *Making Trouble*.

Matthew Hoover furthers the Velorution with everything from choppers to touring bikes in San Francisco.

Dave Horton is an environmental activist, sociologist and founder member of Shifting Ground, a workers' co-operative forging initiatives between activists and academics (see www.shiftingground.org). He lives in Lancaster, England.

Michael Humphries, British national, has worked in the UK, France, Denmark and Germany. He is currently a lecturer, translator, and freelance journalist.

Adam Kessel is a law student at Northeastern University who eventually will be able to help keep all of us out of jail. He has worked in the labor and environmental movements, and got started with Critical Mass in Chicago. He rides daily and celebrates monthly on the streets of Boston.

Michael Klett lives in San Francisco. He supports his long time bicycling habit by working as an IT consultant.

Charles Komanoff is active in the pedestrian and cyclist movement in NYC as a founder of Right Of Way, as "re-founder" of Transportation Alternatives, and as editor and author of the *Bicycle Blueprint* and *Killed By Automobile*.

Daniel Kopald is a multimedia developer currently living in Chicago. Today Daniel is active in the Chicago Critical Mass scene making fliers and keeping a photo journal of all the Critical Mass rides he has been on.

Marina Lazzara is a poet and musician in SF. She rides a '76 brown Raleigh 3 speed, that she loves.

Jason Meggs has been spearheading car-free campaigns in the Bay Area for over a decade. His radio, video, xerocracy, street theatre, advocacy and action legacy with others merits a book in itself.

Megulon 5 is a soldier from the post-apocalyptic future who can sometimes be seen on the streets of Portland with his companions, the riders of C.H.U.N.K. 666. He records their works for future generations in print and on the web (http://www.dclxvi.org/chunk).

Peter Meitzler: current NYC and former Cal. resident; NY Transportation Alternatives, Bay Area Bicycle Action (BABA), S.F. Bicycle Coalition *Tubular Times*; Time's Up! (NYC); operator Manhattan Rickshaw (pedicab) Company; various & ongoing photo exhibitions of & assistance with NYC street memorial project, pedestrian protests, street vendor protests, and Critical Mass. Currently working on photo project of early days of SFBC and BABA.

Jeremy Murphy toured with the Climate Change Caravan and continues to promote sustainable living in his everyday life and by encouraging Canadians to join The BET!

Fred Nemo is a long-time single parent and grandparent, multi-media collaborationist, archivist, performance artist, and all-round agitator.

Giovanni Pesce, aged 31, born and bred in Milan, never owned a car. Worked as a copy writer for Fiat ad agency and Fiat radio station. Fed up with Fiat, he now works as press officer for environmental NGO *Legambiente*. For Critical Mass in Milan, he works on press relations, ad busting and media jamming actions.

Joel Pomerantz is a freelance project manager who helped to create Critical Mass, the SF Bike Coalition, the Duboce Bikeway Mural and the annual international festival known as BikeSummer.

Ben Salzberg is a cycling fanatic in Portland OR, whose web pages do an OK job of illustrating his obsessions: http://www.arborrhythms.com/~ben

Benjamin Shepard is coeditor of *From ACT UP to the WTO: Urban Protest and Community Building in the Era of Globalization* (Verso, 2002). **Kelly Moore** is the author of *Disrupting Power: Political Activism and the Transformation of American Science, 1955-2000* (Princeton Univ. Press, forthcoming, 2003). We worked together in the Lower East Side Collective (disbanded summer 2000). Since then, Ben's been working with RTS, and Kelly has been doing bike activism.

David Snyder has served as Executive Director of the San Francisco Bicycle Coalition since July 1991. Snyder established the SFBC to bridge the gap between bicycle advocates within city government and those from the city's grassroots constituencies.

Anna Sojourner has loved public transportation since she was a small child.

Darren Stehr first began photographing bicycle races in the late '80s. Shortly after starting to commute on bicycle, he discovered Toronto's CM ride. Since 1997 he has been photographing each CM while riding and posting the images to www.torontocranks.com.

Bill Stender probably should have been working more diligently in his sign shop where he has earned his pay for the last 20 years instead of penning this and other seditious opinions.

Steven Stevenson was born in Melbourne in 1960, wasted a lot of time, stopped wasting as much time and now sometimes write articles for www.melbourne.indymedia.org.

Jim Swanson is an award-winning filmmaker, animator and illustrator. He helped start Critical Mass in San Francisco, and his illustrations have become icons of the movement internationally.

Joshua Switzky is an urban planner in San Francisco. He has lived car-free for 10 years. Josh co-organized Bike Summer in San Francisco in 1999 and is on the Board of Directors of Walk SF, a pedestrian advocacy group, and Transportation for a Livable City.

Sam Tracy is author of *How To Rock and Roll, A City Rider's Repair Manual*, available through shops or online at www.howtorockandroll.net. Excepting a brief stint editing the *Auto-Free Times* in 1998, he has been a bike messenger or bike mechanic since 1993. He lives in Minneapolis.

Beth Verdekal recently moved from San Francisco to Marin (just across the Golden Gate Bridge) after 12 years in SF. Two years ago, she started a career as healer. She wants to learn how to wheelie, surf and play surf guitar.

Victor Veysey is the founder of the Bike Hut at Pier 40 in S.F., where he mentors kids from poorer SF neighborhoods to become bicycle mechanics. He is also an accomplished songwriter, scribe, masseur, cook, and civic gadfly.

Howard A. Williams, 50, has been a messenger in San Francisco since 1982 and has been active in the courier industry union effort. He also was an aid worker in travels to Pakistan and Afghanistan from 1989 to 1997. He participated in the first Critical Mass of 9/92 and in such notable Masses as the 8/96, 7/97 and 12/99 rides.

Ted White is an independent filmmaker and glorifier of the new bicycle renaissance. Two of his most formative bicycle advocate years were spent working with Jan VanderTuin at the Center for Approriate Transport in Eugene, Oregon. More information on his bikeumentaries can be found by visiting www.tedwhitegreenlight.com

Josh Wilson is a journalist working in nonprofit media in San Francisco.

INDEX